D0819999

THE ASSISTED LIVING RESIDENCE

THE ASSISTED LIVING RESIDENCE

A Vision for the Future

Edited by

STEPHEN M. GOLANT
Professor
Department of Geography
University of Florida
Gainesville, Florida

and

JOAN HYDE
Chief Executive Officer
Ivy Hall Senior Living
and Senior Fellow, Gerontology Institute
University of Massachusetts
Boston, Massachusetts

The Johns Hopkins University Press
Baltimore

© 2008 The Johns Hopkins University Press
All rights reserved. Published 2008
Printed in the United States of America on acid-free paper
9   8   7   6   5   4   3   2   1

The Johns Hopkins University Press
2715 North Charles Street
Baltimore, Maryland 21218-4363
www.press.jhu.edu

Library of Congress Cataloging-in-Publication Data

The assisted living residence : a vision for the future / edited by Stephen M.
Golant and Joan Hyde.
   p. ; cm.
  Includes bibliographical references and index.
  ISBN-13: 978-0-8018-8817-5 (hardcover : alk. paper)
  ISBN-10: 0-8018-8817-4 (hardcover : alk. paper)
  1. Older people—Housing. 2. Older people—Housing—Economic
aspects. 3. Congregate housing. 4. Older people—Care. 5. Long-term care
facilities. I. Golant, Stephen M. II. Hyde, Joan.
HV1454.A87 2008
362.61—dc22   2007038403

A catalog record for this book is available from the British Library.

Special discounts are available for bulk purchases of this book.
For more information, please contact Special Sales at 410-516-6936 or
specialsales@press.jhu.edu.

The Johns Hopkins University Press uses environmentally friendly book
materials, including recycled text paper that is composed of at least 30
percent post-consumer waste, whenever possible. All of our book papers are
acid-free, and our jackets and covers are printed on paper with recycled
content.

CONTENTS

FOREWORD

Nothing about the past, present, or future of assisted living is clear-cut. For almost any statement that may be made about assisted living, one can find an equally well founded exception or contradiction. Perhaps not surprisingly, then, consumers, family members, state and federal policy makers, and researchers often express varying degrees of confusion about this long-term care option. Although most people have opinions about what assisted living means, they are often based on a generalized notion of what it may or should mean, on a particular company's model, or on a specific state's regulatory model or practice. This book seeks to understand these complex and competing visions of the future of assisted living and its potential to serve elders who are now aging in place in ordinary dwellings, who have nursing home trajectories, and who need assistance but lack financial resources. The contributors to this volume advance considerably the discussion about the factors likely to shape the future of assisted living and how this long-term care alternative might look and operate two or three decades from now.

Ambiguities about how it should be defined and what its future holds have not stopped its growth. The number of licensed assisted living residence units grew dramatically, 33 percent, between 1998 and 2000 and then slowed to 13 percent between 2000 and 2002 and to 3 percent between 2002 and 2004; but between 2004 and 2007, the growth rate accelerated to 6 percent. By 2007 there were 974,585 units in 38,373 licensed facilities. The supply is primarily affected by market forces, because few states regulate the size of the assisted living industry. After a decade of rapid change and growth, it is appropriate to pause and reflect on the multiple issues that will affect changes in the future.

Even though the term *assisted living* has existed for at least twenty years, it remains difficult to define. In the late 1980s and early 1990s, assisted living appeared as a new housing and services model based on a philosophy that promoted individual autonomy and decision making. Although by 2004, forty-one states and the District of Columbia used the term *assisted living,* it is still known by other names: residential care, adult care homes, personal care homes, homes for the aged, and even adult family care. More important, there is no national consensus or even federal guidelines governing who can be served, what services can be provided, whether the staff can assist with or administer medications, what constitutes minimum staffing standards, or any other aspect of assisted living. And there are different views within the industry itself about what assisted living is, should be, or will become.

The difficulty finding consensus was apparent during the deliberations of the Assisted Living Workgroup (ALW) convened by the U.S. Senate Special Committee on Aging to develop recommendations designed to ensure more consistent quality in assisted living services. The workgroup included more than fifty organizations representing a variety of interests, including industry associations, professional organizations, consumer and advocacy groups, and regulators. Discussion about how to define the assisted living option led the members of the workgroup to deliberate about three separate components: what services it should offer and the extent of regulatory oversight, whether it should be required to offer private units (that is, no sharing of bedrooms and bathrooms), and whether states should establish at least two levels of care based on the acuity of residents' needs—but their views on nearly all of these topics differed.

This lack of consensus is reflected in the regulations and oversight of assisted living, which differ significantly from state to state. The absence of uniform standards may be viewed as a weakness, but it may also be considered a strength. There are good arguments for flexible and changing state licensing requirements because they define the environment in which assisted living operates and therefore have a major role in shaping the industry. Public policies and regulators must strive to keep pace with the dynamic development of the industry as it grows and adapts to consumer and business expectations. For their part, operators seek the ability to respond differently to the changing operating environments of assisted living properties and test new ideas.

At any given time over the past decade, about half the states have been reviewing, updating, or issuing new regulations, often forming task forces to consider proposed changes or make recommendations for improving regulations. Some states have substituted *assisted living* for other terms in

existing regulations governing long-term care without significantly changing the regulations themselves; others have added assisted living as a separate category while retaining existing categories. The latter approach typically establishes more homelike, residential requirements for assisted
living than other categories of long-term care, which are likely to affect
newer residences. States that want to require apartment-style units must
maintain separate standards for residences that offer shared units in more
institutional settings.

States may take one of three approaches when licensing assisted living
residences: the institutional approach, the housing and services approach,
or the service model approach. The institutional approach permits residences to offer shared bedrooms without attached baths. The housing and
services approach requires apartment settings and allows facilities to admit and retain residents with a range of service needs. The service model
approach licenses the provider of the service and regulates the building
itself through existing building codes and requirements. This approach
may define which buildings (or apartment units or living spaces) qualify
as assisted living but not otherwise define the building's characteristics.
All three approaches incorporate into law or regulation a statement of
philosophy. States that take the housing and services approach may include a philosophy that emphasizes resident autonomy, independence,
dignity, and involvement in making decisions about the services that will
be provided.

Although some observers have bemoaned the absence of a national definition and operating standards, it does not appear that detailed nationwide
regulations will emerge from the federal government. Congressional committees have shown interest in consumer protections and oversight of assisted living, but even if Congress were inclined to set national standards
it is not clear what authority it would have to do so. Medicare is unlikely
to cover services in assisted living settings. Medicaid, which does regulate
a state's long-term care policies for its poor citizens, subsidizes the costs
of services for only a small percentage of residents and lacks enough purchasing power to set standards that would affect the industry.

The diversity of regulatory approaches, definitions, and other features
poses challenges for consumers and family members trying to understand
whether assisted living is the best long-term care option for them and
which residence will best meet their needs. It also challenges owners and
operators, who must keep informed about state licensing requirements,

forms, procedures, and oversight guidelines. All of these groups benefit from the information about assisted living that state licensing agencies disseminate on their Internet sites. A project funded by the Agency for Healthcare Research and Quality, part of the U.S. Department of Health and Human Services, in 2005 investigated the availability of such information. It found that some web sites post information that is directed primarily to consumers and family members, whereas others seem more useful to owners and operators. Nearly every state (forty-eight in all) posts its licensing regulations, and these are usually available on the web site of the licensing agency. Some regulations, however, are available on the web sites of the Office of the Secretary of State or the state legislature. Twenty-six states post information beyond the regulations, primarily for facility owners, administrators, and managers, variously including documents relating to the survey process and operating and staffing guidelines and requirements.

Forty-two states post lists of licensed facilities, sometimes in searchable databases, sometimes in simple files listing the names of properties, addresses, and phone numbers. Fourteen states post consumer guides or lists of questions to help consumers and family understand assisted living and compare and select a residence. Twelve states include information from survey reports and complaint investigations. State monitoring staff prepare survey reports following on-site visits to assess compliance with state licensing requirements.

Information primarily directed to consumers is also available on the web sites of the State Units on Aging (SUAs). SUAs are an important source of information to older adults and families about long-term care services, including assisted living options. Eight SUAs are specifically responsible for licensing assisted living residences. SUAs may be cabinet-level agencies, but most are units within a larger umbrella agency or department. They have broader missions than licensing agencies and are charged under the Older Americans Act with a range of services to older adults "designed to encourage and assist older individuals to use the facilities and services (including information and assistance services) available to them" (Older Americans Act, 42 USC Section 3030D). SUA web sites typically offer general information about state services, Medicare, and resources available through area Agencies on Aging. In 2005, thirty SUA web sites contained information or links to information about assisted living.

Older consumers, however, typically do not look first to assisted living properties when making their long-term care choices. They want an array of options that allow them to "age in place" in their ordinary dwellings. "Aging in place" typically means that individuals who need supports to manage their frailty can receive sufficient assistance—services and personal care—allowing them to remain in their existing housing arrangement. The challenge is to adapt their living environment even as their needed types and frequency of services become more demanding.

It is only when individuals are no longer able to live comfortably or safely in their single-family homes or independent apartments that they seek out the assisted living residence to benefit from an aging-in-place philosophy that ensures their independence, privacy, autonomy, and individualized decision making that they enjoyed in their earlier residences, even as they become more vulnerable. As the General Accounting Office noted in its 1999 report, "Assisted living is often promoted as supporting the concept of 'aging-in-place' that allows residents to remain in a residence as their health condition declines or their needs change." From both a regulatory and an operational perspective, however, this is a complex issue that is difficult to explain and even more difficult to implement.

Regulators, along with other stakeholders, such as adult children and consumer advocates, support—but at the same time—worry about aging in place because it sometimes involves conflicts between offering older individuals more choices and assuring a safe living environment. In practice, however, states respond differently as to how they regulate aging-in-place options. They often cite concerns about potentially unsafe medication practices and the increasing frailty of residents and worry that, to ensure sufficient occupancy rates, properties continue to serve residents with needs that exceed their capacity to provide appropriate care. To determine whether changes in oversight are warranted, states are continually reviewing their regulations governing staffing, training, and services.

Regulatory requirements particularly concern who may be admitted to or remain in assisted living and set the parameters for aging-in-place practices. What is permitted by regulation and how it is implemented often are not clear cut. Opportunities for aging in place, moreover, are not necessarily equitable. If a person lives in his or her own home or independent apartment, the ability to bring in services to support the choice of living arrangement may be limited by cost, health needs, and other factors. If he or she moves to an assisted living residence, aging in place may be encouraged or constrained by the scope of local licensing regulations or the policies of the residence. Some states allow residences to serve residents who have extensive needs with activities of daily living, taking medication, and health-related needs. Others limit who may be served and what services may be offered. Facilities in states with permissive regulations regarding services may be constrained by the interpretation and application of local building codes by fire marshals in their towns or cities, who are concerned about the ability of individuals with greater levels of impairment to evacuate in an emergency.

States typically use one or more of five factors to establish admission/retention policies in assisted living residences: the general condition of the resident, health-related conditions, functional capacity, Alzheimer disease or other dementia, and resident behavior. State licensing regulations define the parameters for who may be served but often allow assisted living residences to set their own admission and retention policies within certain limits. Thus, even when states have permissive regulations, property owners seeking to reduce their risks may decide they will not serve residents with higher levels of need.

For example, some residences do not assist with feeding, provide two-person transfers, or allow staff members to perform subcutaneous injections. One assisted living provider that operates in several states with permissive criteria designed to support aging in place reported that the company offers a minimum to moderate level of care in keeping with its business plan and risk-management strategy. The company does not have sufficient staff to meet the needs of residents with uncontrolled incontinence, who have moderate cognitive impairment, whose behavior poses a threat to themselves, staff, and other residents, or who have more than stage II pressure ulcers. These different practices result in variations in how the aging-in-place needs of different groups are served even among properties within the same state.

State policies on aging in place are often shaped by tragic, well-publicized events. Whether administrators are making correct decisions regarding the admission and retention policies of assisted living residences in their states is often communicated loudly by a news story about an avoidable death, abuse, or poor care. Coverage of major quality-of-care issues galvanizes public opinion and forces regulators and legislators to take steps that might not have been considered in the absence of the event. In some instances, the steps are required to remedy an already-noted weak-

ness in existing regulations or oversight practices and the event is the cata-
lyst for change. Proponents of the autonomy and independence of their
residents worry that an assisted living model that promotes these values
may be compromised by attempts to maximize safety. But advocates for
seniors also worry that limited regulations and oversight may lead to preventable adverse outcomes and poor-quality care.

The tension between consumer preferences and public policy that either
supports or limits aging in place and company policies and practices is
likely to continue. On balance, we predict that state regulators will continue to support flexible policies that allow residences to provide an array
of services that individuals could obtain in their own single-family home
or apartment and that, within a highly competitive assisted living environment, operators will strive to serve consumers and their family as long as
possible.

The cost of services can also be a barrier to aging in place. Most residents
pay with their own funds and assisted living residences are usually inac-
cessible to frail older persons with lower incomes. This is the case even
though it would be an especially valuable resource for those poor older
individuals who have lost their own housing, do not have caregivers able
to provide housing or assistance, or need access to oversight and unscheduled services. Even when individuals can initially afford to enter assisted
living properties, when their needs increase over the course of their occupancy, they may not be able to afford their increased care expenses. States
have many incentives to work with providers to expand access for these
low-income elders. Medicaid supports the cost of services for about 12
percent of today's assisted living residents. With support from the Centers
for Medicare and Medicaid Services (CMS), states are also increasingly
working with lower-income nursing home residents who are interested in
relocating to noninstitutional settings. Texas helped more than ten thousand nursing home residents transition to noninstitutional housing, about
32 percent of whom moved to assisted living residences; however, robust
demand from private-pay residents, concerns about inadequate Medicaid
payment rates, and limitations on the number of people who can be served
under Medicaid waivers for home- and community-based services may
limit the potential for further growth of affordable assisted living.

It is noteworthy that Congress passed the new "Money Follows the
Person" Demonstration Grant program as part of the Deficit Reduction Act

of 2005 to encourage the relocation of Medicaid nursing home residents to community settings. The act, however, excluded residential settings serving five or more individuals.

What lies ahead? Although a great deal of information is available about assisted living, charting a path for the future is fraught with uncertainty. Tomorrow's market forces, changing technology, and the balance of activity and influence by stakeholders are difficult to predict and will play out differently throughout the country. What is clear, however, is that state regulators, state legislatures, owners and operators of assisted living, and consumers will all play key roles in shaping the future of assisted living. On the one hand, these stakeholders can take the better-known path. It is well traveled, with all of its limitations, standards, and oversight practices. It combines national standards and fairly rigorous oversight practices, but it does not always achieve the high expectations for quality that they all seek. On the other hand, they could chart a new course. Someone will attempt to lead the way, but not everyone will follow once a leader or leaders emerge. In fact, opposition may be sufficient to impede or halt the process. Anyone who has participated in a group discussion to seek consensus on a new approach appreciates how difficult it is to create new versions of an accepted alternative.

The research community will also be influential through its collection, analysis, dissemination, and translation of data about assisted living. Many key questions must be answered. Does the housing and services approach that supports aging in place and higher levels of care have better outcomes than other approaches? Do stricter regulations reduce negative outcomes and poor quality? Does imposing special requirements for residences that serve people with dementia ensure better care for these individuals? Can technology safely help promote independence? Should state regulations be permissive or restrictive regarding the level of service and admission and retention requirements of assisted living properties? The chapters in this book offer a rich variety of perspectives and possibilities for what the future holds.

Predictions about the future of assisted living differ dramatically. There are multiple layers and perspectives. Our task is to begin assembling information that will shape the future; to collect and translate information in a timely manner that reflects the public policy process and the need for useful information when policy decisions are being made; and to make the best use of the limited windows of opportunity that arise in the public policy arena that may close before we have the information to contribute to the process.

Robert L. Mollica, Ed.D.
Senior Program Director
National Academy for State Health Policy
Portland, Maine

PREFACE

This book brings to bear the knowledge and views of nationally recognized leaders in gerontology and long-term care services, crystallized around the task of using their particular expertise to speculate on the future of assisted living. Many of the social issues facing our society in the coming decades intersect with and inform this inquiry.

The chapters are grouped into three parts. Chapters in part I focus on the "big picture" and consider the overall influences that will shape the future of assisted living and how it will look and operate. Stephen Golant's vision for the future is dominated by uncertainty, and he discusses the likely influences that may temper optimistic expectations. He envisions that the industry will have higher operating costs and that larger provider and management groups will dominate; thus, he predicts the demise of small mom-and-pop board-and-care homes. The prospects for serving greater numbers of low-income residents will depend on the willingness of public programs to increase subsidies and reimbursement rates, a difficult task in view of budget constraints and the focus on curbing public spending.

Joan Hyde, Rosa Perez, and Peter Reed emphasize that all long-term care providers will face challenges serving the growing number of people with serious physical and cognitive impairments and that assisted living providers will evolve in order to be able to serve this population competently. They expect more pressure from family members and government oversight agencies intent on creating secure, safe, and high-quality living while maintaining a residential, homelike environment.

Margaret Calkins and William Keane expect that differences between assisted living and nursing homes will blur as nursing home operators begin to mirror operational practices and physical features of assisted living facilities. They point to various examples of the transformation of nursing homes. Sheryl Zimmerman, Philip Sloane, and Susan Fletcher also describe how care and outcomes in assisted living differ from nursing homes. Public perceptions and research findings about the quality of care may be the single most important influence on future standards and the direction the industry will take. Zimmerman, Sloane, and Fletcher, however, emphasize that conducting quality of care assessments is seldom a straightforward exercise and will require the collaboration of all involved stakeholders.

Paula Carder, Leslie Morgan, and Kevin Eckert consider the future viability of small board-and-care facilities—sometimes referred to as the poor population's assisted living—given tomorrow's large and corporate-run competitive assisted living market. They worry about the marginal place of small board-and-care homes in the public policy arena and the competition from large corporate-operated assisted living properties.

Part II covers the private sector factors that will affect the appearance and operation of future assisted living residences. Margaret Wylde argues that consumers may have the most influence on changes in assisted living. Consumers will continue to expect a safe and secure environment and service levels that meet increasing needs in an appealing residential setting. Anticipating changing consumer expectations and developing an appealing product will challenge operators. Douglas Wolf and Carol Jenkins describe the changing role of family caregivers and how the availability of this informal care will influence the future desirability of assisted living. They argue for the continued importance of family members as caregivers but consider the pressures that will limit their ability to provide care and, thus, might result in a greater demand for assisted living. David Kutzik, Anthony Glascock, Lydia Lundberg, and Jack York offer an overview of the unpredictable world of technology and how innovations may substantially change the way tomorrow's assisted living properties will operate on a daily basis.

Douglas Pace and Karen Love explore how stakeholder organizations with very different interests—provider, professional, worker, and consumer—will likely influence the design, operation, and oversight of assisted living residences and particularly how their initiatives might help shape how state governments regulate these settings.

Providers' ability to respond to changing market expectations depends largely on the availability of financing. Anthony Mullen and Harvey Singer contend that large companies with successful track records will be able to attract the financing needed to create products that meet changing preferences. The cautious nature of lenders may limit financing for new ap-proaches in favor of tried-and-true models even as they become outdated.

Part III focuses on the expected influences from the public sector on the future of assisted living. Pamela Doty anticipates that changes in the availability, types, and funding of home and community-based services for low-income residents will affect assisted living providers. She examines the complex historical roles that have been played by federal programs—especially Medicaid—in the evolution of both assisted living and nursing homes, along with new influences played by private sector long-term care insurance products. State Medicaid policy decisions concerning the scope of coverage and reimbursement rates will determine how many low-income individuals are likely to be served, but she is not optimistic about future prospects. Robyn Stone, Mary Harahan, and Alisha Sanders consider the multiple ways that housing providers can provide services to low-income elders with impairments and health needs. Generally not licensed by state agencies, housing with services programs occupy one of the many gray areas in oversight of assisted living, even as they offer valuable assistance to low-income and frail older persons. Robert Newcomer, Cristina Flores, and Mauro Hernandez speculate about the potential federal roles as Medicaid coverage expands, as well as the expected direction and impact of state regulation on the affordability, demand, and quality of care. Keren Brown Wilson discusses the gap between the long-term care expectations of low-income consumers and what public policies can deliver. She considers the challenges faced by the public sector seeking to offer assisted living settings with privacy, choice, and flexible services and offers different scenarios that may frame future debates. Finally, Larry Polivka and Jennifer Salmon's chapter describes assisted living's strong potential as an alternative to entering a nursing home or living with risk in one's own home. They articulate the essence of the assisted living alternative, focusing on its values, physical design, operational characteristics, and performance standards and the steps that will be needed to assure its integrity into the future.

CONTRIBUTORS

Margaret P. Calkins, Ph.D., president, I.D.E.A.S., Inc., Kirtland, Ohio

Paula C. Carder, Ph.D., assistant professor, Institute on Aging, School of Community Health, Portland State University

Pamela Doty, Ph.D., senior policy analyst, Office of the Assistant Secretary for Planning and Evaluation, Office of Disability, Aging and Long-Term Care Policy, U.S. Department of Health and Human Services, Washington, D.C.

J. Kevin Eckert, Ph.D., dean and professor, Erickson School and director, Center for Aging Studies, University of Maryland, Baltimore County, Baltimore, Maryland

Susan K. Fletcher, M.S.W., University of North Carolina at Chapel Hill, Chapel Hill, North Carolina

Cristina Flores, Ph.D., R.N., Nursing Health Policy Program, Department of Social and Behavioral Sciences, University of California, San Francisco, California

Anthony P. Glascock, Ph.D., professor of anthropology, Drexel University, Philadelphia, Pennsylvania and president, Behavioral Informatics, Inc., Media, Pennsylvania

Mary Harahan, M.A., senior advisor, Institute for the Future of Aging Services, Greensboro, North Carolina

Mauro Hernandez, Ph.D., research associate, Department of Social and Behavioral Sciences, University of California, San Francisco, California

Carol Jenkins, Ph.D., associate professor, School of Social Work and associate director for Educational Programs, Center on Aging, East Carolina University, Greenville, North Carolina

William Keane, M.S., M.B.A., LNHA, consultant in aging, Chicago, Illinois

David M. Kutzik, Ph.D., associate professor of sociology, Drexel University, Philadelphia, Pennsylvania and vice president, Behavioral Informatics, Inc., Media, Pennsylvania

Karen Love, B.S., founder, Consumer Consortium on Assisted Living and Managing Director, Center for Excellence in Assisted Living, Falls Church, Virginia

Lydia Lundberg, founder and owner, Elite Care/Oatfield Estates, Milwaukie, Oregon

Leslie A. Morgan, Ph.D., professor and associate dean, Erickson School, University of Maryland, Baltimore County, Baltimore, Maryland

Anthony J. Mullen, M.S., senior fellow, National Investment Center for the Seniors Housing & Care Industry, Havertown, Pennsylvania

Robert Newcomer, Ph.D., professor, Department of Social and Behavioral Sciences, University of California, San Francisco, California

Douglas D. Pace, NHA, executive director, National Commission for Quality Long-term Care, Washington, D.C.

Rosa Perez, M.Ed., project coordinator, Center for Aging Studies, University of Maryland, Baltimore County, Baltimore, Maryland

Larry Polivka, Ph.D., associate professor and associate director, School of Aging Studies, College of Arts and Sciences, and Director, Florida Policy Exchange Center on Aging, University of South Florida, Tampa, Florida

Peter S. Reed, Ph.D., M.P.H., senior director, programs and outreach, Alzheimer's Association, National Office, Chicago, Illinois

Jennifer R. Salmon, Ph.D., consultant, Aging Research Group, Gulfport, Florida

Alisha Sanders, M.P.Aff., Policy Research Associate, American Association of Homes and Services for the Aging, Institute for the Future of Aging Services, Washington, D.C.

Harvey N. Singer, M.B.A., principal, REDMARK Economics for Real Estate Development and Market Research, Annapolis, Maryland

Philip D. Sloane, M.D., M.P.H., professor, School of Medicine, University of North Carolina, Chapel Hill, North Carolina

Robyn I. Stone, Dr.P.H., executive director, American Association of Homes and Services for the Aging, Institute for the Future of Aging Services, Washington, D.C.

Keren Brown Wilson, Ph.D., president, Jessie F. Richardson Foundation, Clackamas, Oregon

Douglas A. Wolf, Ph.D., Gerald B. Cramer Professor of Aging Studies, Maxwell School of Citizenship and Public Affairs, Syracuse University, Syracuse, New York

Margaret A. Wylde, Ph.D., president and CEO, ProMatura Group, LLC, Oxford, Mississippi

Jack York, B.S., founder and CEO, It's Never 2 Late, Englewood, Colorado

Sheryl Zimmerman, Ph.D., professor and director of aging research, School of Social Work; co-director, Interdisciplinary Center for Aging Research; and co-director, Program on Aging, Disability and Long-Term Care, Cecil G. Sheps Center for Health Services Research, University of North Carolina at Chapel Hill, Chapel Hill, North Carolina

PART I

LOOKING TOWARD THE FUTURE

CHAPTER 1

The Future of Assisted Living Residences

A Response to Uncertainty

STEPHEN M. GOLANT, PH.D.

Assisted living residences in the United States have become important long-term living arrangements that offer shelter and care to physically and cognitively frail older persons, typically in their eighties or older. These purposively designed group residential settings offer a protected residential living arrangement with 24-hour awake staff, meals, a congenial social situation, scheduled and unscheduled help with everyday activities (e.g., bathing, dressing, grooming, mobility, and eating), medication management, and sometimes health- or nursing-related services. These predominantly private-pay options are mostly marketed to higher-income or asset-rich older persons, who are unable to live safely or comfortably on their own in their ordinary dwellings even with the assistance of family members but seek to avoid entering a nursing home. The most exemplary properties look more like well-designed apartment buildings or even hotels than institutions and have architecturally attractive lobbies, common areas, and apartment suites. The best of these alternatives also try to integrate humanely their shelter and care by respecting their occupants' distinctive lifestyles, their individual care needs, and their desire to remain as independent as possible.

Nonetheless, even as its most ardent advocates argue that assisted living will be part of our future, they at the same time express uncertainty concerning the role it will play in the arena of options for long-term care. And not all experts, professionals, or consumers agree that assisted living is the most desirable way to accommodate frail older persons. Making definitive predictions about the future turns out to be especially complicated because the properties that today refer to themselves as "assisted living" can be very different from one another. This diversity partly reflects the varied care missions of their owners and their idiosyncratic design and operation features. Just as important, their variability reflects the diversity of state governmental regulation (Mollica & Johnson-Lamarche, 2005).

Our current knowledge simply does not allow us to draw definitive conclusions about the myriad factors that will influence the availability of assisted living options and how they will look and operate in the future. The unknowns include:

- The size and growth of the future older market for assisted living;
- The extent to which assisted living properties will primarily serve older persons needing high-acuity, as opposed to light, care—and thus constitute a substitute for nursing homes;
- Whether older consumers will prefer properties that physically stand alone over those that are part of more extensive long-term care complexes that offer many different types of care and services;
- Whether older consumers will be disposed to living in group housing arrangements with other older persons;
- What role family members will play in the long-term care decisions of older persons;
- The strength of competing long-term care alternatives—the familiar homes and apartments of older persons and, perhaps surprisingly, even nursing homes;
- The extent that new caregiving technologies will favor ordinary dwellings or assisted living residences as places to live;
- Whether long-term care insurance will become a more important funding source to pay for assisted living stays—and thus enlarge the potential older consumer market;

- How expensive assisted living properties will be and the extent to which older consumers will be able to afford their costs;
- The cost-competitiveness of assisted living compared to emerging long-term care alternatives;
- The extent to which state governments will increase their regulatory oversight to ensure better-quality care;
- How assisted living providers will change their business models to cope with tomorrow's uncertain consumer markets;
- What operating models of assisted living will thrive in the future;
- The extent to which developers seeking financing for their assisted living products can compete with other uses of capital and its overall cost;
- The extent to which federal or state governments will try to make assisted living properties affordable to lower-income older persons; and
- Whether mom-and-pop board-and-care facilities will survive.

This chapter attempts to shed light on these questions and reflects critically on what the next two or three decades will hold for assisted living. Its core argument is that the most important determinant of the status of tomorrow's assisted living industry will be the efforts of its developers, owners, and managers to cope with an uncertain future.

We predict that the most successful assisted living providers will respond by continuing their current practice of steadily increasing the critical mass or the scope of their operations to achieve greater economies of scale. Thus, they will try to capture a diverse population of older consumers, who have both lower- and higher-acuity care needs, and will back state legislation that makes it economically attractive for them to serve both lower- and higher-income consumers. We predict that assisted living will predominantly be the province of large corporate chains that own or manage multiple properties and offer the full continuum of care to residents, whatever their needs. The business models that drive their operations will allow their owners to respond readily to changes in consumer demand and to fend off competition from other care alternatives.

We also expect that a confluence of factors will make the development and operation of assisted living options more expensive and will require the public sector to find imaginative ways to make them more affordable not only to very low-income, but also to moderate-income, frail seniors. This will not be an altruistic response, but one driven by government agencies believing that there are fiscal advantages to subsidizing the costs of assisted living residences as opposed to other shelter-and-care alternatives. Not all types of assisted living residences will thrive in this new climate, and we predict the demise of small board-and-care residences, sometimes considered a poor person's assisted living because it is dominated by occupants receiving federal and state government assistance (see chapter 5).

A Complex, Moving Target

Predicting the future from even a known present is always a perilous exercise. When the phenomenon at hand is as eclectic as assisted living, gazing into the crystal ball becomes especially difficult. Unambiguous portrayals are difficult, because "assisted living" has come to refer to such a wide range of integrated housing and long-term care arrangements that can assist older persons with a wide range of vulnerabilities.

There is no fundamental unanimity about the desirability of assisted living options as long-term care settings, now occupied by more than a million seniors. On the one hand, there are experts, professionals, and practitioners—probably the majority—who laud the mission of these settings and their quality of life and care. They would endorse (albeit perhaps not as enthusiastically) the following views expressed by the CEO of the industry's major professional association—ALFA, or the Assisted Living Federation of America: "Assisted living communities operated by ALFA members are professionally managed, warm, welcoming, and comfortable homes to thousands of seniors who need some assistance in daily living. And they bring peace of mind to the families of their loved ones—knowing that they are safe and secure under the thoughtful supervision and care of their staff" (Grimes, 2006, p. 5).

On the other hand, uncomplimentary government assessments of quality of care in assisted living and press stories about how residences have failed consumers are not hard to find (U.S. General Accounting Office, 1999). A prominent geriatrician, for example, offered this unequivocally negative assessment: "Assisted living is the grayest of options, neither fish nor fowl and tends to be inflexible and unimaginative about tailoring care to individual needs. . . . Residents are rushed off in ambulances for minor ailments and accidents because the staff is not medically qualified and afraid of liability. . . . Each hospitalization [for my mother] made things worse, forcing her eventual transfer to a nursing home" (Gross, 2005).

Furthermore, these disparate positions, particularly the unfavorable, have the power to sway public opinion. The best advertising for assisted living options is satisfied consumers and complimentary "word of mouth" communications—and their absence has serious consequences for influencing demand and public policy responses. Thus, the same CEO's future concerns are well founded: "Over time, a poor public image (perpetuated by the media) can eat away at public confidence, which in turn can lead to political opportunism, which in turn can produce onerous legislation and regulations ostensibly intended to 'protect' our residents from the fictional depictions of assisted living in the media" (Grimes, 2006, p. 5).

The many different products and service arrangements that today pass as assisted living make simple generalizations about either their physical settings or their care environments particularly challenging—and inevitably contribute to consumer confusion. Some are stand-alone buildings in which a relatively narrow range of care is provided throughout; others are physically and organizationally subdivided by floors or sections—sometimes into different buildings—each designed and staffed to provide different levels of care. Many assisted living residences more resemble upscale hotels than caregiving facilities because of their attractive dwelling and building designs and their more flexible person-centered care environments (see chapter 3). Others more resemble nursing homes because of their medical, hospital-like ambience, nursing stations, long, sterile corridors, or shared rooms and bathrooms.

Assisted living properties are also not occupied by residents with similar vulnerability profiles. Some assisted living arrangements accept residents who are almost as cognitively and physically impaired as those in nursing homes. These professionally managed assisted living residences are staffed by workers who may provide nursing services as complex as wound care and intravenous medication and who may offer therapeutic responses to the wandering and inappropriate behaviors of their residents with dementia (Golant, 2004). The high-acuity care offered in such residences can make it possible for their elder occupants never to have to move again. Other assisted living facilities offer primarily low-acuity or light care and cater to residents who are only minimally dependent and frail. This is often true of affordable rental apartment complexes—sometimes

TABLE 1.1
Categories of Service Capacity in Assisted Living/Residential Care

Service Category	Basic	Moderate	High
Personal care	Supervision, reminders, and some assistance with bathing, dressing, and hygiene	Assistance with bathing, dressing, and hygiene, plus limited assistance with toileting, ambulation, and eating	Assistance with all ADLs, including regular incontinence care, transferring, and feeding
Nursing	Coordination with third-party provider	Consultation, coordination, assessment, and episodic direct care (e.g., catheter reinsertion)	Regularly scheduled direct care (e.g., wound care)
Orientation/behaviors	Occasional reminders; infrequent behavioral interventions	Regular reminders, prompting, and direction; managing occasional episodes of disruptive or intrusive behavior	Structured programming; behavior plans to manage occasional, potentially unsafe behaviors

Source: Hernandez (2005), p. 20. Reprinted with permission from *Generations*, 29, no. 4, p. 20, 2005. Copyright © 2005 American Society on Aging, San Francisco, California. www.asaging.org.

given an assisted residence label—which limit their services to congregate meals and the information, service referral, and monitoring assistance offered by an on-site service coordinator (Table 1.1) (see chapter 12).

Furthermore, the appearance and operations of assisted living properties are continually in flux because providers change their business models or state governments change what they allow under their assisted living regulations. More than ever, assisted living residences are admitting and retaining chronologically older residents with more demanding impairments and, in particular, larger shares of residents with cognitive deficits (see chapter 2). One recent survey reported that 61 percent of assisted living residences now provide dementia care (Metlife Mature Market Institute, 2006).

The care boundaries of assisted living residences have become increasingly blurred. A growing share of assisted living arrangements rely on outsourced home care assistance brought into their properties, which can cater to very impaired older persons. Now, when residents become more functionally dependent in senior housing arrangements not staffed with persons offering heavier care, they do not necessarily have to relocate to other long-term care facilities offering more extensive care—such as other assisted living properties, nursing homes, or rehabilitation centers (Golant,

2004). These *movable* service delivery strategies make it increasingly difficult to simply characterize assisted living properties as providing either "heavy" or "light" care.

The costs of occupying assisted living residences can also differ greatly, reflecting how much high-acuity care they offer, the luxuriousness of their quarters, and whether they are located in higher-priced housing markets. Although the more costly residences are occupied primarily by older persons with higher incomes and above-average wealth, these properties also are occupied by residents with moderate incomes. Seniors in these places receive financial assistance from their families or have used the equity generated from selling their homes (Promatura Group, 1999). About 3 percent are able to afford these accommodations because they are covered by long-term care insurance (Bersani, 2007). A small share of assisted living units (just over one in ten) is also occupied by very poor seniors whose costs are subsidized by government programs (including Supplemental Security Income [SSI] and Medicaid). Another small, distinctive group includes low-income seniors who occupy government-subsidized rental buildings offering supportive services (e.g., Public Housing projects or privately owned rent-assisted HUD properties [Department of Housing and Urban Development]) that are licensed as assisted living residences (see chapter 12).

State governments regulate the 38,373 assisted living properties in the United States (as of 2007; Robert Mollica, personal communication), but far from uniformly, as evidenced by the annually produced 100-plus-page manuals that detail their very different requirements (Mollica & Johnson-Lamarche, 2005). Legislators must decide on the care role their assisted living properties will play in their long-term care networks, especially in comparison with nursing homes, and the extent to which they believe they should or can influence residents' safety and quality of care. State regulations often dictate the physical or architectural requirements of assisted living properties (e.g., the size and design of their dwelling units and common areas) and their allowable admission and retention policies for residents with high-acuity needs. Some states have a dedicated licensing category reserved for assisted living residences; others refer to similar facilities by different labels; still others have multiple licensing categories, each differently reserved for assisted living residences based on allowable services and the severity of residents' impairments. Some providers operate properties that function like assisted living residences but are not licensed by their state regulations. They rely on various subcontracted or outsourced licensed vendors from whom they purchase the same services offered by state-regulated properties (Mollica & Johnson-Lamarche, 2005). Local building codes, however, may restrict occupancy to persons who can exit a building on their own in the case of a fire or other disaster (see chapter 13). Adding to the complexity are the presence of individual- or family-operated board-and-care and foster-care facilities, typically occupied by fewer than 20 residents, that are affordable to the poorest segments of the old who often receive federal SSI payments, supplemented by State Supplementary Payments (SSP), and, less often, Medicaid assistance. Although some states regulate these properties under their assisted living licensure category, other states include them under other licensing categories, and in other states they are unregulated. Moreover, assisted living professional organizations often do not recognize these smaller residences as part of their membership (National Investment Center, 2001).

Factors Influencing the Future: Uncertain Assumptions and Predictions

It is straightforward enough to identify the factors that will influence the future availability and attributes of assisted living residences. It is far more difficult, however, to predict how these influences will unfold over time and thus shape the next generations of this long-term care option. These challenges are exemplified by the past prediction efforts of the National Investment Center (2001), an organization dedicated to providing financially reliable data to the seniors housing industry and its investors. Its growth projections for the assisted living market between 2000 and 2020 ranged widely, from 32 to 71 percent, depending on the sets of assumptions. Those presumably closely monitoring the preferences of consumers have also revealed the fallibility of prediction. During the period 1998–2002, assisted living developers overestimated the demand by older persons for their products and services, resulting in a multiyear period of overbuilt and oversaturated markets (see chapter 10).

Predicting the future would be simpler if we only had to foresee the demographics of tomorrow's older population, but such changes alone offer an incomplete and sometimes superficial glimpse into the future (Friedland & Summer, 1999). Only a subset of the aging baby boomer bulge will have disabilities that will put its members at risk of needing the care offered in assisted living residences. Even then, the duration and trajectory of their vulnerabilities are uncertain—some will experience improvements, some will remain stable, whereas others will decline. Moreover, not all of those who would be candidates for assisted living will have the necessary income and assets to afford them.

It is also unclear whether assisted living solutions will be considered viable and attractive options by future elderly persons (and their family members) given their often difficult-to-predict idiosyncratic housing and care preferences. We do not know with any certainty, for example, whether they will be more open to an age-homogeneous social context—consisting of other frail older persons—that differs spectacularly from their past household-oriented living arrangements (Knickman & Snell, 2002). Indeed, the most difficult challenge for the futurist is to judge what share of older consumers will opt for assisted living residences as opposed to other housing and care alternatives. Competing options include the informal assistance offered by family members in their ordinary homes and apartments (see chapter 7); the supportive services offered by independent living or congregate housing centers, and the skilled nursing home (see chapters 3 and 11).

The future is also clouded because, as already pointed out, almost all of today's long-term care options, including assisted living residences and nursing homes, are unlikely to look and operate similarly three decades from now (see chapters 3 and 11). The private sector is unlikely to offer today's residential care products to tomorrow's older consumers. It is difficult to foresee the future regulatory policies of state governments and whether they will be receptive to assisted living residences accommodating older persons with more serious physical or cognitive disabilities and chronic health conditions. It is also difficult to know whether the public sector will feel it necessary to impose new layers of regulation on assisted living residences that will be designed to assure quality and protect the consumer but that will also likely influence both the supply of these options and the costs to build and operate them (see chapter 13). Finally, it is not easy to predict whether new government initiatives will make it easier for lower-income elders to afford future assisted living options (see chapter 11).

To shed light on these issues, we examine nine of the most important factors that are likely to influence the future status of assisted living residences. We make predictions and assumptions regarding the future when they appear warranted by current research, but more often than not focus on the uncertainties that cloud their effects.

Growth Demographics

The projected growth of the U.S. older population is the least uncertain trend influencing the future demand for assisted living residences. After 2020, driven by the aging of the baby boom cohort, the population age 75 or older—the most likely users of assisted living—will grow in size and constitute a larger share of the overall elderly population (Morgan, 1998). During the first decade of this century (2000–2010), the age 75–84 group will increase by 4 percent, the age 85+ group by 44 percent, and the overall age 75+ group by 14 percent. Between 2010 and 2030, the age 75–84 group will increase by more than 86 percent, the age 85+ group by 57 percent, and the overall age 75+ group by 77 percent (U.S. Census Bureau, 2004).

Uncertainty still remains because even large numbers by themselves do not equate simply with a greater risk of need. The emergence of an unexpected new medical or rehabilitation breakthrough—a cure, or the discovery of a disease-controlling pharmaceutical, for Alzheimer disease—could result in substantial declines in the numbers of elderly Americans who need different supportive services. By contrast, even small increases in life expectancy could substantially inflate these estimates because larger numbers of the disabled oldest old would survive longer (Cohen, Weinrobe, Miller & Ingoldsby, 2005). The result would be more older persons coping for longer periods with their disabilities and chronic health problems and increased needs for high-acuity care (Kemper, Komisar & Alecxih, 2005).

Thus, a prediction of larger numbers of frail elderly people is reasonably certain unless there are major medical or therapeutic breakthroughs (Cohen, Weinrobe, Miller & Ingoldsby, 2005). Even as the disability rates of recent generations of older persons declined between the mid-1980s and mid-1990s, for example, the population with chronic disabilities still increased substantially (Spillman & Black, 2005).

(1) A large increase in the numbers of older persons at risk of needing the supportive services offered in assisted living residences is relatively certain.

Prevalence of Need

Although the numbers are likely to be larger, estimates of the potential demand for assisted living will be significantly influenced by the share (or prevalence) of tomorrow's elders that have difficulties living independently because of their disabilities or chronic health problems. People, especially women who live beyond the age of 75, have a relatively high probability of becoming frail at some point (Cohen, Weinrobe, Miller & Ingoldsby, 2005; Knickman & Snell, 2002). Currently, the prevalence of disability increases with age—from 9 percent among individuals aged 75–79 to 35 percent among individuals aged 85 and older. It is estimated that about 58 percent of men and 79 percent of women who turn age 65 today will need some combination of family or professional care during the remaining years of their lives to address their impairments. Forty-eight percent of these men and 63 percent of these women will need this care for at least two years. Furthermore, based on current patterns, about two-thirds of the years in which they need long-term care will be spent in their ordinary dwellings (Kemper, Komisar, & Alecxih, 2005).

These estimates, however, are not carved in stone. Experts cannot agree if future older Americans will experience the same risk of having disabilities after they turn 65 (Kemper, Komisar & Alecxih, 2005). Optimists point to the declines in the disability rates already experienced by the most recent generation of older persons. They further emphasize that the future benefits of advances in disease prevention and management, pharmaceuticals, assistive and monitoring devices, and surgical treatments (Knickman & Snell, 2002) should guarantee declines in the rates of disability. Indeed, most projections of long-term care have built this assumption into their models (Kemper, Komisar, & Alecxih, 2005; Knickman & Snell, 2002). Other experts, however, are less confident about declining levels of need (Wolf, Hunt, & Knickman, 2005) and observe that the improvements in mobility were primarily experienced by the least disabled older population, those having only limitations in IADLs or instrumental activities of daily living (e.g., shopping, housework, and managing money) as opposed to ADLs or activities of daily living (e.g., bathing, eating, transferring, grooming, walking). They also note that between 1984 and 1999 declines in disability rates were small (Spillman & Black, 2005). All of these predictions may be inaccurate to the extent that the growing numbers (and prevalence) of foreign-born older persons have different disability (and mortality) risk rates.

Other speculations are more foreboding. One study notes that the "prevalence of persons with three or four ADL limitations actually rose, from 3.0 percent of the over-65 population in 1982 to 3.5 percent in 1999" (Wolf, Hunt, & Knickman, 2005, p. 368). Other experts predict that tomorrow's older population will experience an increased prevalence of chronic diseases and poor health conditions (e.g., obesity, high blood pressure, and diabetes) that will lead to increases in chronic health problems and impairment levels (Wolf, Hunt, & Knickman, 2005). Altogether, these conflicting research findings make it difficult to predict with any certainty the relative size of the future market of older persons with disabilities.

> *(2) The prevalence of or share of future older persons with cognitive and physical impairments and chronic health problems that make them candidates for assisted living cannot be predicted with any certainty.*

Progression of Need

Another factor that will shape the future market for assisted living is how fluctuations in the needs for assistance will change over the remaining lives of frail older persons (see chapter 2). Deliberations of older persons (and their family members) about the need for care often depend on whether the symptoms or behavioral outcomes of a chronic health problem or disability are likely to remain the same, improve, or worsen—and at what rate and for what duration? Not all older persons who experience the onset of disability will progress to having more serious acuity needs. Even older persons who enter a nursing home can display stable ADL abilities, whereas others can experience improved functioning (Li, 2005). For example, some older persons who become disabled because of a stroke can regain many of their original abilities with appropriate rehabilitation therapies.

These fluctuations in need are played out frequently in long-term care settings. They are manifested by the short-term stays of older persons in nursing homes or rehabilitation centers and the moves by older persons from the assisted living to the nursing home quarters of continuing-care retirement communities (that offer multiple levels of care). Nursing home and assisted living residents may experience "many transitions between and among different types of care" (Cohen, Weinrobe, Miller, & Ingoldsby, 2005, p. 20) and "projecting specific service use patterns is much less precise than predicting disability itself" (Cohen, Weinrobe, Miller, & Ingoldsby, 2005, p. 21).

Addressing this issue is obviously central because today's older persons often must make a pivotal care decision. On the one hand, when they currently have minor disabilities, they can stay put in their current households, move into the dwellings of a family member, or move into a residential care setting that offers lower-acuity care. Older persons moving into these less institutional options may guarantee themselves a more familiar and desirable quality of life, but they must contemplate the possibility that their current abilities will deteriorate shortly and necessitate another disruptive move. On the other hand, older persons can immediately move into a setting in which higher-acuity care is available, because they assume they will eventually need it, although this residence has a less desirable quality of life because of its more institutional ambience. As we improve treatments for older persons with acute health problems and make further therapeutic advances in long-term care, a higher share of elders will face these uncertain trajectories of change and enter these revolving assistance doors. This may contribute to their demanding assisted living settings where they have the opportunity to access all levels of care. For their part, providers must decide whether it is in their best interests to offer a wider selection of care levels as a way to respond to the vagaries of disability trajectories and increase their chances of capturing a wider market.

(3) Trajectories and durations of change in frailty defining lifetime needs will be more variable and less predictable.

Long-Term Care Options

Predicting whether older Americans will opt to occupy assisted living residences would remain difficult even if we could predict accurately the numbers and percentages at risk of needing long-term care. This is because long-term care can be delivered conveniently and safely in almost all kinds of shelter-and-care arrangements if family assistance, appropriate medical equipment, assistive devices, monitoring approaches, professional staff,

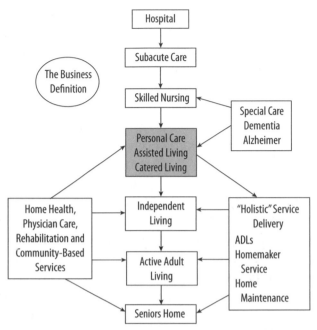

Figure 1.1. The vertical continuum of housing and care arrangements for older adults. *Source:* Modified from Moore (2001), p. 17.

and quality controls are available (Figure 1.1). There are few care-related factors—except perhaps displays of physically aggressive and disruptive behavioral disorders, and frequent wandering behaviors—that unequivocally account for why older persons will have to occupy one long-term care alternative as opposed to another.

Research findings, however, continually remind us that older persons prefer to age in place in their homes and apartments (American Association of Retired People [AARP], 2000). Thus, it is not surprising that we find older persons in ordinary dwellings who are just as frail as those in nursing homes, especially when they receive extensive assistance from family members or paid caregivers or regularly attend a nearby adult day center offering them both long-term and acute care on a 9-to-5 basis (e.g., services offered by Program of All-Inclusive Care for the Elderly, or PACE) (O'Brian, 2005). One study found that recipients of such adult day care displayed a very low risk of institutionalization even though all of them were certified (because of their dependencies) to enter nursing homes (Friedman et al., 2005).

It is perhaps surprising that research is not available that systematically identifies the conditions under which it might be "better" (e.g., as measured by quality of life and quality of care indicators) to enter an assisted living residence than to stay put (see chapter 4; Foundation for Accountability, Robert Wood Johnson Foundation, 2001). To the extent that we establish the downsides of dealing with the frailties of old age in ordinary dwellings—and these pronouncements begin to influence consumers—even a small shift in the percentage of older persons changing their aging-in-place preferences would significantly increase the demand for assisted living.

Assisted living residences also compete with other planned group residential care options whose future appeal is uncertain because they are continually transforming their once taken-for-granted long-term care missions. At one end of the spectrum are independent living communities (previously known as "congregate housing"). They seek to make their housing arrangements more architecturally attractive, luxurious, and hotel-like, but at the same time try to capture an older population with more moderate than higher incomes. Although, they were once usually limited to offering shelter, emergency monitoring, meals, housekeeping, and recreation, in an attempt to reach a larger market and keep their residents longer, they are increasingly offering personal assistance and even nursing services to their older occupants. As observed above, rather than offering this assistance with their own paid staff, they rely on an outsourcing model of service delivery whereby direct care workers are brought into their buildings who are hired through home care agencies. To the extent that they can offer shelter-and-care packages at more affordable rates than assisted living, they threaten to capture a larger share of the long-term care market.

At the other end of the long-term care spectrum are nursing homes, distinguished by their sterile, hospital-like, and—to most consumers—unappealing institutional qualities. Even though state governments regulate them more stringently than assisted living residences, they are often found to offer poor quality care (Mor et al., 2004). Their proponents argue that this is because they predominantly accommodate lower-income older persons covered under the Medicaid program, which offers inadequate provider reimbursements paling in comparison to the fees commanded by higher-end, private-pay facilities (see chapter 11).

These venerable settings, however, are also reinventing themselves. Every year brings new examples of nursing homes transforming themselves into more humane and person-centered long-term care settings (see chapter 3) and moving away "from the traditional medical model of health care toward a more social, resident-centered model of care" (Utz, 2003, p. 381). Facilities identified under such rubrics as the Eden Alternative, the Pioneer Network, Green Houses, and other consumer-friendly labels have emerged that appear and operate more like contemporary assisted living residences than traditional old-age institutions (Rabig et al., 2006). Although these new prototypes are still very much in the minority, their supporters are enthusiastic about their potential (Robert Jenkens, personal communication) as more consumer-friendly long-term care options, even as others are skeptical about their staying power and their quality of care and quality of life claims (Robyn Stone, personal communication).

If, however, most nursing homes come to embrace a social model of care (see chapters 3 and 15), will they really be different from assisted living residences? Moreover, will such a makeover substantially change how tomorrow's mainstream population of older Americans, particularly those with higher incomes, respond to this new generation of redesigned settings? Indeed, one can imagine a future scenario in which assisted living residences no longer have a monopoly on its now distinctive brand of care. The increasingly blurred boundaries between long-term care settings will simply disappear, and what we now know as nursing homes—as least as they are currently understood—will cease to exist. Assisted living residences and nursing homes will become indistinguishable. Some further believe that tomorrow's so-called nursing homes will operate more like hospitals or rehabilitation centers—as is increasingly true today—because they will predominantly serve older persons with shorter-term subacute or postacute needs (Decker, 2005).

Predicting the future is difficult because responses by assisted living properties to these sources of competition are also clouding our view of long-term care. Even as nursing homes continue serving older persons who, on average, have more serious chronic health problems and disabilities overall, national surveys confirm that a significant and increasing share of assisted living facilities are offering comparable care (Golant, 1998; Spillman, Liu & McGilliard, 2002; Waidmann, 2003; Rosenblatt et al., 2004). It is not uncommon for operators of assisted living residences to dedicate a floor or wing—or their entire buildings—for example, for older persons with late-stage Alzheimer disease (Rosenblatt et al., 2004). Even palliative or hospice care is increasingly delivered in assisted living settings (Jerant, 2004).

Federal and state governments are also contributing to these trends through programmatic initiatives designed to help accelerate the substitutability of nursing homes with assisted living residences for their very frail and low-income elderly constituencies. With the goal of slowing the growth of their Medicaid program expenditures, these efforts have succeeded in moving, or *transitioning*, older nursing home residents into community settings, including assisted living. Related *diversion* programs have offered community-based options, including assisted living, to frail seniors now living in their ordinary homes, making it possible for them to avoid a nursing home stay (Summer, 2005).

In light of these developments, it is not surprising that assisted living residences have siphoned off older persons who earlier would have entered these institutions (Bishop, 1999; see also chapters 11 and 13). Moreover, research on care outcomes offers little reason to question these trends. Studies offer little evidence that when the older occupants of assisted living residences are very frail they receive less adequate care than the comparable occupants of nursing homes. Findings show that they do not experience significantly different downward changes in their ability to perform ADLs or negative changes in their experiences of pain, discomfort, and psychological well-being (Frytak et al., 2001).

These trends, however, raise a troubling question. If the individuals occupying assisted living residences need full assistance with their activities of daily living, require 24-hour nursing care, nursing home–like equipment (e.g., Hoyer lifts), and the skilled nursing staff dominates the managerial climate, is it possible for these housing arrangements to be anything but nursing home–like? Expressed more simply, can a long-term care setting serve a group of older residents with high-acuity and significant medical needs and still offer a design- and staff-friendly social model of care?

(4) As traditional boundaries separating long-term care settings continue to blur, older persons and their families will have more shelter-and-care choices and it becomes more difficult to predict whether they will occupy assisted living residences.

Caregiving by Family Members

The bulk of caregiving takes place in ordinary houses and apartments and depends heavily on the assistance of family members—predominantly spouses, daughters, and daughters-in-law—sometimes assisted by paid caregivers (see chapter 7). These "informal care" arrangements constitute the greatest competitor of assisted living residences (Golant, 2008a, forthcoming). Even when older persons are receiving assistance from government-sponsored or private-pay programs that offer home- or community-based services, the success of these responses depends heavily on whether family members are also there to assist. When, for various reasons, they cannot count on their own families, older persons are more likely to seek the care offered by assisted living residences and nursing homes.

What the future holds for the viability of family members as caregivers, however, is uncertain. This was the conclusion of a comprehensive assessment that looked at the future availability of adult children and spouses as influenced by marriage and divorce rates, women's greater participation in the labor force, later childbearing, rates of childlessness, and the age structure of spouses (Wolf, Hunt, & Knickman, 2005; see also chapter 7). Other analyses offer decidedly pessimistic scenarios. One recent study showed that between 1982 and 1999 family members became "a relatively less prominent source of elder care" than had previously been the norm (Wolf, Hunt, & Knickman, 2005, p. 381). To the extent that large geographical distances increasingly separate the residential locations of younger and older generations, such a trend may be heightened going forward.

Despite the emphasis of research on the demographics of the informal support network, the availability of family members as caregivers will probably more depend on how future generations of women view their family obligations. Just as women no longer feel compelled to be "stay-at-home" moms to care for even their youngest children, in the future, they will feel much less obligated to provide the bulk of the assistance to their frail older parents or even their frail spouses. Many reasons may contribute to these changing female role expectations. There is already cumulating evidence pointing to the tremendous physical and emotional toll of caregiving, and family members are increasingly being accused of physical, psychological, and financial abuses against those in their care (Johnson & Wiener, 2006). Reinforcing these predictions of a weaker female caregiving role is what we can term the selfishness factor. Three decades from now women will want to spend less time fulfilling their traditional filial and spousal responsibilities and rather seek to practice more independent lifestyles and expand their roles in the labor force.

Absent this critical source of informal care, older households may find that aging in place is a less attractive option. This assessment may be even stronger to the extent that family members find that getting in-home assistance from paid professionals is increasingly prohibitive because of labor shortages and higher wage rates. Under these circumstances, they will look more favorably on assisted living properties as the primary source of their long-term care. The income and assets (including the owned home) of older persons that might have passed to these younger family members as inheritance will be used to pay for their assisted living expenses.

Not all experts, however, agree that aging in place will erode as an alternative. Many predict that assistive devices, technological monitoring approaches, and even robots will make it possible for older persons to be less physically (perhaps even less emotionally) dependent on family members or on paid caregivers in their ordinary dwellings (Spillman & Black, 2005; Summer, 2003). Other research points to the much greater likelihood that tomorrow's older households will consist of ethnic minorities (e.g., Asians and Hispanics) who will benefit from family networks that have traditionally consisted of more dedicated caregivers. Still, the skeptics counter that as these families become assimilated into American culture, they will become more reluctant caregivers.

One trend may tip the balance in favor of the family becoming a more important source of informal care. As discussed below, we expect that the cost of occupying assisted living residences, along with other long-term care options, will rise substantially (much faster than consumer incomes) in the future. When older persons and their families are less able to avail themselves of affordable assisted living options, they may be more inclined to assume the long-term care burden—even though it will be more out of financial necessity than "love." They will rationalize their decisions by pointing to the savings in shelter costs (as opposed to service costs) that result from themselves caring for an older family member either in their own or in the older person's home.

(5) The availability of family as providers of long-term care is uncertain.

Seniors' Social Lifestyle Preferences

The social setting that seniors envision for themselves as they age will also play an important role in defining the future of assisted living. The typically homogenous age composition of assisted living residences and the possibility that a significant share of their neighbors will be very frail makes for a distinctive social context. How tomorrow's baby boomers will feel about living in such residential settings is uncertain. Early in their history, age-segregated residential settings were characterized as places with isolated older populations abandoned by their families. In contrast, now most of the literature emphasizes the supportive interpersonal relationships found in these settings, their more protective environments, and the overall higher residential satisfaction of their older occupants (Golant, 1998; Mitchell & Kemp, 2000).

There are reasons to predict that future populations of older adults will be more favorably disposed to living with others in their age group. Today, larger-than-ever numbers of persons in their sixties and early seventies—the average age of entry of persons into assisted living is 83 (American Association of Homes and Services for the Aging, 2006)—are now satisfied occupants of either planned or unplanned active adult–oriented communities or senior apartments or are familiar with persons who are enjoying living in such places. The favorable attitudes to these settings held by the next wave of older adults are further suggested by opinion polls reporting that about 47 percent of today's age 50- to 69-year-old adults would definitely or likely consider moving into an active adult community (Harris Interactive Market Research, 2005). These late-middle-aged persons are part of a generation that throughout their lives have enjoyed living arrangements where they shared accommodations with persons of their own age—as students occupying dormitories or sororities, summer campers, young professionals occupying "singles' buildings," younger married couples in neighborhoods dominated by school-age children; middle-aged "empty nest" couples in gated subdivisions; and as late-adult residents in working- and middle-class neighborhoods.

The identity of the next generation of older Americans as "older baby boomers" rather than "older adults" may also contribute to their being more favorably disposed to living in age-homogeneous enclaves. Although "boomers" display a great deal of social, economic, and political diversity (Hughes & O'Rand, 2005), they will be one of the best-educated generations of older persons and the mass marketing and advertising media have consistently celebrated their positive, upbeat, healthy self-images. One national polling study characterized them as "confident, independent, [and] optimistic" (Roper Starch Worldwide, 1999). These positive portrayals of old age are echoed by the builders of age-targeted or age-restricted "active adult" communities (Hairston, 2006). Thus, there is good reason to assume that tomorrow's elders will think more highly of themselves and will associate "being old" with positive attributes such as maturity, competence, sophistication, and self-reliance. Conversely, they will be less inclined to think of old age as a period linked with decline, loneliness, loss of status, and poor self-esteem (Golant, 2002b). If these assumptions are correct, they may well be more favorably disposed toward living with others who share their elevated status (Golant, 2002a) and less likely to attach a negative stigma to occupying age-homogeneous housing arrangements such as assisted living residences.

The ageist responses of tomorrow's younger population may also be influential, and it will not be surprising to hear them argue that older persons do not deserve their federal entitlement benefits. These assaults, however, may have unintentional consequences. They may produce a more cohesive and stronger older subculture—its members uniting in response to these verbal attacks. In this event, older persons will seek to live in residential arrangements dominated by their age group, not only for their dependable services and their beneficial social and psychological supports but also as means to avoid confronting such ageist responses and finding comfort in living with others who share their values and beliefs (Binstock, 2005).

Equivocation is, nevertheless, warranted. The members of the up-and-coming generation of older persons have spent a considerable amount of their time and energy trying to look and feel young and want others to share their perceptions. The members of this future "Botox generation" may therefore not look favorably on living in a setting—like assisted living residences—that is dominated by persons whom they consider far "older" and frailer than themselves. Not wanting to be associated with vulnerable elders and thus being defined as a member of such a group, they will avoid places like assisted living settings—or at the least delay entering them until they are very old and frail.

(6) It is unclear to what extent tomorrow's seniors will be more positively disposed to the prospects of living in a social context like assisted living that is occupied only by persons their own age who may also be very frail.

Consumers' Shelter-and-Care Preferences

Tomorrow's older consumers are likely to hold more strongly held beliefs about the characteristics they seek in their future housing and long-term care arrangements. Overall, this will be a better-educated group, more accustomed to living in higher-end housing, and generally more knowledgeable about their options than previous generations. Their family members—also more likely to come from higher socioeconomic backgrounds—will often be key participants in their decision making, a market reality that distinguishes assisted living properties from other housing arrangements.

When older consumers (and their families) are ready for the services and care offered by assisted living residences, they will demand more luxurious residential-style settings—such as, more architecturally attractive atriums, larger private dwellings, gourmet dining, concierge services, Internet and other wireless technologies—offering higher-quality and more personalized care (see chapter 6). Most future occupants will have been homeowners and, unlike their renter counterparts, will not be accustomed to having property managers dictate their residential behaviors and experiences. They will also have been nurtured in a culture offering everything from multiyear maintenance contracts on equipment and products to consumer hotlines allowing spontaneous expressions of discontent with defective merchandise or services. They will disproportionately be women who have had more extensive work histories than previous generations and who consequently will have experienced the independence, challenges, and trouble-shooting aspects of workforce participation. Consequently, they will be less reticent about criticizing the inadequacies of their accommodations.

Thus, tomorrow's elders will be inclined to reject settings that are reminiscent of the controlling and impersonal environment of the nursing home and will be less willing to trade their previously comfortable residential worlds simply for the guarantees of a more protective environment and ongoing assistance. They will want the best of worlds: a setting that is secure, safe, supportive, and comfortable but does not assault their individuality and autonomy. Future attitudinal guideposts are indicated by reports from builders of active adult communities who emphasize that today's market of younger retirees is seeking more architecturally upscale features in more spacious dwellings than prior generations, even as they seek residential settings that are easier to maintain (Webb, 2004).

As already suggested, tomorrow's older consumers will also seek out turnkey assistance solutions that allow them to access (when needed) care environments that can (eventually) respond to their high-acuity needs so that they can age in place even as their dependencies worsen. They will also be less hesitant to accuse providers of violating federal antidiscrimination laws (Americans with Disabilities Act; Fair Housing Act) when they refuse to accommodate their chronic health problems and severe disabilities and instead ask them to move to more supportive residential arrangements elsewhere (Carlson, 2005).

Overall, therefore, tomorrow's generation of older consumers—and their families—will be more demanding, less trusting, and potentially more critical of the assisted living products offered to them than have their predecessors and they will not view decline "as an inevitable consequence of aging that must be borne with equanimity" and thus will not be willing to "accept less, and hence to demand less" (Kane & Kane, 2005, p. 52). It will be the difficult task of assisted living providers to respond effectively to these more complex—and thus less predictable—consumer needs.

(7) It is likely that older consumers and their family members will be more demanding and less compromising in their long-term care selections than prior generations of seniors.

Ability to Pay for Assisted Living

The price and thus the affordability of tomorrow's assisted living product will influence the size of the future elderly consumer market (Hughes & O'Rand, 2005). Based on their future estimates of real wage growth and the overall expansion of the American economy, Knickman and Snell (2002) estimate that a greater share of seniors will be able to afford the assisted living alternative in 2030 than can today.

Knickman and Snell distinguish three current (year 2000) income-wealth groups: the poorest, that is, those who are Medicaid bound; the "Tweeners," the middle class who have adequate lifetime income and wealth but cannot handle long-term care costs; and the financially independent, who have income and wealth to handle three years of long-term care costs. They predict optimistically that the financially independent will constitute a greater share of the elderly in year 2030 compared with year 2000 (rising to 38 percent from 27 percent) and the Medicaid bound a smaller share (declining from 45 percent to 39 percent). They also predict pessimistically, however, that a greater share of the older population will consist of Tweeners (33 percent compared to 28 percent in 2000).

Even if the assumptions underlying these estimates are correct, the actual affordability of tomorrow's assisted living residences will depend on the uncertain answers to five other critical questions: (1) How disposed will tomorrow's older homeowners be to draw on the financial wealth tied up in their home equity to pay for their long-term costs? (2) How willing (able) will be the subset of economically successful adult children of tomorrow's poor or near-poor old to help defray their parents' long-term care bill? (3) How likely will it be that older persons will even ask their adult children for financial assistance (Harris Interactive Market Research, 2005)? (4) What share of seniors will be covered by long-term care insurance that could defray the costs of tomorrow's assisted living products? And (5) to what extent will public subsidies, such as Medicaid, defray the costs of tomorrow's assisted living residences (see chapters 7 and 11)?

(8) The ability of tomorrow's older consumer to pay for assisted living products is uncertain.

State Regulation of Assisted Living Residences

State governments will continue to have the major role regulating future assisted living residences; however, the agencies charged with this responsibility will confront many more types of housing and long-term care settings under their jurisdiction that offer both low- and high-acuity care. The labels we typically rely on today, such as congregate housing, assisted living, and nursing homes, which imply that there is a clear-cut continuum from low- to high-acuity care among shelter-and-care options, will increasingly become obsolete.

Most state governments will respond (as many have today) by allowing assisted living residences to operate under different licensing categories based on the level of needs of their residents and the extent to which they provide personal care and nursing and medical assistance. Few if any states will rely on a single licensing standard that imposes a "one size fits all" set of standards on all of its assisted living properties. Providers will thus have the option of catering to older persons who need either low- or high-acuity care (Carlson, 2005).

At the same time, state governments will also feel compelled to require assisted living settings to offer more protections for their elderly residents. These regulatory responses will be driven by an inevitable surge in reports by more vigilant, more informed, and better-educated older consumers (and their family members) that they have received incompetent care. This is entirely likely if only because we expect that the older population found in assisted living residences will become more physically and cognitively vulnerable. States will respond by imposing more stringent regulatory controls and will require greater accountability from the operators of assisted living residences. Quality-of-care assessments will be more detailed and comprehensive; staffing requirements will be more specifically defined and more demanding (with respect to both hours and training); negotiated risk agreements will become more standardized; and there will be more formal mechanisms required for mediation and conflict resolution (see chapter 4). Operators will have greater disclosure requirements (regarding the rules, costs, and care constraints of assisted living operations); states will impose stronger enforcement procedures; and together these responses will strengthen family advocacy rights. There will be far more regulatory oversight of outcomes of care and more demanding monitoring approaches, independent of how the delivery of care is organized (e.g., whether by professional staff hired by assisted living operator to work in a designated part of a facility or by contracted outsourced vendors).

This is a scenario that many stakeholders will find objectionable (see chapters 4, 13, and 15). More demanding state regulatory environments will initially draw criticism from assisted living advocates, who will be quick to reference the nursing home model as an example of how excessive rules and regulations can create an "institutionalized" environment that stifles residents' autonomy and dignity without guaranteeing an acceptable quality of care. State governments, however, will stop short of calling for rules and regulations as extensive as those now governing nursing homes for fear of alienating consumers who strongly dislike the institutional model. Professional associations representing the assisted living industry will help slow, but not stop, this push for a more regulated assisted living setting by trying to encourage greater numbers of their members to police themselves (see chapter 9).

Those stakeholders who endorse more regulations will have different motivations (Assisted Living Workgroup Steering Committee, 2003). For example, nursing home providers will seek to restrict the ability of assisted living residences to provide high-acuity care because of their continuing concern about losing market share, especially if government programs begin to subsidize the occupancy and care costs of assisted living residences (see chapter 15).

In addition, a wide-ranging group of medical, rehabilitation, and therapeutic professionals will push for greater regulation of assisted living and a more medical model of care (Assisted Living Workgroup Steering Committee, 2003). They will be motivated in part by their legitimate skepticism that it is not possible to offer nursing-related services competently in settings for which there are no uniform standards regarding staff training and qualifications. They will also be concerned that a less regulated assisted living option will reduce the certainty that residents will be offered a predetermined number of hours of their services—thus jeopardizing their own livelihoods.

The financial community will equate a more regulated long-term care setting with greater certainty of product performance—thus fewer financial surprises and overall a more predictable return on their investment. Underwriters of various types of insurance products will similarly view more regulation as a means to reduce unforeseen resident accidents and abuses and thus their liability exposure.

Even as the family members of older persons have increasingly shunned the overregulated and institutionalized nursing home alternative, they will be at the vanguard of groups demanding more government oversight of tomorrow's assisted living products. Although they may be more open to relinquishing their own caregiving responsibilities, it will not mean that they will experience less guilt or fewer worries regarding their decisions. They will thereby feel more comfortable when they perceive that their loved ones are in more protected and, by inference, more predictable care environments. To receive ongoing feedback on their status, they will demand that assisted living providers rely on more sophisticated monitoring techniques and provide up-to-date reports on their care responses (see chapter 8). Adult children willing to divest themselves of their caregiving roles will have witnessed a lifetime of corporate abuses that have harmed consumers and employees alike. In this context, it seems unreasonable to expect that they will trust (what will become increasingly large and complex) corporate entities that provide long-term care. This greater consumer vigilance will undoubtedly be accompanied by more frequent disclosures of quality-of-care lapses and horror stories as the industry expands and matures, particularly as less experienced companies try to capitalize on the growing assisted living market. A more regulated assisted living product will inevitably expose the less competent practices of this small subset of providers.

Large assisted living corporations that own or manage facilities in multiple states may also view stepped-up regulations as a positive development. As public policy expert Barbara Manard (1997) has reported, assisted living providers will be willing to accept more oversight as long as states are not "heavy-handed about it." In particular, new regulatory requirements that are similar across states will enable providers to deal with more geographically uniform construction, admitting, and operating standards (e.g., common resident and staff assessment tools). Thus, they will look positively on the prospects of not having 50 different state-focused management and staff handbooks and construe such imposed standardization as making it easier to monitor care across all their properties. They will also interpret more regulation as a means to drive away—or at least equalize—the competition of less competent providers who have been unwilling to meet agreed-upon voluntary professional association standards, but as a result could offer less expensive accommodations (see chapter 9). They will also consider the departure from the marketplace of these competitors as a means to insure an overall better product image and thus to present older consumers a less ambiguous product line. Finally, they will believe that by acceding to somewhat less burdensome state regulations, they will fend off potentially far more imposing federal oversight and at the same time better protect themselves against insurance liability claims, which in turn should keep their insurance rates lower. By contrast, smaller assisted living (board and care) providers may resist being more heavily regulated because they will be less able to absorb the extra costs of compliance (Mollica & Johnson-Lamarche, 2005).

(9) States will recognize more diverse types of assisted living properties but will regulate them more stringently.

Response to Uncertainty: The Business Models of Tomorrow's Assisted Living Residences

Business models designed to thrive in a climate of uncertainty will drive the look and functioning of tomorrow's assisted living residences. Providers will have to grapple with four fundamental questions: (1) What will be the most desirable number and case mix of high- and low-acuity residents in our properties, and should we attempt to capture greater shares of older consumers who are at the extreme ends of the frailty continuum—that is, who require both heavy and light care? (2) How can we design, manage, and market our properties to compete more effectively for older consumers—at both ends of the care continuum—who are opting to age in place in their ordinary dwellings? (3) To what extent can our lobbying efforts and those of our professional associations contribute to public policies that make our properties more accessible to low- and moderate-income older persons yet at the same time allow us to price units consistent with our cost realities? (4) To what extent will our potential market of older consumers favor assisted living residences from which they do not have to move again even as their physical and cognitive impairments worsen?

We predict that two broad goals will guide assisted living providers as they seek to cope with tomorrow's uncertain business climate. First, they will continue to increase the critical mass or scope of their operations in order to achieve greater economies of scale by serving a larger and more diverse market of older consumers. Second, they will attempt to create a more flexible and fluid model of assistance and care that will enable their properties to quickly respond to unexpected changes in consumer markets or by the competition.

These strategies will be propelled by studies showing that, if properties are appropriately designed and staffed, they can competently serve older persons with both low- and high-acuity needs. There is simply little research evidence reporting that the quality-of-life and care outcomes of residents are linked to the size, age, ownership status, or operations style of their assisted living properties (Zimmerman et al., 2005; see also chapter 4). As a result, cost and profit concerns, consumer preferences, and sound management principles will shape the business models that drive the look and operations of assisted living. Assisted living operators will respond by increasing both the vertical and horizontal integration of their businesses, which in turn will result in the continuation and acceleration of current merger and acquisition trends.

Vertically Integrated Assisted Living Residences

A more vertically integrated assisted living industry will be dominated by fewer but more diversified corporations, each of which will be more likely to own or manage properties running the gamut of long-term care alternatives: subacute care settings, nursing homes, assisted living residences, home care agencies, and independent living (congregate) housing sites (or their merged or morphed versions). Corporate providers will seek to integrate their operations seamlessly to eliminate consumer anxiety over dealing with different long-term care providers and of having to relocate (except perhaps to a nearby building) when their impairment and needs for assistance change. The most recent and notable evidence of assisting living providers expanding their marketing reach is for them to deliver their services and assistance right into the ordinary residences of frail older persons who are trying to avoid relocating elsewhere.

Assisted living providers will rely more heavily on outsourcing and partnership relationships with firms offering services that they can readily introduce or stop as residents' frailty needs change. This will enable providers to offer their residents more individualized care and give them ever more options to bundle together idiosyncratically those services specifically tailored to their individual disability profiles and lifestyle needs. These operations will mimic the just-in-time manufacturing processes of many of today's computer companies, whereby their managements can quickly modify the manufacturing schedule and components of products to respond to changes in consumer demand.

Future assisted living providers will increasingly introduce architectural, technological, and organizational innovations to enable their properties to accommodate simultaneously both the least and most impaired older residents. Properties will be distinguished by their chameleon-like appearance and operations—operating over one period of time as independent living centers (serving seniors who are less frail) and over another as assisted living communities (serving seniors who are more frail). To execute this more complex business model, we expect that providers will incorporate more architecturally flexible strategies for interior building design, initiate staffing practices malleable enough to accommodate a broad case-mix of residents, and depend far more on computer-assisted care and monitoring regimens to respond quickly to the more complex array of resident needs.

They will be inspired by the successes of the Green House project (see chapter 3) and its podlike or modular shelter-and-care organization, which consist of multiple residential buildings (mini-board-and-care properties?) that each accommodates about ten occupants. The pods of tomorrow's assisted living providers—which often will consist of larger and more luxurious residential buildings than the Green House fare—will each be able to accommodate a homogeneous cluster of residents who require comparable levels of care and/or share similar cultural backgrounds. This will enable providers to accommodate consumer groups with various distinctive lifestyle and competence needs, yet make it possible for residents to associate primarily with persons like themselves. Research has pointed to the downsides of mixing residents in the same quarters with different levels of impairment or lifestyles. A pod design allows providers to create separate living and eating areas to ensure boundaries between these resident groups (Golant, 1998). This will avoid such problems as more impaired residents feeling overly challenged in a setting geared to more active residents; conflicts arising from cognitively intact older residents interacting with persons having dementia; and less impaired residents having to be reminded of their own prospective vulnerability. Overall, vertically integrated assisted living residences offer various advantages to assisted living providers:

- Capture higher shares of both the low- and high-acuity consumer markets and thus reduce the downsides of inaccurate demand predictions. It will be easier to own or manage the long-term care component that unpredictably becomes your major competition.
- Offer older consumers more flexible alternatives tailored to specific lifestyles (ethnic, religious, occupational) and levels of wealth.
- Obtain resident referrals from all properties along the care continuum. As one consultant expressed it, "Most savvy developers recognize that combining levels of care is the best way to guarantee a feeder market and maximize tenant retention" (Gerard, 2000, p. 2).
- Cope more effectively with predicted shortages of both unskilled and professional long-term care workers—and with the higher labor

costs that result (Toossi, 2005; U.S. Congressional Budget Office, 2004). Vertically integrated corporations will have the expertise and financial means to substitute technological inputs for labor inputs (monitoring, diagnosing, controlling ambient environment, communicating needs); be able to share more effectively their operations staff, care personnel, and overall management resources with other properties they own; and will organize their own training programs through outsourcing arrangements with third-party organizations (which they will often own) to ensure that their staffs receive the most specialized and up-to-date training.

- Achieve greater corporate visibility overall and become identified by more nationally known brand names. Brand loyalty will become a marketing tool. Although today we are not accustomed to assisted living providers marketing on national media or consumers receiving frequent flier miles when they pay for their long-term care bill, these will become mainstream marketing approaches in the future.

Horizontally Integrated Assisted Living Residences

Vertically integrated corporate entities will also seek to integrate their business operations horizontally. Assisted living corporate chains will own or manage clusters of assisted living properties, along with other components of their vertically integrated long-term care operation, within a relatively proximate or compact geographic area (e.g., on the same campus setting, within adjacent counties, or within a group of transportation-linked metropolitan areas).

These spatial agglomerations of long-term care settings will offer multiple advantages:

- The sharing of material resources (vans, buses, staffing, equipment).
- The negotiation of more favorable local pricing contracts with food, pharmacy, and home-care providers resulting in lower operating costs per unit or bed.
- The sharing of advertising, marketing, and client assessment costs (Redding, 2005).
- The ability to build or acquire assisted living properties with smaller tenant populations, which in total, however, will still achieve the same economies of scale advantages as larger facilities. These smaller

buildings will again give their operators various competitive ad-vantages. Here residents can realize more personalized and hands-on staffing assistance (equivalent to the luxury bed-and-breakfast inn). In turn, smaller projects will allow for the more effective sepa-ration of older occupants by impairment level, because with smaller numbers it is easier to achieve homogeneity. They also allow provid-ers to more readily "transform" their accommodations to fit the dif-ferent long-term care needs of their diverse consumer market (Red-ding, 2005).

The Continuing-Care Retirement Communities (CCRCs) of Tomorrow

The adoption of a horizontally and vertically integrated business model for assisted living has an important and successful precedent in today's senior housing industry—the CCRC that offers the full gamut of low- to high-acuity care, including assisted living, often sited on a campus-like setting but sometimes also dispersed among different floors of a high-rise building.

CCRCs distinguish themselves by the payment plans and types of con-tracts they offer their residents. Almost 80 percent of these communities charge an up-front entrance fee (that may be up to 100 percent refundable to older person or estate), in addition to charging monthly service fees (American Seniors Housing Association, 2004). Close to half of the CCRCs require their residents to sign full or modified life-care contracts that obli-gate them to provide a guaranteed level of assisted living or nursing home care at discounted prices over the course of their remaining lives. Others offer fee-for-service contracts (typically, monthly rents and service fees) that do not include any promise of discounted prices for their other levels of care; these CCRCs may also charge an entrance fee.

We predict that fee-for-service occupancy agreements (monthly rental payment contracts) will become more prevalent in the future and that tomorrow's CCRCs will be less likely to require that their occupants sign life-care contracts or hand over large up-front entrance fees. Property own-ers will offer their residents considerable flexibility as to how they bundle together personally tailored packages of services to match their distinctive lifestyles and care needs. We also expect to see more ownership-oriented CCRCs than are found today, with residents negotiating separate contracts

for their long-term care. Providers, however, will demand carefully exe-
cuted estate plans from this new generation of "owners" to ensure smooth
property transfers upon their deaths.

The most visible of these future exemplars, which we refer to as "elder
parks" (Golant, 2002a), will be sited on large and attractive, upscale campus-like complexes reminiscent of our current office and industrial parks.
In these complexes will be located a wide variety of housing arrangements
and long-term care establishments that will cater to everyone from young
elders, who are healthy and independent, to those who are very old and
frail. Elder parks, owned by corporate conglomerates and large nonprofits,
will be architecturally well designed, with much open space, and taste-
fully landscaped to showcase their establishments.

More Expensive Assisted Living Products and the Government's Response

As discussed above, a significant share of tomorrow's seniors (or their
families) will find it impossible to afford the costs of occupying future
assisted living options. This will be even more likely if our predictions are
correct that providers will confront higher costs of building and operating
their properties. The ability of lower- and moderate-income older persons
to access these alternatives will depend on whether state and federal governments provide funding to make them affordable.

More Expensive Assisted Living Products

In 2007, the average annual cost to occupy a one-bedroom unit in an
assisted living residence in the United States was about $32,500, still con-
siderably less than the $75,000 annual cost for a private room at a nursing
home (Genworth Financial, 2007). Average prices can be deceptive, however, and costs can be substantially higher in states and metropolitan areas
with pricier housing markets. Many assisted living residences also charge
substantially more than the average because of their architecturally more
luxurious properties and their provision of higher-acuity care to a population of more vulnerable residents (Genworth Financial, 2007).

The costs of building and operating assisted living residences are expected to rise significantly faster than the general inflation rate (assumed
to be 3 percent annually) over the next two or three decades (Kemper,

Komisar, & Alecxih, 2005). Builders of these properties are predicted to confront higher borrowing costs because the U.S. economy will have to finance the costs of the burgeoning demand for Medicaid and Medicare services and the large Social Security expenditures linked with the retirement of the baby boomers (Holtz-Eakin, 2005). Efforts by state and local governments to contain urban sprawl and thus to reduce the availability of developable land will also put upward pressure on land costs and property taxes. Much higher costs for building materials and construction labor will also be contributing factors. The continuing efforts of local governments to pass on to developers the costs of funding basic infrastructures (roads, sewers, utilities) in the form of impact or user fees are specifically likely to add to building costs. Development costs will also increase as both state and local governments make greater demands on assisted living residences to satisfy more stringent architectural design requirements and security precautions (see chapter 13).

In their efforts to curb these increasing costs, assisted living developers will favor exurban areas on the perimeters of expanding metropolitan areas as locations for their new vertically and horizontally integrated developments. Lower land costs, the ability to assemble large tracts of land, the absence of NIMBY (not in my back yard) protests, the proximity of large consumer markets of older persons, including their children (who want to live near the assisted living residences of their loved ones), and less restrictive building constraints will be the benefits. Developers will still favor sites, however, that are readily accessible by car or rail to ensure their accessibility to visiting family members. Assisted living providers will market the "closeness to nature" of their properties as an amenity unattainable in more urban locations.

Higher operating costs will be a likely consequence of state governments regulating assisted living residences more stringently to ensure the delivery of good quality of care—for example, by establishing minimum staffing ratios, requiring more staff training, and more strictly defining the scope of practice of staff members. As residents needing higher-acuity care increasingly enter assisted living, providers will need staff (whom they hire or outsource) who have more nursing care skills and who have the training to operate sophisticated assistive technology and monitoring equipment. Operating cost increases may be especially high if predictions are accurate regarding a future labor shortage linked to tightened federal immigration laws and a smaller cohort of working-age individuals that will drive both wages and fringe benefits higher (Friedland, 2004; Kemper, Komisar, & Alecxih, 2005; Toossi, 2005; U.S. Congressional Budget Office, 2004).

Consumers themselves will also play a role in driving up the cost of assisted living. First, their higher-income older occupants will demand higher-quality, more luxurious, and thus more expensive products. Second, in the absence of adequate government subsidies to make assisted living properties affordable, family members will assume more of the costs of long-term care for their loved ones, which will enable assisted living providers to charge a higher price for their properties. Third, compared to other generations of older Americans, tomorrow's residents of assisted living properties will have owned the historically largest and highest-valued dwellings and it will be common practice for them to sell their properties to pay for their long-term care rather than transfer their "housing" wealth to their children. Fourth, and finally, although still in the minority, a larger share of future older consumers will be self-insured, relying on their long-term care insurance to cover their assisted living expenses (see chapter 11).

Assisted Living for Poor and Frail Elders

These projected higher prices will make most assisted living properties unaffordable to a significant share of tomorrow's older population in the lower- and moderate-income brackets—the aforementioned Medicaid bound, but also the near-poor or Tweener group. If the public sector does not change its current policies, today's shortfall of affordable assisted living will undoubtedly worsen in the future (Golant, 2002c).

It is easy to be pessimistic about the role that government will play in helping the poor afford assisted living. As others remind us (chapters 11, 12, 14, and 15), it is extraordinarily difficult to predict the extent to which the public sector will respond to the long-term care needs of this country's economically deprived elders. Currently, state Medicaid programs remain heavily biased toward subsidizing nursing home care of our poor. By 2004, only 36 percent of the long-term care expenditures of Medicaid were paying for care outside of nursing homes, although this was up from 14 percent in 1991 (Shirk, 2006). Moreover, many states are reluctant to move away from the institutional model. Older persons in only about 12 percent of the nation's private-pay assisted living units received Medicaid (waiver) funding to defray their costs of care (see "Foreword"), although most of this group occupied smaller board-and-care facilities rather than professionally managed properties (Kitchener, Hernandez, Ng, & Harrington, 2006). Substantial changes in the administration of the Medicaid program will be necessary if it is to continue to move away from its institutional bias (Mollica & Johnson-Lamarche, 2005; Shirk, 2006; Spillman, Liu, & McGilliard, 2002).

State governments, however, will confront continued pressure to reduce their already swollen Medicaid budgets. Federal budget deficits are likely to offer further catalysts for such reductions given our country's future obligations to finance our large entitlement programs of Social Security and Medicare. In the worst case scenario, the fiscal demands of these programs will be so burdensome that they sharply reduce the availability of subsidies for all other types of affordable housing and long-term care options. Furthermore, it is likely that an even larger share of the American public than today will be hostile to the idea of the government subsidizing the occupancy and care costs of assisted living to make it affordable for the poor. The public will be much more inclined to demand that tomorrow's aging baby boomers protect against catastrophic long-term care costs by acquiring insurance or alternatively that the families of impaired elders assume more of the financial costs of their care.

Nonetheless, both the federal and state governments will still feel pressured to offer community-based shelter-and-care assistance to low-income seniors who cannot count on their family members. Assisted living alternatives will increasingly be viewed as the most attractive long-term strategy, not only when compared with nursing homes but also with home- and community-based care delivered to a geographically spread out population of older recipients. Research will convincingly show that assisted living residences offer various advantages over these alternatives for delivering long-term care, based on indicators such as labor productivity, unit care costs, access to advanced technology, and quality of care outcomes.

The Demise of the Small Board-and-Care Option

Smaller, less professionally managed, and often family-run residential care facilities, primarily occupied by low-income older persons, often identified as board-and-care facilities (see chapter 5), will be substantially disadvantaged by these assisted living trends. They will experience more difficulties absorbing the overall increases in the cost of doing business and will be less able to pass their higher operating costs on to their consumers. In particular, they will have poor access to capital markets to obtain new construction or rehabilitation loans, be less able to benefit from the economies of scale enjoyed by corporate entities, and have more difficulty complying with the costs of a more demanding regulatory environment. Financial constraints will further limit their ability to offer state of the art technological responses to tomorrow's impaired and chronically ill seniors. Furthermore, as state governments look to corporate-managed assisted living properties to increase the stock of affordable units, small board-and-care facilities will be the losers. The economics of the real estate market will offer a further incentive for their owners to cease their operations. Many operators will be able to realize high selling prices for their properties because they will be sited on valuable real estate for which prospective buyers will envision more profitable uses (Morgan, Eckert, Gruber-Baldini, & Zimmerman, 2004; Thomassy, 2000). (There is anecdotal evidence that once profitable bed-and-breakfasts are experiencing the same economic incentives.) Confronted with these challenges, a significant share of today's board-and-care facilities will close.

Two unique features of these small residences, however, may play havoc with this prediction. Most board-and-care facilities—at least at the small end of the continuum—are able to fill their rooms because state governments have relied on these options to accommodate poor and frail elders who would otherwise end up in nursing home rooms subsidized by far more expensive Medicaid dollars. Most occupants of today's board-and-care options are SSI recipients who also benefit from additional subsidies though state supplements to this federal program as well as Medicaid reimbursements. Thus, the financial viability—indeed, the existence—of the board-and-care option owes much to federal and state government transfer payments targeted to poor older persons.

State governments have the power to strengthen or weaken the competitive position of this option. For example, they can create a licensing category under which "board-and-care" facilities are required to satisfy less demanding regulatory criteria in the recognition that they cannot afford the staffing and care requirements imposed on larger, corporate-run properties (see chapter 5). How state governments respond will depend on whether it is in their fiscal interests to maintain small board-and-care residences as a haven for their poor elderly constituencies. They must confront the risk that, with the demise of this option, they would end up with higher long-term care bills because of their need to care for this vulnerable group in more expensive facilities. We predict, however, that state leaders will favor larger and corporate-managed assisted living residences as more cost-effective approaches to achieve affordable shelter and care.

Some board-and-care facilities, however, might persist for a different reason. Many current providers could adopt a high-end, boutique model of long-term care. Such residences could conceivably be operated through franchising or chain business arrangements and would cater to a wealthy clientele. These persons would welcome a setting offering around-the-clock staffing and care, including nursing services, and be willing to pay these higher costs in return for enjoying a highly personalized care arrangement. Thus, the future small board-and-care facility could reinvent itself by catering to a very small but ultra-wealthy niche market that parallels the elite services offered, for example, in small cruise ships, small hotels, small, luxurious, private retail stores, and small, high-end restaurants.

Conclusions and Implications for the Future

The factors that can influence the availability and attributes of tomorrow's assisted living options are well known. Almost all them, however, ranging from the disability profiles of older persons to the competitive appeal and public support of long-term care alternatives, have uncertain future trajectories. Although assisted living providers may be able to count on generally larger numbers of future frail and disabled older persons as potential consumers, almost all other determinants of their operations are difficult to predict. Thus, coping with uncertainty is likely to drive the future business models of assisted living stakeholders.

This chapter has predicted that the assisted living industry will cope with these pervasive unknowns by continuing the current trend of adopting highly vertically and horizontally integrated business models. These strategies will maximize their flexibility to capture a market of older persons who need both low- and high-acuity care, allow them to respond quickly to the vagaries of consumer demand, and make them more adept at reacting to a continually changing competitive environment. Distinctions we now make between housing arrangements, such as congregate (independent) living, assisted living, and nursing homes will become so blurred that tomorrow's assisted living products will emerge as amalgamations or hybrids of these products.

We predict that public programs will tighten their regulatory requirements in response to pressures from multiple stakeholders seeking more predictable quality-of-care outcomes from their assisted living products. At the same time, future regulatory environments will offer private-pay providers considerable flexibility as to how they tailor their assisted living operations to fit their markets of elderly consumers—likely to consist of larger shares of older persons with high-acuity needs.

A more stringently regulated assisted living product will be but one of the factors that will drive up the occupancy price of assisted living and increasingly put it out of financial reach of most older Americans. In response, the public sector will be under more pressure to allocate larger amounts of funding to make private pay assisted living residences affordable (Golant, 2008b, forthcoming). The future role of the government as a provider of affordable shelter and care, however, is difficult to predict, and there is good reason to be pessimistic about its future commitments (Golant, 2003). In all likelihood, family members will assume a larger share of the financial burden of long-term care and middle-aged and young-old persons will feel more pressure to take out long-term care insurance coverage. Nonetheless, even in the face of more limited fiscal commitments, assisted living residences will be considered one of the most cost-effective strategies by which to provide affordable long-term care.

On the one hand, most small board-and-care facilities will be the casualties of these changes, because they will have greater difficulty competing with the more regulated and comprehensive assisted living products that benefit from operating economies of scale and more flexible business models. Their future viability will wane as public programs less frequently offer them favorable subsidies. On the other hand, some share of board-and-care facilities will repackage themselves as niche or boutique products offering highly personalized care to the very wealthy.

REFERENCES

AARP. 2000. *Fixing to Stay: A national survey on housing and home modification issues.* Washington, DC: AARP.

American Association of Homes and Services for the Aging. 2006. *2006 Overview of assisted living*. Washington, DC: American Association of Homes and Services for the Aging.

American Seniors Housing Association. 2004. *The state of seniors housing*. Washington, DC: American Seniors Housing Association.

Assisted Living Workgroup Steering Committee. 2003. *Assuring quality in assisted living: Guidelines for federal and state policy, state regulations, and operations: A report to the U.S. Special Committee on Aging from the Assisted Living Group*. Washington, DC: American Association of Homes and Services for the Aging.

Bersani, M. 2007. Tackling the new political landscape. *Assisted Living Executive* January/February, 29–30.

Binstock, R. H. 2005. Old-age policies, politics, and ageism. *Generations 29* (1), 73–78.

Bishop, C. E. 1999. Where are the missing elders? The decline in nursing home use, 1985 and 1995. *Health Affairs 18* (4), 146–55.

Carlson, E. M. 2005. *Critical issues in assisted living*. Washington, DC: National Senior Citizens Law Center.

Cohen, M. A., Weinrobe, M., Miller, J., & Ingoldsby, A. 2005. *Becoming disabled after age 65: The expected lifetime costs of independent living*. Washington, DC: AARP.

Decker, F. H. 2005. *Nursing homes, 1977–99: What has changed, what has not?* Hyattsville, MD: National Center for Health Statistics.

Friedland, R. B. 2004. *Caregivers and long-term care needs in the 21st century: Will public policy meet the challenge? Issue Brief*. Washington, DC: Georgetown University, Long-Term Care Financing Project.

Friedland, R. B., & Summer, L. 1999. *Demography is not destiny*. Washington, DC: National Academy on an Aging Society, Gerontological Society of America.

Friedman, S. M., Steinwachs, D. M., Rathouz, P. J., Burton, L. C., & Mukamel, D. B. 2005. Characteristics predicting nursing home admission in the program of all-inclusive care for elderly people. *Gerontologist 45* (2), 157–66.

Frytak, J. R., Kane, R. A., Finch, M. D., Kane, R. L., & Maude-Griffin, R. 2001. Outcome trajectories for assisted living and nursing facility residents in Oregon. *Health Services Research 36* (1 Pt. 1), 91–111.

Foundation for Accountability and the Robert Wood Johnson Foundation. 2001. *A portrait of informal caregivers in America, 2001*. Portland, OR: Foundation for Accountability.

Genworth Financial. 2007. *Genworth Financial 2007 cost of care survey*. New York: Genworth Financial.

Gerard, A. 2000. Taking the temperature of seniors' housing. *National Association of Home Builders News*.

Golant, S. M. 1998. The promise of assisted living as a shelter and care alternative for frail American elders: A cautionary essay. In B. Schwarz & R. Brent (Eds.),

Aging, autonomy, and architecture: Advances in assisted living (pp. 32–59). Baltimore: John Hopkins University Press.

Golant, S. M. 2002a. Deciding where to live: The emerging residential settlement patterns of retired Americans. *Generations 26* (11), 66–73.

Golant, S. M. 2002b. Geographic inequalities in the availability of government-subsidized rental housing for low-income older persons in Florida. *Gerontologist 42* (1), 100–108.

Golant, S. M. 2002c. The housing problems of the future elderly population, appendix G-1. In Commission on Affordable Housing and Health Facility Needs for Seniors in the 21st Century (Ed.), *A quiet crisis in America: A report to Congress* (pp. 189–370). Washington, DC: American Association of Homes and Services for the Aging.

Golant, S. M. 2003. Political and organizational barriers to satisfying low-income U.S. seniors need for affordable rental housing with supportive services. *Journal of Aging and Social Policy 12* (2), 36–57.

Golant, S. M. 2004. Do impaired older persons with health care needs occupy U.S. assisted living facilities? *Journal of Gerontology: Social Sciences 59* (2), S68–79.

Golant, S. M. 2008a, forthcoming. Irrational exuberance for the aging in place of vulnerable low-income older homeowners: A commentary. *Journal of Aging and Social Policy 20* (4).

Golant, S. M. 2008b, forthcoming. Affordable clustered housing-care: A category of long-term care options for the elderly poor. *Journal of Housing for the Elderly 21* (3).

Grimes, P. 2006. Assisted living image? Positive, mostly. *Assisted Living Executive 13* (1), 5.

Gross, J. 2005. When experts need experts. *New York Times,* November 10.

Hairston, J. B. 2006. Boomer building boom: Generation sets is own course to retirement. *Atlanta Journal-Constitution.* January 13.

Harris Interactive Market Research. 2005. *Pulte homes: baby boomer study, full report.* www.corporate-ir.net/media_files/irol/77/77968/BabyBoomerStudy.pdf.

Hernandez, M. 2005. Assisted living in all its guises. *Generations 29* (4), 16–23.

Holtz-Eakin, D. 2005. *Implications of demographic changes for the budget and the economy.* Washington, DC: Congressional Budget Office.

Hughes, E., & O'Rand, A. M. 2005. *The American People Census, 2000: The lives and times of the baby boomers.* Washington, DC: Population Reference Bureau.

Johnson, R. W., & Wiener, J. M. 2006. *A profile of frail older Americans and their caregivers.* Washington, DC: Urban Institute.

Kane, R. L., & Kane, R. A. 2005. Ageism in health care and long-term care. *Generations 29* (3), 49–54.

Kemper, P., Komisar, H. L., & Alecxih, L. 2005. Long-term care over an uncertain future: what can current retirees expect? *Inquiry 42* (4), 335–50.

Kitchener, M., Hernandez, M., Ng, T., & Harrington, C. 2006. Residential care provision in medicaid home- and community-based waivers: a national study of program trends. *Gerontologist 46* (2), 165–72.

Knickman, J. R., & Snell, E. K. 2002. The 2030 problem: caring for aging baby boomers. *Health Services Research 37* (4), 849–84.

Li, L. W. 2005. Trajectories of ADL disability among community-dwelling frail older persons. *Research on Aging 27* (1), 56–79.

Manard, B. B., & Cameron, R. 1997. *A national study of assisted living for the frail elderly: Report on in-depth interviews with developers*. Washington, DC: U.S. Department of Health and Human Services, Office of the Assistant Secretary for Planning and Evaluation.

Metlife Mature Market Institute. 2005a. *The MetLife market survey of assisted living costs*. Westport, CT: MetLife Mature Market Institute.

Metlife Mature Market Institute. 2005b. *The MetLife market survey of nursing home & home care costs*. Westport, CT: MetLife Mature Market Institute.

Metlife Mature Market Institute. 2006. *Alzheimer's care: Supplemental findings to the 2005 MetLife market surveys of nursing home/home care and assisted living costs*. New York: Metropolitan Life Insurance Company.

Mitchell, J. M., & Kemp, B. J. 2000. Quality of life in assisted living homes: a multidimensional analysis. *Journals of Gerontology, Psychological Sciences and Social Sciences 55* (2), P117–27.

Mollica, R. L., & Johnson-Lamarche, H. 2005. *State residential care and assisted living policy, 2004*. Portland, ME: National Academy for State Health Policy.

Moore, J. 2001. *Assisted living strategies for changing markets*. Fort Worth, TX: Westridge.

Mor, V., Zinn, J., Angelelli, J., Teno, J. M., & Miller, S. C. 2004. Driven to tiers: socioeconomic and racial disparities in the quality of nursing home care. *Milbank Quarterly 82* (2), 227–56.

Morgan, D. L. 1998. Facts and figures about the baby boom. *Generations 22* (1), 10–15.

Morgan, L. A., Eckert, J. K., Gruber-Baldini, A. L., & Zimmerman, S. 2004. Policy and research issues for small assisted living facilities. *Journal of Aging and Social Policy 16* (4), 1–16.

National Investment Center. 2001. *The case for investing in seniors housing and long term care properties*. Annapolis, MD: National Investment Center for the Senior Housing and Care Industries.

O'Brian, E. 2005. *Long-term care: Understanding Medicaid's role for the elderly and disabled*. Washington, DC: Kaiser Commission.

ProMatura Group. 1999. *Income confirmation study of assisted living residents and the age 75+ population*. Annapolis, MD: National Investment Conference for the Senior Housing and Care Industries.

Rabig, J., Thomas, W., Kane, R. A., Cutler, L. J., & McAlilly, S. 2006. Radical redesign of nursing homes: applying the Green House concept in Tupelo, Mississippi. *Gerontologist 46* (4), 533–39.

Redding, W. 2005. When midsize is the right size. *Assisted Living Executive 12* (9), 18–20.

Roper Starch Worldwide. 1999. *Baby boomers envision their retirement: An AARP segmentation analysis.* Washington, DC: AARP.

Rosenblatt, A., Samus, Q. M., Steele, C. D., Baker, A. S., Harper, M. G., Brandt, J., et al. 2004. The Maryland Assisted Living Study: prevalence, recognition, and treatment of dementia and other psychiatric disorders in the assisted living population of central Maryland. *Journal of the American Geriatric Society 52* (10), 1618–25.

Shirk, C. 2006. *Rebalancing long-term care: The role of the Medicaid HCBS Waiver Program.* Washington, DC: National Health Policy Forum.

Spillman, B. C., & Black, K. J. 2005. *Staying the course: Trends in family caregiving.* Washington, DC: AARP, Public Policy Institute.

Spillman, B. C., Liu, L., & McGilliard, C. 2002. *Trends in residential long-term care.* Washington, DC: Urban Institute.

Summer, L. 2003. *Choices and consequences: The availability of community-based long-term care services to the low-income population.* Washington, DC: Georgetown University, Health Policy Institute.

Summer, L. 2005. *Strategies to keep consumers needing long-term care in the community and out of nursing facilities.* Washington, DC: Henry J. Kaiser Family Foundation.

Thomassy, G. E. 2000. For sale: small assisted living facility. *Assisted Living Today 7* (3), 40–43.

Toossi, M. 2005. Labor force projections to 2014: Retiring boomers. *Monthly Labor Review,* November, 25–44.

U.S. Census Bureau. 2004. U.S. interim projections by age, sex, race, and Hispanic origin. www.census.gov/ipc/www/usinterimproj/

U.S. Congressional Budget Office. 2004. *CBO's projections of the labor force.* Washington, DC: Congressional Budget Office.

U.S. General Accounting Office. 1999. *Assisted living: Quality-of-care and consumer protection issues in four states.* Washington, DC: U.S. General Accounting Office.

Utz, R. L. 2003. Assisted living: The philosophical challenges of everyday practice. *Journal of Applied Gerontology 22* (3), 379–404.

Waidmann, T. A. 2003. *Estimates of the risk of long-term care: Assisted living and nursing home facilities.* Washington, DC: Urban Institute.

Webb, D. 2004. *Empty nester syndrome: When the kids go away will boomers play?* Bloomfield Hills, MI: Pulte Homes.

Wolf, D. A., Hunt, K., & Knickman, J. 2005. Perspectives on the recent decline in disability at older ages. *Milbank Quarterly 83* (3), 365–95.

Zimmerman, S., Sloane, P. D., Heck, E., Maslow, K., & Schulz, R. 2005. Introduction: dementia care and quality of life in assisted living and nursing homes. *Gerontologist 45,* special issue, no. 1 (1), 5–7.

CHAPTER 2

The Old Road Is Rapidly Aging

A Social Model for Cognitively or Physically Impaired Elders in Assisted Living's Future

JOAN HYDE, PH.D.
ROSA PEREZ, M.ED.
PETER S. REED, PH.D., M.P.H.

Societal shifts of the twentieth and twenty-first centuries—such as urbanization and suburbanization of the American populace, changes in the roles of women, men, and the family, industrialization, mass education, evolutions in religion and health care, two world wars, the Depression, the postwar boom, the war in Vietnam, the civil rights movement, the creation of entitlement programs, new waves of immigration, globalization, the development of the Internet and other technological innovations, and shifting political alliances—have all shaped and were shaped by those who are now old and by the large cohort of "baby boomers" who will soon be old (Riley, 1997, p. 91).

Assisted living is a cumulative reflection of all these developments. Until recently, people with chronic illnesses, including dementia, were cared for either in their family home or in nursing homes. In the past 15 years a new long-term care setting—generally known as "assisted living," which subscribes to a social model—has emerged as an option for people who want and need assistance.

Many complex and intertwined factors will affect the future of assisted living. They include the change in the profile of residents with regard to chronic diseases (such as multiple sclerosis and dementia) or physically disabling conditions, the growing diversity of the chronically ill population, expectations of the baby boom generation, and the future ability of seniors and others with chronic conditions to afford assisted living. Other options such as supportive housing with the availability of home care services are evolving as well, and their changes will also influence assisted living's future.

Whether assisted living is able to meet the needs of significantly impaired residents will also depend on changing processes of care, such as how technology is integrated into the workflow and how opportunities for social interactions and activities are provided. Of great concern are the issues of staffing shortages, substandard wages, and working conditions for direct-care workers and the ability of assisted living to meet the need for increasing numbers of well-trained and qualified staff.

In this chapter we address the ways in which assisted living, in its role as a major locus for the care of those with considerable levels of sensory or physical impairments, including such chronic conditions as diabetes, arthritis, blindness and low vision, the aftermaths of childhood polio, and of course dementia, both is the result of these societal shifts and will continue to influence them in the coming decades. In particular, we grapple with the radical deviation that assisted living represents in our society's stance toward people with physical, sensory, or cognitive disabilities. This chapter provides background on the fundamental principles of assisted living and on its ability to serve those with the greatest level of impairment. We map the landscape of factors currently enabling or constraining high-quality care for those with the greatest level of impairment and consider how these factors may be organized in a model of assisted living capable of accommodating residents with increasing cognitive or functional needs. We then describe the obstacles on the road to achieving resident autonomy, dignity, and sense of community in assisted living settings in the coming decades. Finally, we consider how evolving regulations and government reimbursement programs could support or undermine the effectiveness of a social model of care. Overall, then, our focus is on the societal forces that will facilitate or impede assisted living's capacity to serve those with the greatest levels of disability and on the structural and process changes that will allow assisted living to provide the services that vulnerable older Americans will want and need.

The fundamental question becomes: "Can assisted living maintain its social model in the face of projected societal and structural changes as it responds to their residents' increased service needs?" Our answer is a conditional yes: assisted living will be able to meet the needs of residents with increased cognitive or physical impairment while maintaining its current respect for residents' dignity and autonomy if specific actions are taken at every level of this multifaceted system and within the context of influences affecting the care it offers.

Background on Assisted Living for Individuals with Cognitive or Physical Impairment
The Social Model

Assisted living is less a set of specific services, building types, or licensure categories than an approach to offering consumer-directed long-term care in a congregate setting. A number of philosophical tenets comprise what we recognize today as assisted living, the central one of which is often described as a "social model." Although this term has been used in a variety of ways, in this chapter it encompasses the following four characteristics:

1. An appreciation for beneficial life circumstances and quality-of-life outcomes as consumers define them. This stands in contrast to a "medical model," in which health care practitioners are the primary decision makers about a person's "needs" and the emphasis is on "good" outcomes, which in the medical model means absence of disease. The social model, by contrast, puts the person first, incorporating a person's medical, psychological, social, and personal needs, as well as strengths, abilities, interests, and preferences— thereby recognizing a person's distinctive life history and set of experiences—all in the context of chronic disease management. Implicit in this model of care is a thorough understanding of the person, infused throughout every aspect of the living experience offered within a thoughtfully constructed community. In an assisted living residence striving to achieve this ideal social model of care, it is imperative that everyone who is a part of the community be invested in the residence's success.

2. The recognition that, despite significant impairment, most people remain capable, both alone and with the support of family members (biological or otherwise) and other representatives, of making appropriate choices about how they live, including what services and care they need and want.

3. The belief that social interactions, which are respectful of an individual's personhood and which value dignity and personal preferences, are intrinsically therapeutic. In addition, meaningful activities, including the residents' self-determined and purposeful activities, are as beneficial as expert-prescribed therapeutic interventions.

4. The commitment to allowing each resident to remain a part of his or her wider social network—loved ones, family, friends, neighbors, local merchants, religious or spiritual community, and trusted health care practitioners. The social model therefore means that the assisted living provider welcomes family and others into the residence and acknowledges their ongoing role and influence in the residents' lives.

Principles Informing the Assisted Living Philosophy: Choice, Autonomy, Dignity

Because the "social model" assumes a high measure of agency on the part of residents, it is natural to ask whether the most cognitively or physically impaired among us are able to or should make decisions on their own behalf. This is an offshoot of a larger philosophical debate regarding autonomy, a concept that has been adopted as a fundamental tenet of American democracy. There are several respects in which perfect "autonomy" is constrained in even the most competent of us: (1) our actions are limited by political and social forces beyond our control; (2) the knowledge necessary to make "perfect" decisions—both knowledge about the effects our actions may have in the larger world and knowledge about our own self-interest—is limited; and (3) our ability to conform our behavior to our perception of the best course of action is imperfect (Buss, 2002).

What is new in assisted living philosophy is the application of the principle of autonomy to people of diminished capacity, including those with dementia, for if people with diminished capacity cannot use their autonomy to further their own best interests as well as the rest of us imperfect people then why grant them autonomy at all? The answer offered by a number of psychologists and philosophers, most notably John Stuart Mill, is that the value of autonomy transcends its specific utility. In this view, autonomy is linked to "the value of self-integration," which is "one element of well-being" (Mill, 1859).

To understand this better, we have only to look at the converse. People who cannot act in concert with their own thoughts and desires, whether due to benign (paternalistic) or malignant interference, and whether because of coercion or manipulation, quickly lose their sense of themselves as valued and free agents in their own lives. Thus, although autonomy is not the only value we hold—others include ethics of virtue, utilitarianism, and care—we must recognize that while interventions that reduce another person's autonomy "might, in the end, be justified, something is lost, and what is lost is a degree of interpersonal respect we owe each other independent of the actual autonomy displayed by the person who is the object of that respect" (Mill, 1859, p. 14).

Assisted living is generally occupied by people who are committed to the principle of maintaining autonomy in the face of significant impairments, to the extent possible. Even the most enthusiastic advocate for autonomy, however, understands that it is "not an all-or-nothing characteristic." Therefore, when it comes to those with the greatest degree of physical or particularly cognitive impairment, much of assisted living is a balancing act between respecting their autonomy and providing protection. In this regard, we can turn to the work of Nobel Prize–winning economist Daniel Kahneman, who in his acceptance speech (2003) said, "Most behavior is intuitive, skilled, unproblematic and successful. . . . Behavior is likely to be anchored in intuitive impressions and intentions even when it is not completely dominated by them." This seems to be true and equally successful (or unsuccessful) regardless of the level of a person's impairment.

From a "commonsense" perspective, as well as from the viewpoint of many adult children, most regulators, and some advocates, it seems obvious that people with dementia may have poor "safety awareness" or are unable to make choices that further their own best interests. Studies of choice among elders with the highest levels of impairment, however, challenge this view. In a study by Fisher, Burgio, Thorn, and Hardin (2006), "a majority of nursing home residents capable of responding to yes-no questions about their daily care could do so accurately." Chu, Schnelle, Cadogan, and Simmons (2004, p. 2059) found that "residents' yes-no responses were significantly similar over a 48-hour time period and interrater reliability among researchers was very high, regardless of resident cognitive status." Feinberg and Whitlatch (2001, p. 380) likewise found that "persons with mild to moderate cognitive impairment (i.e., Mini-Mental Status Examination [or MMSE] from 13 to 26) are able to respond consistently to questions about preferences, choices and their own involvement in decisions about daily living, and provide accurate and reliable responses to questions about their own demographics," concluding that "persons with dementia possess sufficient capacity to state specific preferences and make care-related decisions." Further, in their study of the Cash and Counseling demonstration program—whereby older persons and their families receive subsidies that give them more control over who they hire for assistance—Applebaum, Uman, and Straker (2006) found that

> quality in the program happens because of, not in spite of, consumer choice and control. The shifting roles of regulatory agencies and program staff to accommodate the right of the consumer to be in charge have not created new problems in the areas of quality. . . . Consumers in these programs experience no greater risk and have no higher level of negative outcome than clients in traditional services. In fact, our research thus far suggests that the self-directed consumers report fewer problems and a higher sense of security because they are in charge. In consumer-directed programs, consumers are the agents of quality.

Ultimately, to provide residents with diminished capacity with dignity and a sense of well-being, one must respect their wishes in the present moment. This is not to say that assisted living residents, especially those with dementia or other disorders that limit judgment, necessarily have good safety awareness or that families, informal caregivers, friends, and experienced providers do not also have a role to play in elders' decisions about care. What is at issue is how the individual consumer, his or her representatives, health care professionals, and assisted living providers should best work together to further the interests of cognitively or physically impaired residents.

Today's Assisted Living Population

If we are to understand the future role and impact of assisted living in a changing demographic and regulatory environment, we need to understand how their properties now function and whom they serve. According to the most recent *Overview of Assisted Living* (ALFA, 2006), a periodic industry-wide survey of assisted living providers, nearly everyone who resides in assisted living has one or more chronic conditions and, with an average age of 86, takes an average of 8 medications (both prescription and over-the-counter) daily. Residents typically need help with cooking, cleaning, and taking their medications. Sixty percent require help with bathing, 40 percent with dressing, and 30 percent with toileting (ALFA, 2006). More than half of the 1 million people currently in assisted living residences are cognitively impaired (see Tables 2.1 and 2.2). In addition, as shown in Table 2.3, many residents, both those with and those without dementia, experience multiple health issues and numerous comorbid conditions (Hawes et al., 2003; Leon & Moyer, 1999). More than a quarter of

TABLE 2.1
Prevalence of Dementia in Assisted Living

Author/Principal Investigator	Study Name, Data-Collection Date	Dementia (%)	Comment
Rosenblatt et al. (2004)	Maryland Assisted Living Study, 2001–2002	67	This stratified sample over-sampled smaller homes, which are known to have a higher percentage of dementia.
Sloane, Zimmerman, & Ory (2001)	Collaborative Studies of LTC, 1997–1998	45–63	Prevalence varied with size, where smallest facilities generally serve residents with the most severe cognitive impairment.
Hawes & Phillips (2000)	National Survey of High Service/High Privacy AL, 1998	27 moderate/severe	No information is provided on residents with mild dementia. The ALFA report suggests that an additional 13.5% of residents have "early Alzheimer's" and 21.6% have "mild dementia."
ALFA/NIC/Tingsley (NIC, 2001)	ALFA/Pricewaterhouse Coopers/NIC *Overview*, 1999, 2000	45	This is based on reports of assisted living providers and shows little variation over the four years of the survey or across geographic areas.

TABLE 2.2
Distribution of Dementia Acuity
(%)

Study	Mild	Moderate	Severe
Keene (2003) ($n=532$)	39	46	15
NIC/ALFA (2000) ($n=8,734$)	73	18	9
Leon & Moyer (1998) ($n=161$)	28	34	38
Zimmerman (2005a) ($n=421$)	53 (mild/moderate)	35 (severe)	11 (very severe)
Average across studies	48	33	18

TABLE 2.3
Dementia Residents' Comorbidity Levels

No. of Comorbidities	Nursing Home (%)	Assisted Living (%)
0	2	10
1–2	10	32
3–4	32	30
5–6	38	14
7 or more	18	14
Total	100	100

Source: Data from Leon, Cheng, & Neumann (1998).

assisted living residents generally and nearly half of those in dementia care units will remain in assisted living until the end of their lives, and Rosenblatt et al. (2004), in their research on assessment and treatment of dementia in assisted living settings, suggest that with additional screening and treatment even more assisted living residents would be able to further delay or avoid moving to a nursing home altogether.

These findings suggest that assisted living is now accommodating an even more impaired population than described in Golant's (2004) review. He evaluated some of the major studies of the assisted living population and summarized the extent to which older persons with serious physical or cognitive disabilities and health care problems occupied assisted living residences in the United States. His review used six indicators to determine whether impaired residents occupy assisted living: percentage requiring assistance with activities of daily living or having dementia; average length of stay; reasons for leaving assisted living; percentage admitting residents with impairments; percentage retaining those with impairments; and percentage of freestanding and multilevel properties with different admitting and care patterns. Golant concluded that assisted living residences were more likely to admit frail older persons when they had relatively minor or less serious health care needs or physical or cognitive impairments. These and other findings distinguished assisted living residences from nursing homes that had more highly impaired occupants. Less than 50 percent of the properties referenced in three of the studies would admit older persons if they had any of 14 health conditions, including oxygen supplementation, colostomy care required, behavior problems, and nursing care needed; a similar percentage would not retain older persons if they had any of 10 specific health conditions. Golant (2004, p. 577) concludes that "the finding that assisted living providers retention/discharge policies are more tolerant of higher levels of frailty than their admitting policies is the only evidence of aging-in-place practices in [assisted living facilities]." In summary, nearly all of the 1 million individuals living in assisted living settings as of this writing are quite impaired, and the upper quartiles of residents, as reported by disability level, are very impaired indeed.

Recent reports (ALFA, 2006; Keane, 2003) indicate that about half of the assisted living buildings in the United States are currently either free-standing special care properties or assisted living buildings that include a section specifically designated for those with dementia. Based on a review of the literature (Novartis, 2006), in buildings with a dementia care unit, on average 22 percent of all residents live in the section devoted to dementia care. Residents not in dementia-specific areas are integrated into the general assisted living population. The Assisted Living Federation of America's *Overview* (ALFA, 2006), which surveys assisted living providers regarding their internal data and estimates of building and resident characteristics, reports that staffing in dementia-specific programs is considerably more intensive and residents pay approximately $1,000 more per month than other assisted living residents.

Early Regulations as They Shaped Assisted Living Residences and Services in the Formative Decades of the Industry

Assisted living regulations were initially a response, on the state level, to an industry that was growing up at the fringes of the regulatory structure. As such, early regulations often built on existing "board-and-care" regulations or were adaptations of the nursing home code. This has led to a plethora of regulatory categories and considerable variation from state to state. To some extent, assisted living providers have eschewed serving those with the greatest level of need in order to avoid being categorized as nursing homes or being subjected to the regulations that apply to nursing homes (see chapters 11 and 13).

These regulations nonetheless determine many aspects of the buildings, services, and the level of impairment permitted in assisted living settings. One result is that providers over- or under-serve their residents' needs to comply with regulations. Unlike nursing homes, however, assisted living providers typically have some latitude in the services they are willing to provide, and many discharge residents at a lower level of impairment than allowed by their state's law. Future changes in regulations may thus have a significant impact on both assisted living providers and the characteristics of the residents they serve.

Influences on Assisted Living's Future
The Changing Demographic and Health Context: The Road Is Rapidly Aging

Both the overall numbers of those in assisted living and the proportion with cognitively or physically disabling conditions are likely to grow in the coming two decades, as the percent of individuals over 80, who are at higher risk for developing disabling conditions, increases by 50 percent, from 10.5 million in 2005 to 15.5 million in 2025 (U.S. Census, 2000). According to the Centers for Disease Control and Prevention (2005, p. 9), "The United States is in the midst of a longevity revolution. By 2030, the number of older Americans will have more than doubled to 70 million, or one in every five Americans. The growing number and proportion of older adults places increasing demands on the public health system and on medical and social services. Chronic diseases exact a particularly heavy health and economic burden on older adults due to associated long-term illness, diminished quality of life, and greatly increased health care costs."

Further, the racial and ethnic diversity of seniors, age 65 and older, is projected to change dramatically in the next two decades. In 2003, 17 percent were non-Hispanic whites, but this group is expected to increase to 28 percent by 2030 (Novartis, 2006). Senior blacks, Asians, and Hispanics will all grow substantially. Blacks will increase from 8 percent of seniors to 10 percent and Asians will increase from 3 percent to 5 percent. In particular, Hispanics/Latinos will increase the most, from 6 percent to 11 percent. Based on the projected increase in size and diversity of the older U.S. population, it is likely that the numbers of people needing supportive long-term care services will be markedly greater in the coming decades, and it follows that, along with the entire residential care sector, the assisted living industry will be caring for more racially or ethnically diverse and increasingly impaired residents.

At the same time, with increasing access to information, many seniors who develop chronic conditions may personally manage them more successfully than in the past. This will make a positive contribution, because, as Ekerdt (2005) points out, successful disease management is consistent with the assisted living philosophy of respect for resident choice and empowerment. In a study sponsored by the Agency for Healthcare Research and Quality (2002), older people in the study—who had, on average, more than two chronic conditions—who participated in the Chronic Disease Self-Management Program (CDSMP) increased exercise, had better coping strategies and symptom management, communicated better with their physicians, improved their health self-rating, had more energy, less fatigue, and decreased disability, fewer physician and emergency room visits and hospitalizations, increased self-efficacy, reduced health distress, and had no further increase in disability (AHRQ, 2002; Lorig, Sobel, & Stewart, 1999). Thus, assisted living settings, by facilitating cooperative care, have the potential of meeting the needs of their growing number of residents with multiple chronic conditions.

This is consistent with the findings of Corder and Manton (2001) and Manton, Gu, and Ukraitseva (2005, p. 6), who found "308,000 fewer severely cognitively impaired elderly in 1999 than in 1982. The average decline in prevalence was from 5.7% to 2.9% for this period." Manton et al. (2005, p. 1 [abstract]) further write, "Several possible explanations of such a surprising trend [include] (i) increased proportion of better educated people among the oldest old; (ii) recent declines in stroke rates; (iii) expanding use of neuro-protective medications."

The impact of improved self-management may also be that, despite their disability, many cognitively or physically impaired seniors will be more stable and have fewer negative incidents, such as falls, acute exacerbations, or emergency room visits, of the type that may make them poor candidates for continued occupancy in an assisted living residence. Thus, impaired seniors will be able to "age in place"—not necessarily because the assisted living provider has expanded its available health-related services, but because the residents, with support from a combination of family/informal caregivers, health care providers, and assisted living staff, are able to develop healthier strategies for managing their illness, thus slowing the progression of their chronic diseases. This is consistent with the AARP study "Boomers at Midlife" (2004), which provides indications that the cohort of baby boomers understands that they will need to make lifestyle changes in order to age more successfully. It is also consistent with Golant's (2004, p. 61) conclusion that aging in place does not simply refer to older persons remaining in the same place for a sustained duration but, rather, "involves a proactive response from the older person's residential setting (whether initiated by the older person, significant others, other occupants or providers) that in some way introduces solutions that respond to or compensate for an individuals' functional or physical declines."

The potential for slowing age-related decline by assisted living residents can also be achieved by older persons of lesser economic means. A study comparing low-income older persons in assisted living and community settings found that more than half of those in the former either maintained or improved their level of functioning over two years (Fonda, Clipp & Maddox, 2002).

The Times Are Changing: The Impact of the Baby Boom Generation on Residents' Values and Expectations

The shifting values of the baby boom cohort are likely to be a driving force in the shifting dynamic of residential care as a service option for older adults in the coming decades. Just over a quarter of people in the United States today are baby boomers. In their role as advocates for their parents, and quite often as the visionaries who initiated the assisted living revolution, they are already shaping services for seniors. As boomers become older and are more frequently in need of supportive services themselves we can expect to see changes in the country's long-term care systems that go beyond the impact of their sheer numbers. "Having identified the flaws in this system, some of these so-called 'entitled' consumers are determined to fix what they see as a broken industry" (Novartis, 2006, "Introduction," unnumbered page). Assisted living, with its emphasis on consumer choice and dignity, is uniquely positioned to respond to this emerging customer-centered approach to care. How well a customer-centered approach can be delivered in assisted living settings for the most physically and cognitively impaired will have much to do with the industry's success in the coming decades (see chapter 6).

Just as boomers disabled in the Vietnam War changed our societal response to mobility disabilities, so the baby boomer cohort will change the overall response to chronic physical and cognitive disability in some predictable ways. According to Feld (2006, p. 74), "Many Vietnam War veterans, both those who acquired disabilities in the war and their comrades who did not, became activists in the civil rights movement. The fight for disability rights grew out of opposition to the war in Vietnam and became part of the struggle against racial discrimination, for environmental protection and for women's rights." We are already seeing that response in the shift in the Alzheimer's advocacy movement. Whereas a decade ago supportive services were geared primarily to the needs and perceptions of caregivers, the Alzheimer's Association and others are now addressing the needs of those with dementia themselves. Some key examples of this shift include new initiatives to directly engage people with the disease, including support groups for those with early stage dementia; activities programming that involve even those with serious disabling conditions in setting goals and making progress toward enhancing cognitive, social, and creative functioning; and development of satisfaction and quality-of-life tools that directly capture the experiences of people with dementia. This shift empowers elders, while allowing them to include their healthcare providers, social networks, and family members in a way that is less paternalistic and supports their autonomy.

Part of this trend has been the shift from an emphasis on "healthy aging" to "successful aging." As John Rowe and Robert Kahn wrote in their groundbreaking book, *Successful Aging* (1998), which chronicled the factors associated with a long and productive life, "What really matters is not the number or type of diseases one has but how those problems impact on one's ability to function." Or, as Lisa Gwyther noted in her forward-thinking paper, "The Perspective of the Person with Alzheimer Disease" (1997), "Objective measures of health, wealth and relationships explain less than half the variance in perceived quality of life for most older Americans. What people with Alzheimer disease seem to want is to have their subjective needs for assistance met appropriately and individually rather than being offered too much, too little, or services perceived as irrelevant to self-determined needs or preferences."

Another factor in the trend toward a social model of services for even the most impaired elders among us is the changing diversity—ethnic, racial, and social—of the group who are now aging. The changing role of family is addressed in chapter 7, but it is clear that not only does the family support assisted living residents in ways that differ from their involvement with more traditional long-term care, but that assisted living itself has the potential to enrich the lives of the diverse array of residents' friends and family by bringing them into a meaningful relationship with the assisted living community.

The Evolution of Other Options

As this shift toward consumer-directed care occurs, assisted living stands poised to fill the need for self-directed long-term care services. Assisted living is occasionally referred to as a "step in the long-term care continuum." It is more accurate to characterize it as one among many options that people who need supportive services can choose. When projecting the extent to which assisted living will be used by those who are most physically and cognitively impaired, it is important to consider how well some of the other long-term care options, such as senior housing with the availability of home care services, will be able to meet their needs (see chapter 12).

Only about 30 percent of those with Alzheimer disease or other dementias live in assisted living or nursing homes. The remainder of those with dementia live in the community, including many who live on their own in both subsidized and market rate housing (Evans et al., 1989). Such housing increasingly has formal or informal relationships with home care providers. In some cases the relationship is so seamless that assisted living and "housing with services" are virtually indistinguishable. Also, home care, especially when enhanced with technologies that allow for remote monitoring and "distance medicine," is likely to be popular among those with dementia who have family/informal caregivers available. If the Cash and Counseling programs, which offer older persons and their families more self-determination in how they receive care, become more widely available, it is likely that in-home "long-term care" will compete with assisted living, even for many very physically or cognitively impaired individuals (see chapter 1). Nonetheless, it is a rare supportive housing setting that is able to provide adequate services to residents who develop some of the more troubling symptoms of dementia, such as resistance to help with personal hygiene, physical agitation, or wandering (Kassner, 2006; Schafer, 1999a; Tilley & Weiner, no date).

Nursing homes in particular rival assisted living as the setting of choice for the more severely impaired population. The popularity of this option for the most impaired will be determined by two factors: whether nursing homes continue to receive preferential status from the Medicaid and Medicare programs and whether the culture change movement succeeds in making nursing homes places where people can live out their lives with meaning and satisfaction and they can have more of a voice in the care they receive (see chapter 3).

The Future Ability of Seniors to Afford Assisted Living

The viability of assisted living will also depend on whether the growing senior population is able to afford its accommodations and shelter. The relative lack of third-party reimbursement has resulted in residents who are primarily middle class. Only as their care needs increase, and with it their costs, however, do they sometimes transition to nursing homes, where they are more likely to be eligible for third-party supplementation. Thus, the adequacy of their pensions, Social Security, and income from savings and investments will be key to whether they will be able in the future to pay privately for assisted living, particularly the service-rich assisted living appropriate to their increased needs. We now know, since nearly 50 percent have incomes less than $25,000 per year, that even less cash-wealthy seniors can afford assisted living if they can realize the equity from their owned homes. Although many in the baby-boom generation currently have substantial assets tied up in their homes (Schafer, 1999b, p. 20), it is not clear whether they will be willing to sell their homes or what the value of those homes will be at the time they are ready to downsize or move to assisted living. "The average ratio of homeowner's equity to value, at 55.2 percent, is near its low for the post-war period. A sharp drop in home prices will send this ratio far below its previous low point. Because there are considerable differences in housing markets across the country, if housing prices fall 10 percent nationally, then many regions will see price declines of 20–30 percent. This will create a situation in which millions of families will have little or no equity in their homes, an especially serious issue with the large baby boom cohort nearing retirement. It will also lead to a surge in mortgage default rates, as many homeowners opt not to keep paying a mortgage that exceeds the value of their home." Baker (2002) suggests that this could place serious stress on the financial system.

Another uncertain but critical influence on assisted living's affordability will be the extent that the future older population can depend on long-term care insurance. At present, however, fewer than 10 percent of people age 65 or older, the group most likely to begin to need assisted living services 10 years from now, have purchased long-term care insurance (National Bureau of Economic Research, 2005). In addition, many of the existing policies do not cover assisted living, though limited coverage may be available through a home-care benefit. Another potential complication is that for policies without cost of living riders, the daily benefit may be lower, relative to anticipated assisted living or nursing home costs (see chapter 11). Yet another concern is the uncertainty surrounding pensions, Social Security, and future income from savings and investment. All of these will affect people's ability to pay privately for assisted living, particularly the service-rich assisted living appropriate to their increased needs.

Informal and Family Support for Cognitively or Physically Impaired Assisted Living Residents
The Role of the Family

Family members play several important roles in the lives of assisted living residents: they help residents maintain a sense of community (Kane, 2004); provide a history of residents' lives, especially for residents who are unable to directly communicate this information to the staff and residents in the new setting (Alzheimer's Association, 2005); and help cognitively or physically impaired residents make decisions about their own care. These roles become particularly important to sustaining a social model of care as residents develop significant impairments in the assisted living setting. In his discussion of dementia-care units in assisted living, Chafetz (2001) points out that positive experiences with loved ones may help residents hold on to their identities, which is paramount to the assisted living philosophy.

Family members and other informal caregivers can contribute to both the quality of life and quality of care for residents with cognitive or physical impairments, thereby influencing their ability to age in place. Assisted living can encourage the support and involvement of loved ones and family members to help residents maintain their sense of autonomy, dignity, and sense of community. In their study examining the impact of social involvement, Mitchell & Kemp (2000) found that family contact was significantly correlated with quality-of-life measures and that residents with strong family involvement exhibited fewer symptoms of depression. In a study investigating the process of aging in place in assisted living, Ball et al. (2004) found that support from family members was correlated to increased length of stay.

When asked about their involvement in the care of their loved ones with dementia, family members stated that they sought additional involvement (Port et al. 2005). In addition, family members were found to play a greater role in assisted living than in nursing homes, which perhaps indicates the significance of assisted living's social model of care, which supports each resident to remain a part of his or her social network. With this increased involvement, families can experience a greater burden when their loved ones are in assisted living rather than nursing homes. Despite this increased burden, Singer and Luxenberg (2003), in their report of diagnosing dementia in long-term care, state that families prefer the homier atmosphere of assisted living residences. This may ultimately continue to be a trend that, despite an increased burden, families of people with dementia are choosing assisted living over nursing homes. Kane (2004) points out that 92 percent of assisted living administrators report that residents remain involved in the outside communities primarily through visits with family and friends and that "families are as important as residents" in making assisted living feel like home. This raises the issue of the fate of residents with few or no engaged family or friends or those whose family and friends are not included in the support of their loved ones.

When assisted living residents are seriously impaired and particularly if they have dementia, their families take on the additional role of proxy decision maker. For families who want to maintain resident autonomy, this role can be problematic, as proxy decision makers must struggle to include residents who have difficulty articulating their wishes and who may indicate current preferences that are at odds with their prior habits and inclinations. Neumann, Araki, and Gutterman (2000) write, "In general, studies report fairly good agreement between subjects and proxies in assessments of functioning, physical health, and cognitive status, and fair-to-poor agreement in assessments of psychological well-being. Proxies tend to describe more impairment in functioning and emotional well-being, relative to subjects, a pattern that is particularly marked among persons with cognitive impairment." In a review of the literature, Fisher et al. (2006, p. 9) found that "proxy reports typically do not show good agreement with self-reports." This mixed assessment reinforces the need to let both families and impaired elders have a role in decision making.

Evolution of the Trends in Defining and Addressing Needs of the Family

What effect the evolution of the American family over the coming decades will have on the likelihood that the most impaired elders will reside, and have a high quality of life, in assisted living settings remains unclear. Some trends, such as the increasing numbers of women in the work force, divorce, longer life span, later retirement, fewer and more mobile adult children, increasing numbers of ethnically diverse and non-English-speaking families, and more nontraditional families, are examined in chapter 7 in this book. The effects of some of these trends, especially for those who, because of cognitive impairment or significant health issues, have difficulty speaking for themselves are discussed more specifically here.

Because the older population is becoming racially and ethnically more diverse (Novartis, 2006), assisted living providers will need to expand their capacity to address many groups' distinctive coping strategies, norms of family involvement and values. Newer immigrant groups have historically tended to keep older and disabled family members home longer than more acculturated Americans, so increased numbers of immigrants may lead to higher acuity residents in assisted living.

Research by the Institute of Medicine (2002) demonstrated that racial and ethnic minorities, even when financial situations are equal to those of whites, tend to receive lower-quality care than nonminorities. They also reveal evidence that "health care providers' biases, prejudices, and uncertainty when treating minorities can contribute to health care disparities." In the report on multicultural boomers coping with family and aging issues by AARP (2001, p. 3), there were significant variations in how much stress non-Hispanic whites versus nonwhites felt in the care of their aging parents. For example, Asian Americans were more likely to feel squeezed between caring for their aging parents and children, African Americans expressed a greater sense of being overwhelmed with family caregiving, and Hispanics and Asian Americans were more inclined to want their children to help care for their aging parents than whites and African Americans. Generally, nonwhites are more likely to provide care for their elders. In a study of caregivers of people with dementia, Hinrichsen and Ramirez (1992) report that there are few differences in the ways blacks and whites adapt to dementia caregiving. Black dementia caregivers tended to consist of children, and for white caregivers it was split between children and spouses. These are some of the factors that may influence not only the numbers of minority seniors in assisted living in the coming decades but will also influence the ways assisted living includes the support of loved ones for these cognitively or physically impaired who come from minority backgrounds.

Another emerging concern is properly addressing and involving loved ones constituting spousal equivalents, or what is often referred to as "domestic partners." More and more people reach old age in nontraditional relationships. According to Gallanis (2002) 9.1 percent of households headed by partners in the U.S. 2000 Census have unmarried partners. Of the households headed by unmarried partners, 594,391 (10.9 percent) are headed by partners of the same sex, whereas 4,881,377 (89.1 percent) are headed by partners of the opposite sex. The households headed by same-sex partners, though more numerous in certain parts of the nation than in others, exist in all fifty states and in virtually all counties.

According to Cahill, South, and Spade (2000), a key issue for those with nontraditional families is that "nursing homes and assisted living facilities have ignored the special needs of gay, lesbian, bisexual, and transgender (GLBT) elderly and the dearth of data on old GLBT people makes identifying problems and advocating for solutions very difficult." This relegates the unmarried partners of gays and lesbians, and other spousal equivalents to the "friend" category and therefore does not accurately reflect the caregiving of important members of many residents' families. It also ignores the extended families of members of the GLBT community, which may include close long-term friendships, who are the most familiar with a resident's life and are more able to offer assistance. This is particularly poignant because family members or spousal equivalents of GLBT elders may not be given the opportunity to provide the emotional support and family history needed to help staff contribute to improving the lives of people with dementia in their care. The result as Brotman, Ryan, and Cormier (2003) reported is that many GLBT people, especially those in the current elderly cohort, continue to feel isolated and closeted and therefore a full picture of who they are might not be presented. Their biological family might not be sufficiently close, and this can significantly affect the quality of care and quality of life for these vulnerable elders. It especially poses a challenge for assisted living providers who want to recognize and address the unique needs and rights of all residents with cognitive or physical impairments.

For people who do not sign health-care proxies, the laws in many states only provide for medical decisions to be made by someone in the patient's family. According to Gallanis (2002), the Uniform Health-Care Decisions Act of 1993 states that adults

> may designate any individual to act as surrogate by personally informing the supervising health-care provider. In the absence of a designation, or if the designee is not reasonably available, any member of the following classes of the patient's family who is reasonably available, in descending order of priority, may act as surrogate: (1) the spouse, unless legally separated; (2) an adult child; (3) a parent; or (4) an adult brother or sister. If none of the individuals eligible to act as surrogate under subsection (b) is reasonably available, an adult who has exhibited special care and concern for the patient, who is familiar with the patient's personal values, and who is reasonably available may act as surrogate. The Act embodies a notion of "family"—spouses, children, parents, siblings—yet this conception of family is very traditional. The Act largely ignores the possibility that the patient might have a domestic partner rather than a spouse. Likewise, the statute fails to recognize the possibility that there might be an adult child of the patient's partner, a child whom the patient could not formally adopt. The statute does provide, as a last resort, for decisions to be made by someone who has shown "special care and concern for the patient." However, this clause operates only if no one described in subsection (b) is available, and in any event it is a poor substitute for proper recognition that the patient's family might have a nontraditional structure.

The makeup of assisted living and the issues and challenges of addressing the needs of residents to include family and other informal caregivers including domestic partners and friends will likely change over the coming decades, with the wave of changing populations that assisted living is called on to serve. Increased awareness and inclusion of the needs of elders will help increase the role of their family members, friends, loved ones in supporting their ability to age in place and increasing their quality of life and care. In this way, the social model of care that is intrinsic to assisted living will provide a respectful environment for all residents to be their unique individual selves.

Regulatory Change and Its Potential Impact on the Future of Assisted Living

The very fact that assisted living is serving growing numbers of very impaired residents may hasten changes to the regulatory structure, such as promoting stricter rules designed to protect residents with the highest levels of impairment. Depending on the nature of these changes, future regulations may have the paradoxical effect of reducing the number of those with cognitive or physical impairment who are served in assisted living. This may occur in two distinctly different ways: on the one hand, regulations may further limit the services assisted living providers are able to offer and put strictures on admission and discharge criteria that prevent assisted living from serving those with the highest levels of impairment; on the other hand, increased regulations may well anticipate the needs of those with greater care needs but, by doing so, increase requirements and thus drive up costs, reduce flexibility, and increase the institutional characteristics of assisted living. If this second scenario were to occur, it could lead many of those with significant levels of impairment to choose nursing home care over assisted living, where they are more likely to be eligible for third-party reimbursement. Alternatively, changes to regulations may have the effect of increasing the number of people with the highest levels of need while driving out those who neither need the protection nor desire the increased costs and institutional characteristics such regulations may bring (see chapter 13).

In thinking about the regulatory structures that would both maintain the values unique to assisted living while providing protection to those with the highest level of needs we would advocate for a scheme that focuses on processes rather than health outcomes (see chapter 4). This may seem contrary to the newer regulatory emphasis on outcomes that has been promoted in an effort to humanize nursing homes (see chapter 3; for a fuller discussion, see Institute of Medicine, 1986). Specification and measures of desirable outcomes and demonstration of effective care processes to achieve them are especially difficult, underresearched, and underdeveloped in the multifaceted realm of "quality of life" (National Institute of

TABLE 2.4
Service Domains: Foci in the Medical and Social Models

Service Domain	Medical Model (NH)	Social Model (AL)
Dining	Decreased weight loss 75% of meal consumed	Autonomy maintained in allowing resident to eat preferred food Residents enjoy companionship of table mates
Social activities	Safety, falls reduction Decreased depression	Sense of community Engaged in preferred social interactions and activities
Personal care	Bath completed Successfully toileted	Dignity maintained by allowing resident to self-groom if possible
Family/community involvement	Limited by liability issues	Encouraged

Nursing Research, 2006). We thus support the formulation developed by Frank Caro on "quality of circumstance," about which he writes:

> I have come to use the term "quality of circumstances" to describe largely objective measures of the adequacy of solutions to problems of daily living. (I avoid the term "quality of *life*" because it is typically conceived of as an entirely subjective construct.) Some examples of quality-of-circumstance content may be helpful. In the quality-of-circumstance framework, a highly favorable outcome for assistance with mobility is evidence that the recipient moves around in the living environment *at will* day and night with full access to all rooms in the residence and does so without experiencing injury.

Table 2.4 provides examples of the differences in the quality goals of assisted living regulation, as compared to the health outcome goals typically addressed by nursing home regulations.

In considering their different goals, we do not imply that assisting living and nursing home settings are unaware or unmindful of the range of desirable outcomes. Rather, we are highlighting the difference in *focus* of these two settings and are considering the applicability of outcomes rather than processes as indicators of success. One approach that could address this more complex constellation of quality indicators is offered by Marshall Kapp's article on nursing home regulation (2001). He describes the need to match regulatory mandates with desired results. Unlike the "command-and-control" regulatory approach seen as the key to achieving quality care, he offers the possibility that desired levels of safety and health can be achieved while simultaneously allowing maximum flexibility to all involved parties through what he describes as a "regulatory octopus," which includes a range of players, organizations, and strategies, such as accreditation agencies, quality improvement and assurance organizations, advocacy groups, and reimbursement structures (see chapters 11 and 13).

Approaches to Services for Cognitively or Physically Impaired Residents in Assisted Living

One of the key elements enabling more cognitively or physically impaired residents to remain in assisted living is the availability of appropriate personal care and health-related services, along with social and recreational activities. Depending on state regulations, care-related services may be offered directly by the assisted living provider or they may be available by contract with outside agencies, such as visiting nurses or home health agencies. Whether assisted living is able to meet the needs of those residents with the greatest levels of physical and cognitive impairment will depend on how these services are organized and delivered.

Approaches to Care

Much is known about the needs of people with cognitive or physical disabilities. In her analysis of best practices to reinforce psychosocial care in assisted living, one of this chapter's authors (Hyde, 1995, 1996) outlined the commonalities between dementia care approaches of the Alzheimer's Association's Guidelines for Dignity (1993), the American Association of Homes and Services for the Aging's Best Practices for Special Care Programs for Persons with Alzheimer's Disease or a Related Disorder (no date), and Hearthstone Alzheimer's Care's Life Quality Model for Dementia Care in Residential Settings. Several key themes emerge across these models, including the articulation of a philosophy or mission, the need for assessment and care planning, strategies for behavior and communication, relevance of the environment, and the need for measuring indicators of success. These principles of individualized, resident-focused care likely benefit residents regardless of type of impairment or setting. The contention is that no matter where people fall along the continuum of physical and cognitive impairment, their remaining abilities may be maximized through resident-focused approaches and environmental changes implemented in a manner commensurate with an individual's level of need.

In this context, it is again implied that, although there has been increased emphasis on the use of outcomes to define quality in nursing homes, it may be that processes are more relevant indicators in assisted living settings. As articulated above, this is because many disabled seniors are keenly interested in the manner by which they control their lives and get the services they need and want. Recently the Alzheimer's Association has identified a number of processes reviewed by the Assisted Living Workgroup (2003) that appear to be relevant to the most impaired assisted living residents. Some of these, such as secure exits and overnight awake staff, have not been studied but appear to be commonsense safety measures. Two recommendations deal with resident rights and disclosure. Of the remaining recommendations, the following are consistent with the resident-focused approach discussed above:

- Increasing identification of dementia by having specific procedures in place to increase staff awareness of signs and symptoms of cognitive impairment;
- Carefully constructing care for people with dementia in a way that meets needs while building on strengths and balancing autonomy with safety, with the specific purpose of criteria of any Alzheimer/dementia-specific units clearly defined;
- Accommodating the special needs for daily interaction and social experience of residents with dementia ensuring they are meaningful, appropriate, and respectful.

These recommendations are consistent with Lisa Gwyther's finding (1997) that people with dementia feel better understood if those around them are knowledgeable about and acknowledge their disease process. Throughout each of these recommendations for dementia care in assisted living is a strong focus on persons as individuals and their need for input into the social and community experience, as well as their own care. To implement recommendations such as these properly, one would need a greater focus on processes, rather than on medical outcomes.

Activities Programming

Meaningful social and recreational activities that emphasize resident autonomy and life satisfaction are intrinsic to the assisted living philosophy and are likely to be central to the future ability of assisted living to serve those with physical and cognitive disabilities. It is therefore not surprising that a recent study by Dobbs et al. (2005) reported that assisted living and nursing home residents were more likely to enjoy activities in assisted living or residential care than in nursing homes. They also found that residents with severe cognitive impairment had higher activity involvement in assisted living than in nursing homes.

Most assisted living providers offer a range of formal and informal recreational activities (Kane, 2004), with more informal activities being offered in smaller settings and more large-group and formal activities available in larger and "new model" settings. In general, assisted living residents "vote with their feet" and activities that are not well attended are usually discontinued. At the same time, many assisted living providers, with the expectation that social and physical stimulation helps residents to maintain a higher level of functioning, are motivated to offer therapeutically oriented activities, such as range of motion exercises, even if these activities do not initially appeal to residents.

In its recent practice recommendations (2006, p. 15) the Alzheimer's Association designated "social engagement and involvement in meaningful activities" as an important area of focus and outlined a set of evidence-based recommendations. The Alzheimer's Association recommendations suggest that meaningful activities should respect residents' preferences and should be designed with, not for, residents, whenever possible. They also suggest that the outcome of activities is far less important than the process of participating in an activity.

Intrinsic to the social model of care is the provision of activities geared toward the level of the residents' abilities and increased positive attitudes among people with dementia and other impairments. Among the included activities are music, painting, taking walks, story telling, and gardening. Challenges exist in offering a truly evidence-based set of activities with established efficacy for residents with cognitive or physical disability. In particular, the research basis for specific activity programs to benefit physically impaired assisted living residents appears quite limited. In studying physical, along with cognitive, limitations, Lazowski et al. (1999) found that exercise programs are widely beneficial, including for those who are physically impaired, incontinent, or have dementia. Several researchers have explored the efficacy of various specific activities approaches for individuals with dementia (Hyde, 1995, 1996; Chafetz, 2001; Stasi, 2004) and find that people with dementia may benefit from some basic activities such as meal preparation and laundry. These activities have the potential to awaken former memories and abilities and help those with cognitive or physical impairment communicate in ways that are beneficial to themselves, staff, loved ones, family, friends, and the community at large.

Staffing: Shortages, Consequences, Responses, and Implications for the Future
Staff Shortages and Assisted Living Challenges

The existing and emerging shortage of staff is a major problem for the United States health care delivery system and is especially important for long-term care. According to a report by Biles, Burke, McClosky, and Fitzler (2005), 80 percent of states reported a shortage of registered nurses (RNs) and approximately 60 percent reported a shortage of certified nursing assistants (CNAs). The American Health Care Association ([AHCA] 2004) also cites evidence of a shortage of resident assistants and personal care aides, as well as the fact that 90 percent of long-term care organizations report that they lack sufficient nurse staffing to provide even the most basic of care (Joint Commission on Accreditation of Healthcare Organizations [JCAHO], 2002; National Commission on Nursing Workforce for Long-Term Care, 2005).

According to the U.S. Bureau of Labor Statistics (2003), more than a million new and replacement nurses will be needed by 2012. Several trends that will lead to this situation: (1) the number of people in need of nursing services will increase as the population ages; (2) 400,000 nurses will reach retirement age in the next decade; (3) fewer people are coming forward to fill these positions (JCAHO 2002); with workers between the ages of 25 and 54 declining as a percentage of the workforce, from 71 percent in 2000 to 66 percent in 2012 (AARP, 2005), and (4) nursing institutions are turning away applicants because of insufficient numbers of qualified instructors (ACHA, 2004; American Association of Colleges of Nursing, 2004; JCAHO, 2002). In addition, Buerhaus, Staiger, and Auerbach (2000) hypothesize that, because more career paths are now open to women, fewer women are choosing the woman dominated nursing profession. Finally, Biles et al. (2005) hypothesize that the factors discouraging workers from choosing careers as direct care workers and nurses include the culture of the workplace, lack of career growth opportunities, and salaries that are lower than comparable jobs. Widespread unionization of long-care workers, which is now being promoted by the service workers union

(SEIU) and others, may increase the status, pay, and benefits of long-term care jobs, thereby increasing worker stability and the overall pool of qualified workers in this sector. The downside, however, is that across-the-board wage and benefits increments will also make the long-term care offered by assisted living even less affordable for the middle class. These higher-cost staffing trends may also contribute to the phasing out of some small "mom-and-pop" assisted living residences that serve a population with more cognitive or physical impairments (see chapter 5).

Central to the ability of assisted living properties to serve the most cognitively or physically impaired residents is their hiring of adequate numbers of well-qualified direct care workers and nurses. Though lower than in nursing homes, the rate of staff turnover remains high in assisted living, estimated at 25 percent for all direct care staff during a one-year period (Hawes & Phillips, 2000), and at 21 percent to 135 percent for all staff nationwide (National Center for Assisted Living [NCAL], 2001). Many long-term care providers are incurring direct costs because of this turnover resulting from the need to recruit and train new staff and to hire nurses from staffing agencies (General Accounting Office, 2001). Shortages of both nurses and direct care workers not only challenge assisted living providers but also present challenges for states, staff, families and friends, and, most important, the residents. Better recruitment, retention and training efforts, more adequate wages and benefits, more adequate government funding, and the increased supply of labor through immigration reform would reduce the future magnitude of labor shortages (AHCA, 2004).

Several studies report a correlation between staff stability and positive outcomes among residents (Bowers & Becker, 1992; Bowers, Esmond, & Jacobson, 2000; Cohen-Mansfield, 1997; Schnelle, 1993). A 2003 study by Phillips et al. found that residents were more likely to be able to age in place in buildings with fulltime RNs on staff. Kovner and Harrington (2003) also argue that staffing shortages or increased staffing-related costs may threaten the future ability of impaired residents to age in place. The correlation, however, is far from perfect. Other studies have not always concluded that such extensive nursing staff is needed to ensure that residents' needs are met (Hyde et al., 1998). It is possible that the assisted living provider's philosophy of care more than any specific services can enable people with physical disabilities to age in place (Mitty, 2004).

Issues related to job satisfaction and opportunities for minorities are also of concern in a discussion of staffing shortages. Zimmerman et al.

(2005a) found that staff satisfaction was lower among black workers, who, as shown in a study by Sikorska (2005), represent 34 percent of assisted living staff; however, though prevalent among direct care workers, including personal aides, certified nursing assistants, and other hands-on staff without formal nursing training, minorities are underrepresented in the nursing-specific workforce. Although the percentage has risen in recent years, only 12 percent of nurses are minorities, compared to 30 percent minority representation in the overall population (Spratley et al., 2000). In addition, there is a movement away from training licensed practical nurses (LPNs) and CNAs to become RNs (AHCA, 2005) and because many CNAs are minorities, inequalities may persist and further discourage workers from choosing assisted living as a career option. ACHA and NCAL propose a creative option for recruitment: reauthorizing the Welfare to Work Tax Credit as an incentive for long-care providers to recruit thousands of people from welfare. In addition, NCAL and other groups propose that Congress pass comprehensive immigration reform to help provide an adequate supply of staff in assisted living (Buerhaus, Staiger, & Auerbach, 2003; AHCA, 2004).

Staff Roles and Training

All staff members who interact with residents affect the resident's sense of autonomy and their ability to live with dignity and respect. Direct care workers play a critical role in the lives of the most impaired assisted living residents because they provide the greatest amount of care. Each interaction they have with residents can either positively or negatively impact their quality of life.

The role of staff varies across states and within the various types of assisted living residences. States differ on whether they require a licensed staff person to deliver medications to the residents as well as whether staff can involve residents in activities such as doing laundry. Depending on state-specific regulations, staff that pass medications might be a licensed vocational nurse, a certified medication aide, or other trained and supervised staff (Chafetz, 2001). According to one study (Rosenblatt et al., 2004), assisted living residents with dementia require more than twice the amount of staff time than those without dementia.

Providing appropriate and complete staff training is also a potentially effective strategy for addressing staffing problems and reducing turnover (Winzelberg et al., 2005). Nursing assistants report that they want more training, specifically with regard to dementia care. This training should include helping staff recognize symptoms of dementia with an understanding that losing one's memory is not part of the process of normal aging. In another study in nursing homes, nurse's aides were taught a variety of tasks, though very little was done to help them integrate these tasks. It was therefore difficult to empower the nurses' aides to respond to the demands of their job (Bowers & Becker, 1992).

Zimmerman et al.'s (2005a) study of stress and satisfaction with staff who care for residents with dementia in long-term care, found that attitudes towards dementia care and ongoing training are related to worker satisfaction. A key responsibility of each state and each assisted living residence is to provide appropriate and adequate training for all staff. This is consistent with one of the eight recommendations identified by the Alzheimer's Association to improve dementia care in assisted living. There is evidence that training improves the staff's ability to deliver adequate support to residents with dementia and that staff who are trained to understand the outcomes of cognitive decline are better equipped to care for people with dementia (Singer & Luxenberg, 2003; Alzheimer's Association, 2005).

Empowering staff to maximize their use of their skills and provide adequate training and support also can minimize their stress, thereby presumably reducing turnover and improving care. In their study of nursing assistants in assisted living and nursing homes, Winzelberg et al. (2005) found that nursing assistants' ratings of quality of life for residents with dementia are related to their own attitudes toward residents with dementia and to their own perceived competence to address resident's fundamental care needs. Singer and Luxenberg (2003) reported that staff experience caring for dementia patients is stressful, which leads to staff turnover. They further found that one effective topic for staff training is the understanding of nonverbal cues to detect resident problems. An organizational culture that empowers staff and provides increased training is also important. In a study of assisted living staff with daily contact with residents, including administrative staff, nurses' assistants, and nurses, Sikorska-Simmons et al. (2005) found that residences creating an organizational culture that respects staff members effectively produce higher levels of staff commitment. In addition, higher levels of organizational commitment were associated with greater job satisfaction.

The National Commission on Nursing Workforce for Long-Term Care

(2005), a study of nursing assistants in nursing homes, found that social support can assist nursing assistants in dealing with the most difficult residents. The study also presented recommendations for recruiting and retaining skilled nurses and documenting best practices. They state the retention of nurses will necessitate changes in the organization and operation for the long-term care workplace.

With respect to training, "workers who perceive themselves to be better trained in dementia care are more likely to espouse person-centered care and report more satisfaction" and to have reduced incidence of turnover (Zimmerman et al., 2005a). The Pioneer Network Web site (see chapter 3) further cites various studies reporting on the benefits of training in terms of resident outcomes, including "wandering (Cohen-Mansfield, Werner, Culpepper, Barkeley, 1997), nonverbal communication (Magai, Cohen, Gomberg, 2002), agitation during self-care routines (Roth, Stevens, Burgio and Burgio, 2002), behavioral management (Burgio, Stevens, Burgio, Roth, Paul and Gerstle, 2002), the resident's sleep environment (e.g., reduce noise and waking) (Alessi, Yoon, Schnelle, Al-Samarrai, Cruise, 1999) detecting depression (Wood, Cummings, Schnelle, Stephens, 2002) and other psychiatric needs (Proctor et al., 1999)." Two common concerns about the efficacy of purely educational approaches have been the level of retention of information by staff over time and the integration of the information into actual care routines. Some of the studies mentioned above examine how the delayed effects of training influence staff retention and the application of information on resident care outcomes (Burgio et al., 2002; Cohen-Mansfield et al., 1997; Magai et al., 2002; Wood et al., 2002). Finally, the methodology used to train staff to care for people with depression and dementia may matter as shown by one study that compared training via lectures versus computer-based interactive video (Rosen et al., 2002).

New Technologies and Staff Roles

In addition to providing more training to existing staff, facilities may turn to new technologies to accommodate staff limitations (see also chapter 8). In particular, three types of technological interventions may enhance the ability of assisted living to serve the most impaired residents. These are (1) monitoring, (2) electronic health records and online communications, and (3) interactive entertainment and cognitive strengthening technologies. As resident vital signs and other information, such as whether medications are being taken, can be monitored and transmitted and as health records can be shared among residents, families, assisted living staff and medical providers, given appropriate information privacy controls to meet Health Insurance Portability and Accountability Act requirements, it may become feasible to serve even those with higher level healthcare needs in assisted living. The provision of 24-hour skilled on-site nursing, now primarily available only in nursing homes, may be available remotely for residents who need frequent monitoring. Residents will also be less likely to need to go to a physician's office or emergency room for an un-planned health issue. Monitors of various sorts will reduce the need for time-consuming rounds, especially of the sort that awaken residents at night to check on them. Record keeping may also become more efficient when it can be done electronically and "on the fly." Finally, activity pro-gramming that uses technology, such as customized Internet connections with games, videos, and family interfaces, may replace a small portion of staff-intensive activities programs. If these various staffing solutions are not implemented, and if little is done to rectify the staffing shortage issues, assisted living will have difficulty allowing the most impaired seniors to age-in-place while sustaining a social model of care.

Conclusions and Implications for the Future

During the second half of the twentieth century, people with cognitive or physical disability received care and services either at home with infor-mal caregivers or, increasingly, in nursing homes, where they have been offered a medical model of care. More recently, assisted living, with its "social model" of services, has emerged as an important option for older people who need assistance and also want to maintain their sense of iden-tity and community (Kane, 2004). As large numbers of people live longer with chronic disabilities, however, many will "age in place" in assisted living, making it likely that more will be expected of these settings. Assisted living providers will not only need to make available more health-related services but will also will need to welcome the diversity of residents, as well as their extended community of families and loved ones. The ques-tions we addressed in this chapter were

- What forces are at work that will facilitate or impede assisted liv-ing's capacity to serve those with the greatest disability?
- What structure and process changes, if any, are needed so that as-

sisted living settings are prepared to provide the services that these residents want and need?

- Can assisted living maintain its social model in the face of these changes and their residents' increased service needs?

After reviewing the many evolving factors that affect these issues, we conclude that the keys to successfully serving assisted living residents with serious disabilities are

1. Fostering an environment where residents, their families (in the broadest sense), health-care providers, and assisted living staff can work together to understand and address the needs and wishes of each individual resident.
2. Promoting among the staff a deep appreciation for the autonomy, dignity, needs, and preferences of each resident. This is done through
   a. Processes and organizational factors that empower the staff;
   b. Providing the staff with wages and benefits that support an adequate standard of living;
   c. Training that provides the staff with tools for understanding residents' strengths and needs, including health-related and cognitive conditions, and allows the staff to grow through careers;
3. Focus on processes that support residents' "quality of circumstance" and quality of life.
4. Regulations, financial structures, and third-party payment that ensure appropriate services and safety while sustaining residents' autonomy and dignity.

Looking in our proverbial crystal ball, it appears likely that assisted living will continue to serve those with significant levels of physical and cognitive impairment and will be able to make those changes that will be necessary to adapt to the changing environment and preserve its social model philosophy. To be able to meet the needs of residents with the greatest levels of impairment, it is likely that assisted living residences will add to their staffing and to other structural elements and will be forced to comply with increased regulatory requirements, adding to the cost of assisted living for all.

Despite being strained by increased impairment among resident populations, accommodating shifting family structures, increasing available staff, and designing appropriate regulations to address needed processes of care, the future offers opportunities for assisted living to grow as a care option for people with physical or cognitive impairment.

APPENDIX: THE CASE OF GERALD B.

Mr. B had been followed for "mild cognitive impairment" since his retirement at age 65. Now 72 years old and diagnosed with Alzheimer disease, this otherwise healthy, divorced man decided, with encouragement from his adult children and his girlfriend, to move to the Abbey Road Assisted Living Residence. He is an active member of an Alzheimer's Association early stage group, occasionally serving as a public speaker on his condition. Although he has given up driving and playing bridge, he is playing more golf, joined the choir at his church, and is popular among residents and staff at Abbey Road, where he is on the resident dining review committee and plays drums in a jazz band. Although he understands that his condition will eventually further curtail his activities and affect his health more generally, Mr. B. has developed numerous coping strategies that allow him to remain active. He is also taking a cholinesterase inhibitor, which he feels is helpful in slowing the course of his disease. After his girlfriend moved to California, he focused on organizing his financial affairs, named his oldest son as his health care proxy, and had numerous discussions with his children about his preferences so that he would be able to live out his life in ways that are consistent with his values and allow him as much control and dignity as possible.

Looking ahead eight years, we can imagine Mr. B. still living at Abbey Road, still playing the drums, but in some other ways not nearly as active. His son, now nearing 60 himself, takes Mr. B. out to play golf; they count themselves lucky if he can manage nine holes and lunch. He is crankier, and staff members complain that some days he will not change into a clean shirt and resists a shower. But Mr. B. still has a reasonably clear sense of how he wants to live out his life. His son, daughter-in-law, and daughter support his wishes, even if that includes his taking walks in the neighborhood, walks the staff is hesitant to allow because they are afraid he will fall or have trouble finding his way back, so his children make sure he wears his "dog tag" and buy him a global positioning system–pager that alerts the staff if he stops walking for more than fifteen minutes or if he goes further away from the grounds than they all agree is safe.

Five years further on, now on two cognition-enhancing medications, and engaged in purposeful stimulation activities in small groups and on the computer, Mr. B. struggles to keep up with the world that seems to be flying past him at an ever-faster rate. Besides his cognitive slippage, his arthritis slows him down most days, too, but he and his doctors are managing it with a combination of exercise and nonsteroidal anti-inflammatory medications. His children have retired to Florida, and his grandchildren have taken over as healthcare proxies and frequent visitors. His eighty-fifth birthday party was held as a fundraiser for the Alzheimer's

Association, and he is proud to have his picture used in some of their materials, even though he no longer gives speeches on living with Alzheimer's. He's still popular with the staff, has a lovely new lady friend at Abbey Road, and enjoys visits from his great grandchildren, though he can't quite remember which one is which.

But just after his eighty-sixth birthday Mr. B. had a stroke, which left him greatly weakened on his left side and unable to express himself. After two months of physical therapy he hadn't improved and was beginning to have even more trouble swallowing. Finally, he stopped eating except for small amounts of ice cream if one of his favorite staff members or grandchildren fed him. The family convened an emergency conference, debated whether a feeding tube would be appropriate. But thinking back to their conversations during when he was first diagnosed, Mr. B's children realized that wasn't what he wanted. So they and the staff at Abbey Road arranged for a hospice nurse to come in regularly. Mr. B. died at the assisted living residence among family and friends just short of his eighty-seventh birthday, having received his wish to live out his life with dignity in the setting of his choice.

REFERENCES

Agency for Healthcare Research and Quality. 2002. *Preventing disability in the elderly with chronic disease.* Research in Action, Issue 3. AHRQ Publication No. 02-0018, April. Rockville, MD: AGRQ. www.ahrq.gov/research/elderdis .htm.

Alessi, C. A., Yoon, E. J., Schnelle, J. F., Al-Samarrai, N. R., & Cruise, P. A. 1999. A randomized trial of a combined physical activity and environmental intervention in nursing home residents: do sleep and agitation improve? *Journal of the American Geriatrics Society 47* (7), 784–91.

Alzheimer's Association. 1993. *Guidelines for dignity.* Chicago: Alzheimer's Association.

Alzheimer's Association. 2006. *Dementia care practice recommendations for assisted living residences and nursing homes.* Chicago: Alzheimer's Association.

American Association of Colleges of Nursing. 2004. Enrollment increases at U.S. nursing schools are moderating while thousands of qualified students are turned away. Press release, American Association of Colleges of Nursing, Washington, DC, December 15.

American Association of Homes and Services for the Aging. No date. *Best practices for special care programs for persons with Alzheimer's disease or a related disorder.* Washington, DC: American Association of Homes and Services for the Aging.

American Association of Retired Persons. 2001. *In the middle: A report on multicultural boomers coping with family and aging issues.* Washington, DC: Belden, Russonello & Stewart; Great Falls, VA: Research/Strategy/Management.

American Association of Retired Persons. 2004. *Boomers at midlife.* Washington, DC: American Association of Retired Persons.

American Association of Retired Persons. 2005. *Reimagining America: AARP's blueprint for the future.* Washington, DC: American Association of Retired Persons.

American Health Care Association. 2004. Issue Brief. *Assisted living.* March.

American Health Care Association. 2005. Issue Brief. *Workforce shortage: Who will answer the call button?* June 14.

Applebaum, R. A., Uman, G. C., & Straker, J. K. 2006. Capturing the voice of consumers in long-term care: If you ask them, they will tell. In S. Kunkel. & V. Wellin (Eds.), *Consumer voice and choice in long-term care* (pp. 127–140). New York: Springer.

Assisted Living Federation of America. 2006. *Overview of the assisted living industry.* Alexandria, VA: Assisted Living Federation of America.

Assisted Living Workgroup. 2003. *Assuring quality in assisted living: Guidelines for federal and state policy, state regulations, and operations: Final report to the U.S. Senate Special Committee on Aging.* Washington, DC: Government Printing Office.

Baker, D. 2002. *The run-up in home prices: Is it real or is it another bubble?* Washington, DC: Center for Economic Policy Research.

Ball, M. M., Perkins, M. M., Whittington, F. J., Connell, B. R., Hollingsworth, C., King, S. V., et al. 2004. Managing decline in assisted living: the key to aging in place. *Journals of Gerontology B Psychological Sciences and Social Sciences 59* (4), S202–212.

Biles, B., Burke, R., McCloskey, K., & Fitzler, S. 2005. Developing state partnerships and initiatives to address long-term care nursing workforce challenges. September 30. Grant by the U.S. Department of Labor.

Bowers, B., & Becker, M. 1992. Nurse's aides in nursing homes: the relationship between organization and quality. *Gerontologist 32* (3), 360–366.

Bowers, B., Esmond, S., & Jacobson, N. 2000. The relationship between staffing and quality in long-term care: Exploring the views of nurse aides. *Journal of Nursing Care Quality 14* (4), 55–64.

Brotman, S., Ryan, B., & Cormier, R. 2003. The health and social service needs of gay and lesbian elders and their families in Canada. *Gerontologist 43,* 192–202.

Buerhaus, P. I., Staiger, D. O., & Auerbach, D. I. 2000. Implications of an aging registered nurse workforce. *JAMA 283,* 2948–2954.

Burgio, L. D., Stevens, A., Burgio, K. L., Roth, D. L., Paul, P., & Gerstle, J. 2002. Teaching and maintaining behavior management skills in the nursing home. *Gerontologist 42* (4), 487–496.

Buss, S. 2002. Personal autonomy. In *Stanford encyclopedia of philosophy.* http://plato.stanford.edu/entries/personal-autonomy/.

Cahill, S., South K., & Spade, J. 2000. *Outing age: Public policies affecting gay, lesbian, bisexual and transgender elders.* New York: Policy Institute of the National Gay and Lesbian Task Force Foundation.

Centers for Disease Control and Prevention. 2005. The state of aging and health in America, 2004. Washington, DC: Merck Institute of Aging and Health.

Chafetz, P. K. 2001. Developing dementia care units in assisted living facilities. In K. H. Namazi & P. K. Chafetz (Eds.), *Assisted living: Current issues in facility management and resident care* (pp. 105–125). Westport, CT: Auburn House.

Chu, L., Schnelle, J. F., Cadogan, M. P., & Simmons, S. F. 2004. Using the minimum data set to select nursing home residents for interview about pain. *Journal of the American Geriatrics Society 52* (12), 2057–2061.

Cohen-Mansfield, J. 1997. Turnover among nursing home staff. *Nursing Management 28* (5), 59–64.

Cohen-Mansfield, J., Werner, P., Culpepper, W. J., 2nd, & Barkley, D. 1997. Evaluation of an inservice training program on dementia and wandering. *Journal of Gerontological Nursing 23* (10), 40–47.

Corder, E., & Manton, K. 2001. *Change in the prevalence of severe dementia among older Americans, 1982–1999.* Durham, NC: Duke University Center for Demographic Studies.

Dobbs, D., Munn, J., Zimmerman, S., Boustani, M., Williams, C., Sloane, P., & Reed, P. 2005. Characteristics associated with lower activity involvement in long-term care residents with dementia. *Gerontologist 45,* special issue no. 1, 81–86.

Ekerdt, D. J. 2005. Assisted living: A place to manage uncertainty. *Journal of Gerontological Nursing 31* (1), 38–39.

Evans, D. A., Funkenstein, H. H., Albert, M. S., et al. 1989. Prevalence of Alzheimer's disease in a community population of older persons: Higher than previously reported. *JAMA 262* (18), 2552–2556.

Feinberg, L. F., & Whitlatch, C. J. 2001. Are persons with cognitive impairment able to state consistent choices? *Gerontologist 41* (3), 374–382.

Feld, J. 2006. Some by-products of a vicious war. *Abilities* May.

Fisher, S. E., Burgio, L. D., Thorn, B. E., & Hardin, J. M. 2006. Obtaining self-report data from cognitively impaired elders: methodological issues and clinical implications for nursing home pain assessment. *Gerontologist 46* (1), 81–88.

Fonda, S. J., Clipp, E. C., & Maddox, G. L. 2002. Patterns in functioning among residents of an affordable assisted living housing facility. *Gerontologist 42,* 178–187.

Gallanis, T. P. 2002. Aging and the nontraditional family. 32 *University of Memphis Law Review,* 607. Spring.

General Accounting Office. 2001. *Nursing workforce: Recruitment and retention of nurses and nurses aides is a growing concern.* Report to the Chairman, Subcommittee on Health, Committee on Ways and Means, U.S. House of Representatives, Washington, DC: Government Printing Office.

Golant, S. 2004. Do impaired older persons with health care needs occupy U.S. assisted living facilities? An analysis of six national studies. *Journals of Gerontology Series B: Psychological Sciences and Social Sciences 59,* S68–79

Gwyther, L. P. 1997. The perspective of the person with Alzheimer disease: which outcomes matter in early to middle stages of dementia? *Alzheimer Disease and Associated Disorders 11* (Suppl. 6), 18–24.

Hawes, C., & Phillips, C. D. 2000. *High service or high privacy assisted living facilities, their residents and staff: Results from a national survey.* Washington, DC: Office of Disability, Aging, and Long-Term Care Policy, Office of the Assistant Secretary of Planning and Evaluation, U.S. Department of Health and Human Services.

Hawes, C., Phillips, C. D., Rose, M., Holan, S., & Sherman, M. 2003. A national survey of assisted living facilities. *Gerontologist 43*, 875–882.

Hinrichsen, G. A., & Ramirez, M. 1992. Black and white dementia caregivers: a comparison of their adaptation, adjustment, and service utilization. *Gerontologist 32* (3), 375–381.

Hyde, J. 1995. *Serving people with dementia: Regulating assisted living and residential care settings.* Lexington, MA: Hearthstone Press.

Hyde, J. 1996. Alzheimer's friendly assisted living regulation. *American Journal of Alzheimer's Disease 11* (2), 3–8.

Hyde, J., Segelman, M., Feldman, S., Wilner, M. A., Schmidt, J., & Hunt, J. 1998. Medication management in Massachusetts assisted living settings. *Consultant Pharmacist 13* (9), 1001–1014.

Institute of Medicine. 1986. *Improving the quality of care in nursing homes.* Washington, DC: National Academy Press.

Institute of Medicine. 2002. *Report brief: What health care consumers need to know about racial and ethnic disparities in healthcare.* Washington, DC: National Academy Press.

Joint Commission on Accreditation of Healthcare Organizations. 2002. *Health care at the crossroads: Strategies for addressing the evolving nursing Crisis.* Oakbrook Terrace, IL: Joint Commission on Accreditation of Healthcare Organizations.

Kahneman, D. 2003. A perspective on judgment and choice: Mapping bounded rationality. *American Psychologist 58* (9), 697–720.

Kane, R. A. 2004. *Assisted living as a long-term care option: Transition, continuity, and community.* Fairfax, VA: Assisted Living Research Institute.

Kapp, M. B. 2001. Quality of care and quality of life in nursing facilities: What's regulation got to do with it? *Ethics, Law, and Aging Review 7*, 133–159.

Kassner, E. 2006. *Home and community-based long-term services and supports for older people.* Washington, DC: AARP Public Policy Institute.

Keane, W. 2003. *Assisted living and dementia care: What's working and what's ahead?* Alexandria, VA: Assisted Living Federation of America and the Mather Institute on Aging.

Kovner, C. T., & Harrington, C. 2003. Nursing care in assisted living facilities. *American Journal of Nursing 103* (1), 97–98.

Kuhn, D., Kasayka, R., & Lechner, C. 2002. Behavioral observations and quality of life among persons with dementia in 10 assisted living facilities. *American Journal of Alzheimer's Disease and Other Dementias 17* (5), 291–298.

Lazowski, D. A., Ecclestone, N. A., Myers, A. M., Paterson, D. H., Tudor-Locke, C.,

Fitzgerald, C., Jones, G., Shima, N., & Cunningham, D. A. 1999. A randomized outcome evaluation of group exercise programs in long-term care institutions. *Journals of Gerontology: Medical Sciences 54A*, M621–628.

Leon, J., Cheng, C. K., & Neumann, P. J. 1998. Alzheimer's disease care: costs and potential savings. *Health Affairs 17* (6), 206–216.

Leon, J., & Moyer, D. 1999. Potential cost savings in residential care for Alzheimer's disease patients. *Gerontologist 39* (4), 440–449.

Lorig, K. R., Sobel, D., & Stewart, A. 1999. Evidence suggesting that a chronic disease self-management program can improve health status while reducing hospitalization: A randomized trial. *Medical Care 37* (1), 5–14.

Lyketsos, C., Rosenblatt, A., Steele, C., et al. 2002. Maryland assisted living study: Initial findings from the first 100 cases. Presentation to the Maryland Gerontological Society, Baltimore.

Magai, C., Cohen, C. I., & Gomberg, D. 2002. Impact of training dementia caregivers in sensitivity to nonverbal emotion signals. *International Psychogeriatrics 14* (1), 25–38.

Manton, K. C., Gu, X. L., & Ukraintseva, S. V. 2005. Declining prevalence of dementia in the U.S. elderly population. *Advances in Gerontology 16*, 30–37.

Mill, J. S. 1859. *On liberty.* London: Longman, Roberts & Green, 1859; New York: Bartleby.Com, 1999. www.sacred-texts.com/phi/mill/liberty.txt.

Mitchell, J. M., & Kemp, B. K. 2000. Quality of life in assisted living homes: A multidimensional analysis. *Journals of Gerontology Series B: Psychological Sciences and Social Sciences 55*, 117–127.

Mitty, E. L. 2004. Assisted living: aging in place and palliative care. *Geriatric Nursing 25* (3), 149–156, 163.

Mollica, R. L. 2001. State policy and regulations. In S. Zimmerman, P. D. Sloane, & J. K. Eckert (Eds.), *Assisted living: Needs, practices, and policies in residential care for the elderly* (pp. 9–33). Baltimore: Johns Hopkins University Press.

National Bureau of Economic Research. 2005. *The market for LTC insurance.* www.nber.org/aginghealth/winter05/w10989.html.

National Center for Assisted Living. 2001. *Facts and trends: The assisted living sourcebook.* Washington, DC: National Center for Assisted Living.

National Commission on Nursing Workforce for Long-Term Care. 2005. *Act now for your tomorrow: Final report.* Washington, DC: National Commission on Nursing Workforce for Long-Term Care.

National Institute of Nursing Research. 2006. *Long-term care for older adults: Developing knowledge for practice: Challenges and opportunities.* Bethesda, MD: National Institute of Nursing Research.

Neumann, P. J., Araki, S. S., & Gutterman, E. M. 2000. The use of proxy respondents in studies of older adults: lessons, challenges, and opportunities. *Journal of the American Geriatrics Society 48* (12), 1646–1654.

Novartis. 2006. *The senior care source: Facts, figures, and forecasts.* Vol. 3. Annadale, NJ: Novartis Pharmaceuticals Corporation.

Phillips, C. D., Hawes, C., Spry, K., & Rose, M. 2000. *Residents leaving assisted living: Descriptive and analytic results from a national survey.* Beachwood, OH: Myers Research Institute, Menorah Park Center for Senior Living.

Phillips, C. D., Munoz, Y., Sherman, M., Rose, M., Spector, W., & Hawes, C. 2003. Effects of facility characteristics on departures from assisted living: results from a national study. *Gerontologist 43* (5), 690–696.

Port, C. L., Zimmerman, S., Williams, C. S., Dobbs, D., Preisser, J. S., & Williams, S. W. 2005. Families filling the gap: Comparing family involvement for assisted living and nursing home residents with dementia. *Gerontologist 45*, special issue 1, 87–95.

Powers, B. A. 2005. Everyday ethics in assisted living facilities: A framework for assessing resident-focused issues. *Journal of Gerontological Nursing 31* (1), 31–37.

Proctor, R., Burns, A., Powell, H. S., Tarrier, N., Faragher, B., Richardson, G., Davies, L., & South, B. 1999. Behavioral management in nursing and residential homes: a randomized controlled trial. *Lancet 354* (9172), 26–29.

Riley, M. W. 1997. Commencement address, University at Albany, Albany, NY, May 18.

Rosen, J., Mulsant, B. H., Kollar, M., Kastango, K. B., Mazumdar, S., & Fox, D. 2002. Mental health training for nursing home staff using computer-based interactive video: a six-month randomized trial. *Journal of American Medical Directors Association 3* (5), 291–296.

Rosenblatt, A., Samus, Q. M., Steele, C. D., Baker, A. S., Harper, M. G., Brandt, J., et al. 2004. The Maryland Assisted Living Study: Prevalence, recognition, and treatment of dementia and other psychiatric disorders in the assisted living population of central Maryland. *Journal of the American Geriatrics Society 52* (10), 1618–1625.

Roth, D. L., Stevens, A. B., Burgio, L. D., & Burgio, K. L. 2002. Timed-event sequential analysis of agitation in nursing home residents during personal care interactions with nursing assistants. *Journals of Gerontology B Psychological Sciences and Social Sciences 57* (5), P461–468.

Rowe, J. W., & Kahn, R. L. 1998. *Successful aging.* New York: Pantheon Books.

Schafer, R. 1999a. *America's elderly population and their need for supportive services.* Cambridge, MA: Joint Center for Housing Studies, Harvard University.

Schafer, R. 1999b. *Housing America's seniors.* Cambridge, MA: Joint Center for Housing Studies, Harvard University.

Schnelle, J., McNees, M., Simmons, S., Agnew, M., & Crooks V. 1993. Managing nurse aides to promote quality of care in the nursing home. In L. Rubenstein & D. Wieland (Eds.), *Improving care in the nursing home: Comprehensive reviews of clinical research* (pp. 314–331). Newbury Park, CA: Sage.

Sikorska-Simmons, E. 2005. Predictors of organizational commitment among staff in assisted living. *Gerontologist 45*, 196–205.

Singer, C., & Luxenberg, J. 2003. Diagnosing dementia in long-term care facilities. *Journal of American Medical Directors Association 4* (6), S134–140.

Sloane, P. D., Zimmerman, S., & Ory, M. G. 2001. Care for persons with dementia. In S. Zimmerman, P. D. Sloane, & J. K. Eckert (Eds.), *Assisted living: Needs, practices, and policies in residential care for the elderly* (pp. 242–270). Baltimore: Johns Hopkins University Press.

Spratley, E., Johnson, A., Sochalski, J., Fritz, M., & Spencer, W. 2000. *The registered nurse population: Findings from the National Sample Survey of Registered Nurses.* Washington, DC: U.S. Department of Health and Human Services, Bureau of Health Professions, Division of Nursing, Health Resources and Services Administration. ftp://ftp.hrsa.gov/bhpr/rnsurvey2000/rnsurvey00.pdf.

Stocker, B., & Silverstein, N. 1996. Assisted living residences in Massachusetts: How ready and willing are they to serve people with Alzheimer's or a related disorder? *American Journal of Alzheimer's Disease* March/April, pp. 28–38.

Tilly, J., & Wiener, J. No date. *Consumer-directed home and community services: Policy issues.* Urban Institute occasional paper no. 44. Washington, DC: Urban Institute.

U.S. Department of Health and Human Services, Office of the Assistant Secretary for Planning and Evaluation, the Centers for Medicare and Medicaid Services, and Health Resource and Services Administration and the Department of Labor's Office of the Assistant Secretary for Policy, Bureau of Labor Statistics and Employment and Training Administration. 2003. *The future supply of long-term care workers in relation to the aging baby boom generation: Report to Congress, May 14.* Washington, DC: Government Printing Office.

U.S. Census Bureau. 2000. *United States census, 2000.* Washington, DC: Government Printing Office.

Winzelberg, G. S., Williams, C. S, Preisser, J. S, Zimmerman, S., & Sloane, P. D. 2005. Factors associated with nursing assistant quality-of-life ratings for residents with dementia in long-term care facilities. *Gerontologist 45* (special issue 1), 106–114.

Wood, S., Cummings, J. L., Schnelle, B., & Stephens, M. 2002. A videotape-based training method for improving the detection of depression in residents of long-term care facilities. *Gerontologist 42* (1), 114–121.

Wylde, M., 1998. *National survey of assisted living residents: Who is the customer?* National Investment Conference, Annapolis, MD.

Zimmerman, S., Sloane, P. D., Williams, C. S., Reed, P. S., Preisser, J. S., Eckert, J. K., Boustani, M., & Dobbs, D. 2005a. Dementia care and quality of life in assisted living and nursing homes. *Gerontologist 45*, 133–146.

Zimmerman, S., Williams, C. S., Reed, P. S., Boustani, M., Preisser, J. S., Heck, E., et al. 2005b. Attitudes, stress, and satisfaction of staff who care for residents with dementia. *Gerontologist 45* (special issue 1), 96–105.

CHAPTER 3

Tomorrow's Assisted Living and Nursing Homes

The Converging Worlds of Residential Long-term Care

MARGARET P. CALKINS, PH.D.,
WILLIAM KEANE, M.S., M.P.A., L.N.H.A.

Careful observers are already cognizant of some of the ripples of significant change in how we provide long-term care in the United States. Nursing homes are becoming a less exclusive way by which we care for older persons with high-acuity chronic needs; a small group of nursing homes no longer look like their venerable historical selves; and assisted living residences are increasingly accommodating older persons with more demanding care needs who were once predominantly found in nursing homes. Moreover, both these shared residential settings face formidable competition for their occupants as older persons with even the most severely debilitating physical and cognitive impairments increasingly choose to remain in their familiar homes and apartments.

We offer several alternative scenarios for tomorrow's long-term care landscape. It can be difficult to imagine a time when familiar options like nursing homes and assisted living residences will not look and function as they do today, and one of our future scenarios depicts little change. Two others, however, envision a long-term care landscape two or three decades from now in which the transformations in how these options look and function may be so dramatic that our current nomenclature will no longer accurately describe their missions. One of our scenarios also raises the possibility—perhaps idealistically—that assisted living residences will be widely affordable to lower-income older persons, even as they are now primarily accessible only to those who are financially better off.

The Split Personality of Assisted Living

Despite experiencing some past market downturns, assisted living today thrives as a high-growth option successfully caring for mostly middle- and higher-income older persons who have difficulties living independently because they suffer from physical or cognitive impairments or chronic illnesses. Assisted living has been acclaimed by proponents as a more humane way to deal with the vulnerabilities of old age because of its so-called social model of care. This refers to being more residential-like in physical appearance and more consumer-friendly with respect to its operations and organizational environment. Proponents say that these settings give their residents more choice in their care regimens, are more responsive

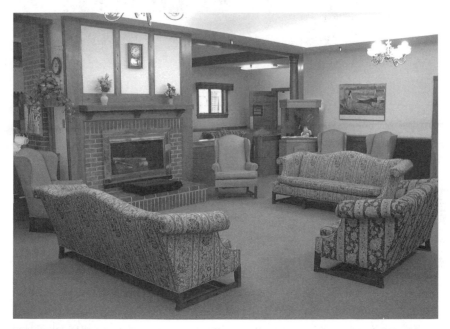

Figure 3.1. Alzheimer's Care Center, Gardner, Maine. *Source:* Maine General Health, Alzheimer's Care Center

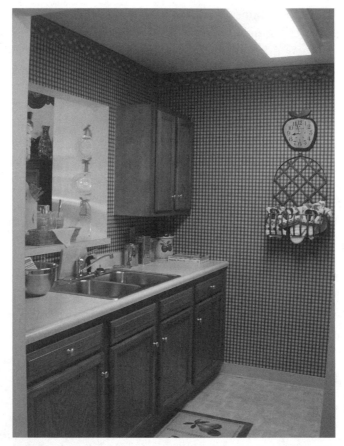

Figure 3.2. Trillium Place, Columbus, Ohio. *Source:* Brookdale Trillium Place

to residents' need for autonomy, and offer greater respect for their individuality. Critics, however, cast doubts on whether it is realistic for assisted living operators to believe that their less regulated and often less professionally staffed options can provide care safely and reliably to older persons with high-acuity needs. They react especially vehemently to those who would suggest that assisted living residences could replace nursing homes (Assisted Living Workgroup Steering Committee, 2003). Some point to assisted living options as an example of the inequities in this country's long-term care system, because (with few exceptions) low-income older persons are unable to afford these residential care alternatives.

These divergent views emphasize what an amorphous option assisted living continues to be. This is also dramatically reflected in how assisted living residences are licensed and regulated by state governments; everything from their physical infrastructure to how they are operated varies significantly from one state to another. Thus, as several chapters in this book point out, assisted living encompasses properties that differ in appearance, operation, and the types of older persons they serve. Part of the reason assisted living belies simple characterizations is because it has roots in two related but distinct traditions.

One group of providers developed this long-term care option to offer "enriched independent living," where less impaired and more cognitively intact older people could live in relatively self-contained apartments, with kitchens, separate bedroom areas, and the capability of locking their doors. Here they could receive some personal care support and assistance with managing their medications (Figures 3.1 to 3.4).

Yet another group of providers, however, a group that appears to be growing in number, developed assisted living as a "nursing home lite," often for people with dementia or who did not need as much *nursing* care but who needed extensive personal care and supervision. The physical

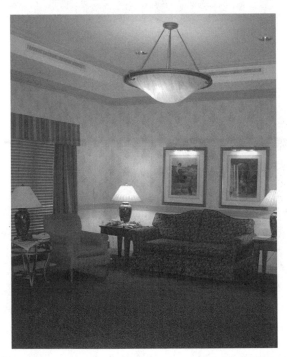

Figure 3.3. Trillium Place, Columbus, Ohio. *Source:* Brookdale Trillium Place

and social design and the organizational environments of these properties were more closely aligned with traditional nursing homes, even as they often employed less highly trained nurses and other professionals. Bedrooms are often shared; there are no kitchens or kitchenettes in residents'

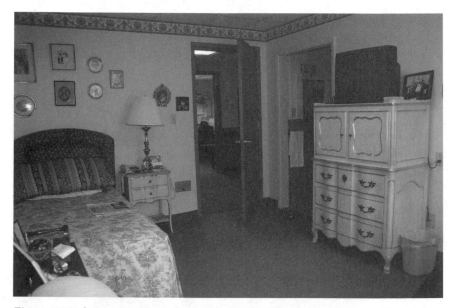

Figure 3.4. Judson at University Circle, Cleveland, Ohio. *Source:* Judson at University Circle

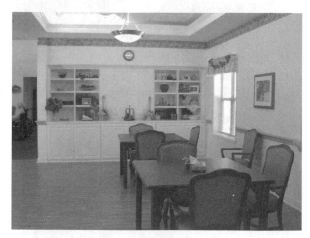

Figure 3.5. Freedom House at Airforce Village, San Antonio, Texas. *Source:* Nelson-Tremain Partnership / RVK Architects

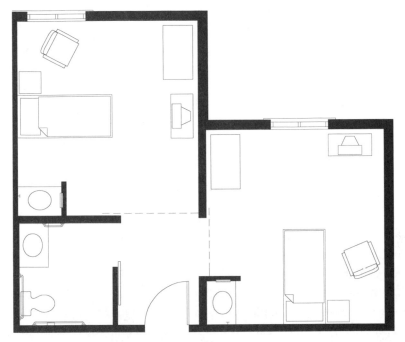

Figure 3.6. Freedom House at Airforce Village, San Antonio, Texas. *Source:* Nelson-Tremain Partnership / RVK Architects

personal spaces and possibly not even in the shared spaces. Although much of the impetus was to serve people with dementia, more recently they have come to serve a more broadly impaired population, including people without cognitive impairments, but who have more serious chronic health problems and multiple disabilities and require more skilled nursing care. More recently, many assisted living residences have struggled to implement a social model of care for mixed populations of residents who differ with respect to age, mental health issues, and acute medical comorbidities (Figures 3.5 and 3.6).

Expanded Home and Community Options

The dual personalities exhibited by assisted living inevitably results in it having to compete with a wide-ranging group of housing and long-term care options that are also catering to both more and less independent elderly consumers. According to most research, the current generation of elders who are having difficulty performing their everyday activities prefers to stay in their conventional community-based homes rather than relocate to a residential care or "institutional" group housing alternative (American Association of Retired Persons, 2005). Although these seniors are on average healthier and less impaired than those opting to live in assisted living or nursing homes, a growing proportion also has significant medical care needs. Those who are more successfully aging in place rely on the assistance of one or more family members or have the financial resources to hire their own private caregivers (O'Brian, 2005). They are also assisted by local grassroots efforts that have helped to create more "livable communities" whereby they can find in their own localities "adequate options for mobility and the various features and services that can facilitate independence and continued engagement in the community's civic and social life" (American Association of Retired Persons, 2005, p. 24). These resources can variously include home repair and upgrading services, personal care, counseling, easy access to key shopping (grocery and pharmacy), and accessible transportation, which are often funded or donated by an eclectic combination of government services, faith-based organizations, and private sector establishments. Sometimes the residents in these communities can rely on adult day centers staffed by persons who can assist them with their everyday needs on a 9-to-5 basis.

A wide array of increasingly popular housing alternatives also now exist—loosely titled "independent living facilities" or "congregate care communities"—where relatively independent elders can receive such services as meals, counseling, preventive health care, and social opportunities in secure, monitored, and well-designed apartment-like settings. Many of these purposely planned communities may provide most of their services with on-site staff; others arrange to receive regular and price-discounted services from banks, restaurants, grocery stores, and health clubs. Confounding this simple portrayal is the increased emergence of apartment-like settings that provide a comparable regimen of services as assisted living but are not licensed by their states. Their operators outsource or subcontract from outside licensed home care agencies and other service establishments a vast array of possible services, encompassing everything from on-demand transportation to nursing services. In many respects, these group housing settings merely mimic the service delivery strategies of older persons who have opted to age in place in their conventional residences but require and can afford to pay for privately hired assistance (see chapter 12).

Other even newer options consist of elders themselves pooling their talents and resources to form co-housing developments where they can live with people of common interests and take greater communal responsibility for their care needs (Durrett, 2005; Golant, 2002). In these developments, everyone has his or her own house or apartment, but residents work together toward various common purposes, whether it be studying or practicing the arts, dedicating their time to a particular cause, or achieving personal growth. In these models, residents might help each other with housekeeping, meals or transportation, and support each other in living in their homes until they die.

Other aggregations of older persons are increasingly found in less intentional housing settings, referred to as "naturally occurring retirement communities" or NORCs (Hunt & Hunt, 1986) and "deliberately occupied but unplanned elder residences" or DOUERs (Golant, 2002). These settings have come to be occupied by a predominantly older tenant population, because the original, once younger residents have aged in place or have been joined by new older tenants deciding to move into these buildings. Through the voluntary efforts of their occupants, often assisted by community-based service organizations, NORCs and DOUERs may introduce a variety of supportive services that are attractive to their residents but without any official oversight from a given provider.

The increasingly muddied boundaries that now separate the care offered in ordinary homes and apartments from that offered in assisted living help to explain why it was so difficult for a representative group of professionals, businesses, and advocates for long-term care interests to reach consensus on definitions of assisted living (Assisted Living Workgroup Steering Committee, 2003). It also explains why there is so much overlap across what people often try to call "distinct" options for care. Consider these estimates (Bishop, 1999; Golant, 2004; Hawes & Phillips, 2000; O'Brian, 2005; Spillman, Liu & McGilliard, 2002; Waidmann, 2003):

- About 20 percent of residents in independent living have some form of dementia.
- More than 40 percent of residents in assisted living have some form of dementia.

- About 20 percent of people cared for in assisted living qualify for nursing home placement.
- From 15 to 20 percent of nursing home residents today could be cared for in assisted living centers.

These percentages vary widely throughout the country, but they point to the overlapping markets served by what were once thought of as very distinctive long-term care options.

Nursing Homes: New Competition and Funding Realities

A consequence of the widespread emergence of these alternative settings during the past two decades is that nursing homes have faced increasing competition for their residents. The nursing home industry has lost important segments of its consumer markets at both ends of the care spectrum. Both older persons who need relatively modest care and those who require significant assistance and/or skilled nursing care now have other options. The meteoric rise of assisted living and the stronger preferences and capabilities of older people to age in place in ordinary dwellings and neighborhoods have steadily eroded the monopoly nursing homes once held in accommodating older persons with modest care needs (Mor et al., 2004), and as state regulators increasingly allow assisted living residences to arrange hospice care or provide more nursing services (Mollica & Johnson-Lamarche, 2005), these facilities are starting to siphon off the heavy-care private-pay clientele that has been the mainstay of nursing homes. Moreover, many assisted living residences now successfully compete with nursing homes for older persons who are coping with mild or moderate dementia (such as Alzheimer disease) and some serve residents who require skilled nursing procedures, such as colostomy care and intravenous feeding (Golant, 2004).

Despite rapidly increasing numbers of frail older persons who would at one time have been considered candidates for nursing home placement, the rate of nursing home use has declined and occupancy rates have been falling even for the oldest old (Alecxi, 2006; Bishop, 1999). Much is at stake. Studies have estimated that the likelihood that persons 65 and older will enter a nursing home at some point in their lives is 35–44 percent. Between 5 and 9 percent of those who enter a nursing home will stay there 5 or more years (Kemper, Komisar, & Alecxih, 2005; Spillman & Lubitz,

2002). The expansion of alternatives, such as assisted living, however, may dramatically change these probabilities.

Another devastating blow to the financial well-being of nursing homes is that low-income seniors, whose shelter and care is often subsidized by the Medicaid program, are an increasing percentage of their resident population. The older persons who could abandon nursing homes were predominantly those with higher incomes, who could themselves pay for their home care or the relatively high costs of private-pay assisted living residences. When this group *did* opt for institutional care, they sometimes occupied nursing homes dominated by private payers (Mor et al., 2004). As Waidmann (2003, p. 11) concludes, "After controlling for health-related factors, [the] finding that high-income persons are significantly less likely to enter nursing homes suggests that high-need individuals who do not rely on Medicaid can make other choices, either assisted living or formal or informal home care." Such a conclusion leads skeptics to argue that what keeps the nursing home industry alive is its ability to offer care to the poorest segments of older persons who simply have fewer affordable long-term care options (Moses, 1995).

It is indeed very expensive to live in a nursing home. In 2006, the average daily rate for a private room in a U.S. nursing home was $206, or $75,190 annually; for a semiprivate room, it was $183 a day, or $66,795 annually (Metlife Mature Market Institute, 2006). Only a minority share of residents, however, pays these rates. Testimony to the importance of the Medicaid program as a financing source of nursing home care is that more than two-thirds of nursing home residents rely on Medicaid to pay their bills. Only 9 percent are Medicare beneficiaries, while 24 percent pay out of pocket or are covered by other sources, such as private insurance (American Health Care Association, 2001). Moreover, as one expert observes, "The wide variation in the number of nursing home beds in parts of the country is not related to variation in the number of old people who might use them, but to different market factors, such as the generosity of Medicaid payments for nursing home care" (O'Brien, 2005, p. 20).

Many experts believe that the quality of care offered by nursing homes has suffered as the industry has become more dependent on Medicaid as a funding source. The average Medicaid reimbursement for nursing home care falls considerably short of the average private pay rate (O'Brian, 2005), even as reimbursement rates vary considerably across the states. Nursing home providers consistently argue that these inadequate subsidies prevent them from offering higher quality of care and from hiring better-trained staff who could be more responsive to individual needs (Spillman, Liu, & McGilliard, 2002). The sad paradox is that federal legislation was intended to address just these problems. The Nursing Home Reform Act, which was part of the Omnibus Budget Reconciliation Act of 1987, imposed more stringent regulatory requirements on nursing home operators, called for better clinical outcomes, and mandated changes ranging from how nursing homes were surveyed to how they were staffed. There was, however, no corresponding Medicaid legislation to offer nursing homes catering to poor elders the financial wherewithal to respond effectively. Residents, family members, the media, and various advocacy groups continued to be dissatisfied with the quality of care and quality of life offered in nursing homes even after the reform act was passed (National Citizens' Coalition for Nursing Home Reform, 2006; Wunderlich & Kohler, 2001).

Some nursing homes are coping better than others, even with low occupancy rates (80–85 percent). Some long-established places have now paid off their mortgages, thus reducing an important monthly financial outlay. Others have more aggressively controlled their payer mix. A example is this hypothetical Illinois nursing home, with 30 percent Medicare at more than $300 per day, 30 percent traditional private pay at $250 per day, and 40 percent Medicaid at $100–$120 per day. The key for these homes is that Medicare rehabilitation and hospice reimbursements in combination with a significant share of private-pay occupants are what pay for their survival.

It would be an overstatement to argue that the poor quality of care and life found in nursing homes is strictly a Medicaid problem. Indeed, one Missouri study found that the cost of providing high-quality care was in fact slightly less than the cost of providing poorer quality care (Rantz, 2004). The homes with better outcomes had leaders who focused especially on quality improvement and on staff practices to achieve it. Nationwide, however, nursing homes generally are inadequately staffed, notably with respect to registered and licensed practical nurses; they experience very high turnover of both managers and direct care workers; and in some states they are burdened by high insurance liability premiums (Harrington et al., 2001). Furthermore, most nursing homes subscribe to a medical model of care that places greater emphasis on curing illness but far less on offering an environment sensitive to the emotional and psychosocial needs and diversity of their residents (Ronch, 2004). As less dependent frail elders have abandoned nursing homes for other alternatives, such as assisted living, the older persons seeking nursing home care have also become increasingly older, sicker, more impaired, and in need of higher levels of care. Many nursing home administrators argue that the more impaired profile of their residents is responsible for the more hospital-like ambience of their facilities (Decker, 2005).

Nursing Homes: Revitalized Competition for Assisted Living?

As these competitive influences eroded the market share of nursing home providers, some recognized that they had to change the way they operated. This was more apparent in some places than in others. For example, in some states, only older persons who require enriched independent living could be admitted or retained in their assisted living residences, such that these options were not infringing on the nursing home market. In other states, such as New Jersey, by contrast, the assisted living regulations were written such that an assisted living home must be prepared to provide a significant amount of nursing care. Moreover, although many of the individuals who moved into assisted living were higher functioning than the typical nursing home resident, as they aged in place, they became frailer and in need of more support—ultimately meeting the criteria for nursing home placement. Yet they were still reluctant to leave. Assisted living residences often were able to retain these residents by their greater use of the services provided by outside licensed home health care and physical therapy agencies (Zimmerman et al., 2003). Faced with this new competition from assisted living, nursing homes reacted in two fundamentally different ways: by tapping an elderly consumer market that could not be served by assisted living and by offering their potential residents not only quality medical care but also a better quality-of-life experience.

The first approach saw some nursing home providers moving back toward their historical roots as an extension of hospital care. Because many nursing homes find Medicaid reimbursement insufficient to cover costs, they instead concentrate on care that is reimbursed by the Medicare program. As a result, some of the most stable and entrepreneurially skilled providers are redefining their businesses and images into high-technology, postacute centers that care for the most medically complex patients who need intensive rehabilitation therapies, dialysis programs, ventilator services, and other specialized care. These providers are exiting their traditional custodial long-term care models for long-stay, chronic care, and dementia residents and competing successfully with medical rehabilitation centers for higher-acuity, short-stay patients. They are also the providers that are buying many of the skilled nursing centers from not-for-profit and continuing-care retirement community providers that are exiting this service to concentrate on independent living and assisted living (Irving Levin Associates, 2005). Nursing homes' greater emphasis on serving Medicare-financed, postacute care residents recovering from a hospital stay is most notably reflected in shorter overall stays for nursing home residents and higher annual discharge rates (Bishop, 1999; Mor et al., 2004).

The second approach was to fundamentally change the nature of nursing homes. A small group of dedicated long-term care professionals belonging to an initiative known as the Pioneer movement began, quietly, to introduce significant changes in nursing home life and to move away from institutional biases that were insensitive to quality-of-life principles, such as privacy, dignity, and choice (Appendix 1). With a few successes, word began to spread, and more nursing homes began to embrace at least some of the principles of what has been most widely known by such names as "culture change," "resident-centered care," "re-engineering," "self-directed"—all embracing the mission to create a new culture of aging in places offering long-term care that is "life-affirming, satisfying, humane, and meaningful" (Misiorski, 2003) (Figures 3.7 and 3.8).

A notable pioneer in this movement is the former medical director of a nursing home in upstate New York, Bill Thomas, M.D., an outspoken critic of nursing homes and cofounder in 1991 of the Eden Alternative: "I'll put the American nursing home on the critical list. It's not going to make it. It's a relic. It's a left-over vestige of a factory, assembly-line approach to care that is just not going to meet the needs of elders in the 21st century. And in fact, I'll do everything that I can to see that, as we move forward, nursing homes cease to exist" (Thomas, 2002, n.p.).

The mission of the Eden Alternative was to change the way that people view long-term care. It was designed to address specifically the boredom, helplessness, and loneliness experienced by nursing home residents and make it possible for the staff working with older persons to make more of the care and organizational decisions (Appendix 2). It is estimated that, by the end of the 1990s, more than 300 nursing homes in the United States had committed in action to the Eden principles (Thomas, 1996).

The most recent approach to accomplishing culture change in the nursing home is far more radical (Appendix 3). It requires nursing homes referred to as "Green Houses" to take on a very different physical layout. Each self-contained house is designed to accommodate 7 to 12 residents and a core group of staff members responsible for multiple tasks, ranging from cooking to personal care (Rabig et al., 2006). There can be 5 to 10 of these houses or homes clustered together or in a community where they are part of a hub nursing care center that is home to the administrative, nursing, and rehabilitation services used by the houses.

The first Green House project was implemented on a campus setting in Tupelo, Mississippi. With support from the Robert Wood Johnson Foundation (RWJF), NCB Capital Impact is providing technical assistance and planning loans to additional organizations interested in creating Green House homes. The goal of the grant funded initiative (see www.ncbcapital impact.org/thegreenhouse) is to create 50 Green House projects in a variety of urban, suburban, and rural settings in as many states as possible by 2010. As of August 2007, 11 projects are open (totaling 31 Green House homes) and 24 projects are under development (representing more than 150 additional Green House homes). More than a thousand groups have registered to learn more about the model and consider it for their organization (Robert Jenkens, personal communication). The Green House Project has certainly garnered the most recent attention, but it is important to recognize that efforts to change the essence of the nursing home have a history that precedes even that of the Pioneer Network, going back to the 1960s and 1970s (Thomas, 1996).

When considered all together, these efforts at transforming the culture of the nursing home display a remarkable similarity with many of the fundamental design and organizational principles of contemporary assisted living residences. The Green House borrows many of the design and care features found in some of the best small, "mom-and-pop" board-and-care facilities (Stephen Golant, personal communication 2006). More generally, these pioneering responses echo the person-centered approach preached by advocates and providers of assisted living. (Appendix 4 offers an abbreviated overview.)

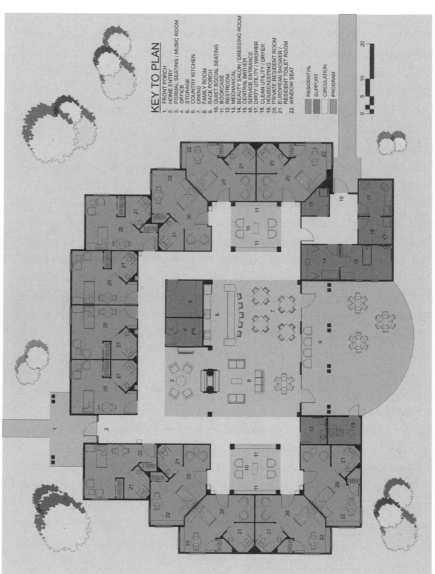

KEY TO PLAN

1. FRONT PORCH
2. HOME ENTRY
3. FORMAL SEATING / MUSIC ROOM
4. OFFICE
5. STORAGE
6. COUNTRY KITCHEN
7. DINING
8. FAMILY ROOM
9. BACK PORCH
10. QUIET SOCIAL SEATING
11. BOOKCASE
12. RESTROOM
13. MECHANICAL
14. BEAUTY SALON / DRESSING ROOM
15. CENTRAL BATHER
16. SERVICE ENTRANCE
17. DIRTY UTILITY / WASHER
18. CLEAN UTILITY / DRYER
19. HOUSEKEEPING
20. PRIVATE RESIDENT ROOM
21. EUROPEAN SHOWER /
    RESIDENT TOILET ROOM
22. WINDOW SEAT

RESIDENTIAL
SUPPORT
CIRCULATION
PROGRAM

0   5   10   20

Figure 3.7. Parkside, Hillsboro, Kansas. *Source:* Studio 360 Architecture

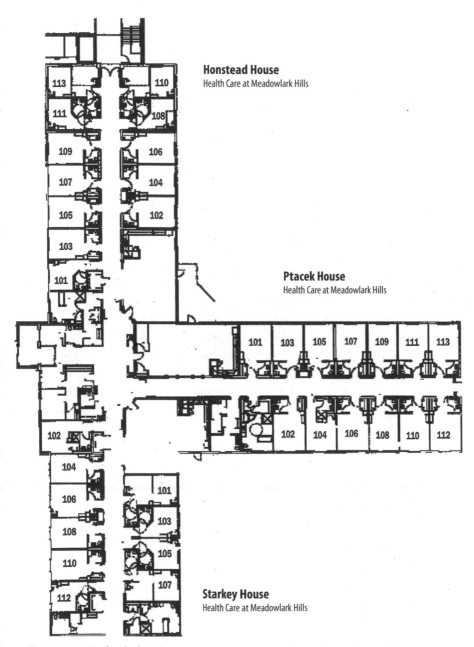

Honstead House
Health Care at Meadowlark Hills

Ptacek House
Health Care at Meadowlark Hills

Starkey House
Health Care at Meadowlark Hills

Figure 3.8. Meadowlark Hills, Manhattan, Kansas. *Source:* Meadowlark Hills

Does Culture Change Work?

How successful have efforts to change the culture of nursing homes been? A growing body of research focused on assisted living, the epitome of culture change, shows that, although there is seldom more "bad" care in newer-model assisted living residences than in the more traditional small board-and-care properties, newer model settings do not necessarily offer better resident outcomes (Zimmerman et al., 2005a). At the same time, research shows that "some people with conditions that could well be served in nursing homes are now in other kinds of residential settings . . . and their outcomes are comparable or better than those of nursing home residents" (Kane 2001, p. 300). More recent research has also found that, when nursing home and assisted living residences serving residents with dementia are compared, "outcomes did not differ significantly across the two types of settings" (Zimmerman et al., 2005b, p. 7).

It is difficult to find scientifically valid assessments of whether culture change in nursing homes yields benefits for the residents or for the organization—or especially for its staff. There is, of course, no shortage of case studies and personal testimonials that point to the improved quality of care and life found in nursing homes that have introduced Eden principles. As one of the earliest and best-known models, it has received more attention and research than some of the other models. It is, however, too early to judge the overall advantages and disadvantages of the more recent Green House option.

At the first nursing home site that implemented the Eden model, research showed lower mortality rates and reductions in the overall number of drug prescriptions, infection rates, and staff turnover. Other Eden nursing homes have reported significant reductions in the number of residents with pressure sores, less use of antidepressant and antianxiety medications, and reduced staff absenteeism. One impressive measure of the success of Eden Alternative homes across the nation is the prevalence of waiting lists for their beds (Thomas, 2006).

Other Eden Alternative nursing homes have reported that residents, family members, and staff hold positive opinions about their operations (Beverly Enterprises, 2000; Rosher & Robinson, 2005) and that residents experience less boredom and helplessness, though not less loneliness (Bergman-Evans, 2004). More recently, preliminary research of the Green

House project in Tupelo found that on virtually all indicators—including quality of life, medical care, staffing attitudes, and costs—the revamped nursing home was performing as well or better than more traditional settings (Rabig et al., 2006). Not all the findings, however, are positive. Two nursing homes operated by the same organization reported greater proportions of residents who had fallen in the past 30 days, more residents with nutritional problems, and more staff terminations after introduction of the Eden principles (Coleman et al., 2002). In one nursing home study, the investigators reported an increase in various types of infectious entities (zoonosis) resulting from the greater presence of pet animals (Guay, 2001).

Is Culture Change Feasible?

There are reasons to be optimistic about the prospect of culture change in the nursing home industry. Our future long-term care will fundamentally depend on what kind of services tomorrow's older consumers will need, prefer, and be able to afford. Most notably, the baby boomers who started turning 60 in 2006 will be a key market to tap in the next 15 years. As adult children, today's boomers demand efficiency and quality for their parents who can no longer live independently at home. They are increasingly turning to professional services and agencies for advice, and, because they are more educated and demanding consumers, they are more discerning of the answers they receive than the elders of the past. If you Google "assisted living" on the Web, you will find more than 13.8 million hits; many of them are consumer advocacy groups, directories, and elder-care-locator or case-management services. Others are informational resources, developed by providers, advocacy groups, or the government to help people become informed consumers about the range of options available. The number of resources reflects the salience of this topic for people who use the Web—most notably adult boomer children.

Boomers will not readily accept the institutional model of traditional nursing homes. They will demand a higher-quality product, and many will have the money to pay for their preferences. But what will they embrace and how far will they go in effecting the deep, systemic changes necessary to achieve it? And will those without adequate financial resources have any real say in system change? Will tomorrow's seniors—rich or poor—subscribe to the theories of "gerotranscendence" proposing that a new sense of life satisfaction and patterns of development can be achieved in the latter decades of life (Tornstam, 1998)? Or will they succumb to the "Botox syndrome," the traditional fears of longevity and the defeatist view of chronic illness? More important, will their values be translated into tomorrow's person-centered assisted living options or perhaps the revamped versions of nursing homes that better fit their views of an ideal old age?

At least one influence would support the opportunity for change. Many facilities in the inventory of the more than 16,000 nursing homes in America will be coming up for either total replacement or major upgrading in the coming decade. It is estimated that the average age of nursing home buildings is approximately 30 years (Lewis, 2005). Although some have been remodeled, much of this aging stock of buildings will need to be replaced in the coming years. Because the building design implications are so very different for different models of care, providers need to determine whether they are moving toward more subacute and rehabilitation services or toward a long-stay facility that must compete with assisted living residences. If they move toward becoming long-stay facilities, it is possible that the current core of traditional nursing home operators will opt to get out of the business or reinvent their physical plants to support a long-term care environment that caters to a whole new image of aging and management of chronic disease.

Despite positive trends, there are probably more reasons to be pessimistic than hopeful about the future for nursing homes. Even those advocates celebrating the person-centered culture changes made by the small group of nursing homes question whether these grass-roots, bottom-up organizational initiatives can lead to revolutionary change in the nursing home industry (Hamilton & Tesh, 2002) in light of the powerful structural constraints that will likely impede change.

Bureaucracy and regulation are likely to be major factors constraining how much and what kind of change is feasible for nursing homes. There are those who believe the two major entitlement programs, Medicare and Medicaid, which so influence the operations and resident composition of nursing homes today, are too large, complicated, and politicized to undergo much change beyond minor tweaking and small add-ons (see chapter 11).

After all, powerful interest groups that are vested in the status quo dominate the nursing home industry. It is second only to the nuclear power industry in terms of its regulatory environment, and with the growing prominence of quality indicators this emphasis on prescriptive regulation will be difficult to change. Regulators have an overriding concern with documentation of care, life safety, and building codes, and lawyers are waiting in the wings to pounce on any incident that is perceived to have been preventable (and even some that are not). There are legitimate fears that a less institutional and more social model of care—sometimes associated with the culture change movement—will lead to an avalanche of episodes of poor and incompetent care, fears that are also continually expressed in response to the emergence of assisted living settings that seek to accommodate a more impaired clientele (Assisted Living Workgroup Steering Committee, 2003).

Thus, despite all this innovative activity to remake the nursing home, some fear that the introduced changes clash too dramatically with its well-entrenched medical model. For example, many view the Eden Alternative as just a "kids, plants and animals" fad and not the basis for sustained "culture change." The net result is that the values and practices of the Pioneer movement might not reach the policymakers, grassroots providers, and practitioners who could create the kind of world that its members seek during the next three decades.

Then there is the matter of finances. The majority of older persons in today's nursing homes receive subsidized shelter and care from the Medicaid program. Thus, their fate and that of their nursing home operators are most directly linked to the status of this federal long-term care and health program. As human service budgets such as Medicaid become the stepchildren to war, terrorism, national disasters, and tax cuts, the resources to implement person-centered care widely may be unavailable. Entitlement spending for Medicare, Medicaid, and Social Security will absorb larger shares of federal revenue and crowd out other spending as the boomers move through their retirement years. This will be the case even as already strained federal and state budgets continue to see an increased demand for long-term care services fueled by the increasing number of disabled elders who will need assistance. The public price tag could reach $379 billion by 2050, with Medicaid as the largest funding source (Allen, 2005). This leads to the following pressing issue: "A matter of compelling interest is whether it is possible for Medicaid to cover assisted living while maintaining the autonomy-enhancing and dignity-enhancing features that appeal to the private market; these may be dismissed as amenities that should not be offered to the poor" (Kane, 2001, p. 300).

In an ageist society wedded to a political system that thinks in short-term actions only to guarantee election results, how do we face the reality

that we see in the demographics and the strains in the current (non)sys-
tems of long-term care? How do we create a willingness to implement *and
sustain* over the long term a national vision of "eldertopia" (Thomas, 2004)
in which entirely new models of assisted living and nursing care may
flourish?

The Look and Functioning of Future Assisted Living

The safest prediction that can be made about the future of assisted living, indeed of the long-term care network generally, is that it will change.
Predicting the "how" is much more difficult. We generally believe that the
fate of assisted living will be intimately linked with how other long-term
care alternatives change. In particular, we expect that the unfolding future
will largely depend on whether the "culture change" now being experienced by a small share of nursing homes will be adopted broadly by the
industry. The most influential future wildcard may be dealt by the federal
government with respect to making assisted living affordable to a vast
potential clientele of low-income older persons (see the discussion of this
possibility in chapter 11). We identify three possible future scenarios, all
of which make critical assumptions that, if they fail to materialize, will
make shambles of our predictions.

Scenario 1: Mostly "Status Quo"

In the first scenario, the majority of nursing homes will continue to
practice their medical and institutionalized model of care. Assisted living
residences will continue to reflect their two distinct etiologies and thus
will function as both enriched independent living and as nursing home
"lite." Assisted living homes will, however, aggressively market to the
more independent, mildly impaired individuals who might otherwise
have remained in their dwellings or would have prematurely entered nursing homes (Mor et al., 2004). At the same time, they will try to keep their
current residents as long as possible even as they need higher levels of
support and their impairment profiles increasingly resemble those found
in nursing homes. They will also increasingly encroach on the nursing
home market by capturing more of their population of highly impaired
older consumers.

Assisted living residences focusing on both of these markets will necessarily target private-pay consumers and thus will mostly exclude low-income seniors because states will allow only a modest number of residents to be subsidized through Medicaid waiver or similar programs. These financial barriers will result in a significant share of impaired low-income seniors in the country occupying nursing homes because they will have no affordable alternatives. Thus, it will increasingly be elders' income status, not their functional abilities, that will dictate where they live. The sorting out of elderly consumers in this way will inevitably result in growing inequalities in the quality of life and care experienced by rich and poor older persons.

The targeting of older persons at both ends of the care need spectrum by assisted living providers will result in the growth of properties providing multiple levels of care. These will increasingly be available within campus-based retirement communities, many of which, however, will offer more flexible monthly contracts without charging up-front entry fees. Ownership options will also increase as a means to reach those older persons who feel more comfortable in this tenure status. The independent living portions of these retirement communities will begin to look more like the assisted living sections of today, because the residents will be older and more impaired before they move into these communities, having clung to their homes in the community as long as possible. If this predicted trend comes to pass, tomorrow's retirement communities will diverge significantly from the status quo. The net result will be retirement communities in which a higher share of older persons will occupy assisted living apartments, and this population will be more likely to resemble the very impaired seniors who now occupy our nursing homes.

The major regulatory difference will be that states will grant assisted living residences more flexibility in admitting and retaining older persons who need higher-acuity care. Most other regulatory changes will consist of modest fixes, not wholesale differences between the present and the future.

Some stakeholders may be reluctant to embrace these trends and may even consider them irresponsible. They will argue that it is unrealistic to expect that less-regulated settings, such as assisted living, can be depended on to offer the quality of care demanded by older persons with higher-acuity needs. Moreover, they will cynically argue that a tipping point is often reached at which an assisted living residence begins to assume all the physical and organizational trappings of a traditional nursing home when it begins to care for a larger number of older persons with serious impairments and chronic health problems. More skilled nurses are needed, more sophisticated, hospital-like equipment is brought in, more restrictions are established, and the overall ambience changes. The net result, these critics will argue, is that the so-called social model practiced by the assisted living residence will look increasingly like the medical model practiced in the conventional nursing home.

Scenario 2: Culture Change Mostly Takes Hold

In the second scenario, it will be impossible to conceive of nursing homes as some monolithic category, and indeed at least three distinctive prototypes will emerge, the second of which may be so similar in look and functioning to today's assisted living residences that it may not even be given the nursing home label.

Nursing homes in the first group will be outgrowths of what is now an emerging trend, the transformation of these institutions into postacute or subacute centers. Nursing homes of this type will predominantly serve patients recovering from strokes, accidents, or surgery who need intensive therapy services or those who are medically unstable but not acutely ill. Their occupants will have relatively short lengths of stay, except possibly for those with medically complex, chronic conditions, such as the requirement of a ventilator or a feeding tube.

Nursing homes in the second category will morph into assisted living residences, adopt the person-centered principles now associated with today's emerging culture change, and serve predominantly private-pay seniors. Indeed, they will in all likelihood cease to be known as nursing homes. Rather, they will probably be considered assisted living residences because the majority of states will have designated a "nursing home–like" assisted living legislative category whereby properties can serve more impaired seniors needing high-acuity care. The nursing homes of the future that do not adopt this more person-directed model of care will lose their private-pay consumer market and many will be forced to close. We are already seeing signs of this trend in New York state, among other places, where the governor has allowed nursing homes to decertify their unused beds and permitted them to function as assisted living centers.

A third group of nursing homes will continue to function largely unchanged from today's institutional prototype and its medical model of care. These will predominantly accommodate lower-income seniors and other special needs populations occupying Medicaid-subsidized beds. Because of the poverty and lack of influence of their residents, these homes will operate under separate agreements within Medicaid guidelines, providing a very basic level of care and support. Because their minimalist budgets will not permit implementation of best practices in culture change, these homes will continue to be at risk of offering poor quality living environments and care.

Scenario 3: Affordable Assisted Living Hybrids

The most radical scenario may be more hopeful than realistic, but it envisions widespread emergence of assisted living settings that provide options of both high-acuity care *and* enriched independent living. It draws on the arguments made by many advocates that even the most impaired group of older persons can be accommodated in assisted living residences that adhere to a social model of care. It is further buttressed by research showing that nursing home–eligible low-income or Medicaid-qualified older persons can be accommodated less expensively in these person-centered settings (Jenkens, Carder, & Maher, 2004).

With the large growth of the boomer population—a significant share of whom will be poor—this scenario predicts that the federal government will be pressured to increase funding options for assisted living, as the preferred long-term care setting for high-acuity care and as a lower-cost alternative to nursing homes. Currently, only about 12 percent of assisted living units are subsidized under the Medicaid program, often through their states' Medicaid waiver program and, to a lesser extent, under their state plan's personal care services (Mollica & Johnson-Lamarche, 2005). Thus, this future scenario envisions a large expansion of assisted living units accessible to poor seniors and at the same time the demise of most nursing homes now accommodating low-income seniors subsidized by Medicaid. This might be accomplished through such things as tax incentives to develop more affordable projects, capping the number of Medicaid-eligible residents who can be served in any one residence, thus forcing the provider to market to a wider community, and requiring family participation in the monthly payment. The Medicaid program—or some new federal program—will also be expanded to make it possible for some share of NORCs, DOUERs, cohousing, and rent-assisted government rental options to accommodate older persons who need affordable long-term care. These will compete with assisted living centers for low-income seniors who need "light" nursing care or enriched independent living.

Two potentially large obstacles may stand in the way of any scenario that predicts the expansion of government financing of long-term care for poor people. First, there is the fear that Medicaid coverage for assisted living will bring millions of people "out of the woodwork" of self-pay onto the public dole. Many critics would argue that policies that support such a program are fiscally irresponsible and will bankrupt the nation. Second, the prospect of widely available affordable assisted living is objectionable to many who believe that Medicaid should function as a safety net to be used only as a last resort, not as an entitlement program that could irresponsibly be used by higher-income seniors who "make themselves poor" to avoid responsibility to pay for their own long-term care (Moses, 2004).

Conclusions and Implications for the Future

Our examination of the future of long-term care has revolved around some key issues: first, culture change and the emerging dominance of person-centered principles in the construction and operation of long-term care residential options; second, the capacity of assisted living residences that adopt person-centered principles to serve the seniors with highest acuity needs; and, third, the expansion of affordable assisted living opportunities that give people the option to be served in the setting that is most appropriate for their needs, regardless of their ability to pay. The future will depend on how our society and its major stakeholders grapple with the desirability of these changes and the complex challenges of implementing them.

APPENDIX 1. THE EDEN ALTERNATIVE

The Eden Alternative was created in 1991 by Dr. William H. Thomas and wife, Judy Meyers Thomas, along with the administrative team at Chase Memorial Nursing Home in upstate New York. Administrators from more than 300 nursing homes have been trained to operate the principles of its fundamental mission. This model aims to combat what its originators identified as the three plagues accounting for most of the suffering among the nursing home population: loneliness, helplessness, and boredom. To address these ills, the Eden Alternative encouraged bringing in pets and involving children more frequently in everyday activities at facilities, introducing plants into facilities, and making vegetable gardens that could be tended to by the residents. But Eden's mission was much broader: to deinstitutionalize nursing home culture. The most important aspects of its organizational philosophy included the following (National Center on Accessibility, 2003; Beverly Enterprises, 2000; Thomas, 1996):

- Achieve a strong sense of community and connectedness among all participants in nursing homes, including both residents and staff.
- Provide residents with opportunities to experience variety and spontaneity in their daily life by creating an environment in which unexpected and unpredictable interactions and happenings can take place.
- Provide opportunities for meaningful activity.
- Avoid sameness among residents' rooms.
- Minimize top-down bureaucratic authority and place the maximum possible decision-making authority in the hands of the older residents or in the hands of those closest to them. Thus, staff working with older persons should be given more opportunities to make care decisions. Key to the person-centered approach is the creation of permanent nursing home teams encompassing all persons who come into contact with the residents (including housekeepers, maintenance staff, rehabilitation staff, and certified nurse assistants). Each team is responsible for a small number of residents, to replicate the informal family network. In this organizational environment, certified nursing assistants are given greater control over schedules and responsibilities.
- Treat staff more humanely; in turn, they will treat older residents more humanely.
- Give older residents more decision-making power so that they have more of a voice in their daily routine and life.
- Assume that even the frailest, most demented, and most feeble elder can achieve self-growth and self-fulfillment.

APPENDIX 2. THE PIONEER NETWORK

The Pioneer Network originated as a grassroots organization of 33 long-term care professionals who formally assembled in 1997 in Rochester, New York, helped with funding from the Daisy Marquis Jones Foundation. Members disseminated ideas through forums and conferences. Later, in 2000, this group was instrumental in establishing an umbrella organization united in efforts to "transform the culture of aging in America." Their mission was to change prevailing institutional culture in the following ways (Misiorski, 2003, p. 26):

INSTITUTION-DIRECTED CULTURE

- Staff provides standardized "treatments" based on medical diagnosis.
- Schedules and routines are designed by the institution and staff, and residents must comply.
- Work is task-oriented and staff rotates assignments. As long as staff know how to perform a task, they can perform it "on any patient" in the home.
- Decision making is centralized.
- There is a hospital environment.
- Structured activities are available when the activity director is on duty.
- There is a sense of isolation and loneliness.

RESIDENT-DIRECTED CULTURE

- Staff enters into a relationship with the elder based on individualized care needs and personal desires.
- Residents and staff design schedules that reflect their personal needs and desires.
- Work is relationship-centered, and staff has consistent assignments. Staff brings their personal knowledge of residents into the caregiving process.
- Decision making is as close to the resident as possible.
- The environment reflects the comforts of home.
- Spontaneous activities are available around the clock.
- There is a sense of community and belonging.

APPENDIX 3. THE GREEN HOUSE

The Green House was originally articulated by William Thomas as a nursing home without institutional qualities. In 2002, Mississippi Methodist Services in Tupelo, Mississippi (a rural setting), became the first organization to implement the model (Rabig et al., 2006; Thomas, 2004). Green Houses can be built on a nursing home campus, long-term care multipurpose campus, or scattered throughout a residential community. Although they can vary in size, physical design, and service configurations, they are designed to serve a high-acuity population currently found in nursing homes. In states where assisted living services are funded by adequate Medicaid reimbursements, organizations may operate Green Houses under assisted living licenses. The following aspects distinguish them:

- Purpose-built and operated residence (as opposed to an adaptation of an existing nursing home structure or organization), designed like a self-contained private home that typically accommodates 7–12 occupants.
- Overall nursing home complex typically consists of small cluster (4 or more) of these Green Houses.
- Operationalize a social as opposed to a medical model philosophy of care

and thus is largely consistent with missions of the Eden Alternative and the Pioneer Network.

- Emphasize quality-of-life outcomes identified by Kane (2001), including assurances of security and safety; promoting functional competence and physical comfort; fostering enjoyment and opportunities for meaningful activity; conveying the importance of an individual's dignity, and privacy; recognizing and valuing individuality; honoring autonomy and choice; and enhancing spiritual well-being.
- Each Green House attempts to resemble external and internal architectural style of houses in a conventional community and thus avoid architecture and symbols of the traditional nursing home:
  - Overall small in size, consisting of living room, hearth, family dining area, farm house kitchen, laundry area, and porch.
  - No long hallways
  - Residential-like, as opposed to institutional, furnishings and decorations.
  - All residents have private rooms with full bathrooms
  - Share common kitchen, eating area, living room with fireplace
  - Wireless call systems
  - No nurses' stations or medication or treatment carts
  - Innovative assistive technology
  - Bedroom with track for a ceiling lift
  - Smart house technology (e.g., unobtrusive monitoring devices)
- Each Green House has its own dedicated direct care staff.
- The core persons in this team are the "universal workers," or "Shahbazim," certified nursing assistants who work closely with their elders and are trained to support a wide range of individual needs and routines that includes the provision of personal care, implementing health care plan of a clinical support team, and habilitation resource, but also, cooking, cleaning, doing laundry and shopping. Staff is responsible to Green House administrator (guide).
- Elders have meals, receive personal care, sleep, rest, and engage in activities whenever they choose.
- Caregiving staff and elders are expected to eat, talk, and make decisions together.
- Green Houses are linked administratively to constitute a nursing facility of sufficient size to operate economically and to be organizationally efficient.
- Each Green House is served by a clinical support team (e.g., nurses, medical director, social worker, dieticians, and therapists) that would be found in a traditional nursing home. These professionals are situated in another building in the complex and visit each Green House according to a schedule determined by residents' needs and regulatory requirements.

APPENDIX 4. IDEAL PERSON-CENTERED CARE APPROACH OF ASSISTED LIVING RESIDENCES

INDIVIDUAL EXPERIENCES AND ACTIVITIES

- *Daily routines* that focus on the choices and preferences of the elders, remembering they had pasts with idiosyncratic styles of living.
- *Individualized activities* that reflect the interests, past lifestyles, and life histories of the elders.
- *Involvement of residents* in the design and operation of the home.
- *Maximal functional independence* supported as much as possible within the constraints of regulatory requirements.
- *Choices,* in terms of such options as where the residents can spend their time and enjoy different experiences, when they can eat their meals, and when and how often they are bathed.
- *Personal possessions* of the residents are everywhere.
- *Alternative, therapeutic experiences* around holistic well-being, spirituality, physical exercise, the enjoyment of animals, continued learning, and opportunities to develop.
- *Productive contributions* that reinforce a person's self-esteem are encouraged and facilitated as much as possible.
- *Dining experiences* resembling those occurring in conventional homes (such as in conventional kitchens) that go beyond the nutrition requirements and become an event to anticipate every day.
- *Aromas* of food or flowers are those that would be found in conventional residences.
- *Fun experiences* are encouraged, such as by having pets and visits by children.
- *Privacy* is maximized as much as possible in both shared or common areas and personal spaces of the building, such as bedrooms.

DESIGN OF THE PHYSICAL AND PROXIMATE NATURAL SETTINGS

- *Carefully designed spaces,* which reflect public, semi-private, and private needs. A major illustration is the breaking down of large 40–60-bed units into smaller clusters—usually called "households" or "neighborhoods," with kitchens, dining rooms, and living rooms instead of the ubiquitous multipurpose day room.
- *Buildings and spaces* are smaller scaled and thus accommodate fewer residents, but in more intimate and friendly settings.
- *Richly textured interior spaces* with different characters and styles counter one of the hallmarks of an "institutional" environment—namely, the sameness of everything, chairs, color palette, only soft and muted colors. This helps people feel they have a choice of where to spend time.

- *Orientation in space* is achieved. This means more than a few signs directing residents to the dining room. Rather, layering as many cues as possible to distinguish different sides of a building. For instance, two parallel corridors are visibly different—color, art, theme, and what is visible at the ends.
- *Nonglare and indirect lighting* should be incorporated throughout setting.
- *Institution-like paraphernalia* is eliminated or minimized, everything from the large nursing station to carts in the hallways. Medications do not have to come from a huge cart rolled down the hall by nurses, which sits in the dining room during all meals. There are systems where medications are kept in the residents' rooms, or where the cart is more like a piece of furniture and is restocked by the night shift.
- *Natural outdoor environments* that are accessible to both residents and staff and have a variety of uses.

STAFFING ENVIRONMENT
- *Staff teams* that include the elder and family in decision making and planning. Staff is well-trained, consistently assigned to promote relationships and have career ladder opportunities for growth.
- *Staff teams* respect residents' individualized needs, especially for autonomy.
- *Direct care workers,* usually referred to as CNA (certified nursing assistant) or STNA (state-tested nursing assistant) and traditionally looked down on as the least knowledgeable and capable people receive more training and assume more responsibility for supporting residents' decisions about daily routine and care.
- *Electronic charting,* which eliminates the need for a large central nursing station that usually separates staff from residents.
- *Performance is evaluated* on not only how much care is delivered, but also the extent to which staff supports these person-centered care principles.

CONNECTIONS WITH FAMILY AND COMMUNITY
- *Family and community connectedness* is nurtured such as family participation in the daily life of the home. Family members participate in joint activities with other residents and families. Residents are still considered active members of the community and are encouraged to participate in community-based events.
- *End-of-life care* is dignified and inclusive of all members of the community, celebrating life and honoring the experience of grief.

REFERENCES

American Association of Retired Persons. 2005. *Reimagining America.* Washington, DC: American Association of Retired Persons.

Alecxi, L. 2006. *Nursing home use by "oldest old" sharply declines.* Washington, DC: Lewin Group.

Allen, K. 2005. *Long term care financing: Growing demand and cost of services are straining federal and state budgets: Testimony before the Subcommittee on Health, Committee on Energy and Commerce, House of Representatives.* Washington, DC: Government Printing Office.

American Health Care Association. 2001. *Facts and trends: The nursing facility sourcebook.* Washington, DC: American Health Care Association.

Assisted Living Workgroup Steering Committee. 2003. *Assuring quality in assisted living: Guidelines for federal and state policy, state regulations, and operations: A report to the U.S. Special Committee on Aging from the Assisted Living Group.* Washington, DC: American Association of Homes and Services for the Aging.

Bergman-Evans, B. 2004. Beyond the basics: Effects of the Eden Alternative model on quality of life issues. *Journal of Gerontological Nursing 30* (6), 27–34.

Beverly Enterprises. 2000. *The human side of the enterprise.* Pasadena, CA: Beverly Foundation.

Bishop, C. E. 1999. Where are the missing elders? The decline in nursing home use, 1985 and 1995. *Health Affairs 18* (4), 146–55.

Coleman, M. T., Looney, S., O'Brien, J., Ziegler, C., Pastorino, C. A., & Turner, C. 2002. The Eden Alternative: Findings after 1 year of implementation. *Journal of Gerontology: Medical Sciences 57* (7), M422–427.

Decker, F. H. 2005. *Nursing homes, 1977–99: What has changed, what has not?* Hyattsville, MD: National Center for Health Statistics.

Durrett, C. 2005. *Senior cohousing: A community approach to independent living.* Berkeley, CA: Habitat Press.

Golant, S. M. 2002. Deciding where to live: The emerging residential settlement patterns of retired Americans. *Generations 26* (11), 66–73.

Golant, S. M. 2004. Do impaired older persons with health care needs occupy U.S. assisted living facilities? *Journal of Gerontology: Social Sciences 59* (2), S68–79.

Guay, D. R. 2001. Pet-assisted therapy in the nursing home setting: Potential for zoonosis. *American Journal of Infection Control 29* (3), 178–86.

Hamilton, N., & Tesh, A. S. 2002. The North Carolina Eden Coalition: Facilitating environmental transformation. *Journal of Gerontological Nursing 28* (3), 35–40.

Harrington, C., Woolhandler, S., Mullan, J., Carrillo, H., & Himmelstein, D. U. 2001. Does investor ownership of nursing homes compromise the quality of care? *American Journal of Public Health 91* (9), 1452–55.

Hawes, C., & Phillips, C. D. 2000. *High service or high privacy assisted living facilities, their residents and staff: Results from a national survey.* Washington, DC: U.S. Department of Health and Human Services, Office of the Assistant Secretary for Planning and Evaluation, Office of Disability, Aging, and Long-Term Care Policy.

Hunt, M., & Hunt, G. 1986. Naturally occurring retirement communities. *Journal of Housing for the Elderly 3* (3/4), 3–21.

Irving Levin Associates. 2005. *The SeniorCare Acquisition Report.* 10th ed. Norwalk, CT: Irving Levin Associates.

Jenkens, R., Carder, P. C., & Maher, L. 2004. The coming home program: Creating a state road map for affordable assisted living policy, programs, and demonstrations. *Journal of Housing for the Elderly 18* (3/4), 179–201.

Kane, R. A. 2001. Long-term care and a good quality of life: bringing them closer together. *Gerontologist 41* (3), 293–304.

Kemper, P., Komisar, H. L., & Alecxih, L. 2005. Long-term care over an uncertain future: what can current retirees expect? *Inquiry 42* (4), 335–50.

Lewis, R. 2005. SNF's need to tough it out for the first part of 2005. *Nursing homes and long-term care management 53* (3), 62–63.

Metlife Mature Market Institute. 2006. *The MetLife market survey of nursing home and home care costs.* Westport, CT: MetLife Mature Market Institute.

Misiorski, S. 2003. Pioneering culture change. *Nursing Homes and Long-term Care Management 52* (10), 25–26.

Mollica, R. L., & Johnson-Lamarche, H. 2005. *State residential care and assisted living policy, 2004.* Portland, ME: National Academy for State Health Policy.

Mor, V., Zinn, J., Angelelli, J., Teno, J. M., & Miller, S. C. 2004. Driven to tiers: socioeconomic and racial disparities in the quality of nursing home care. *Milbank Quarterly 82* (2), 227–56.

Moses, S. A. 1995. *Long-term care public policy and the future of seniors housing.* Washington, DC: American Seniors Housing Association.

Moses, S. A. 2004. *The realist's guide to Medicaid and long-term care.* Seattle: Center for Long-Term Care Financing.

National Center on Accessibility. 2003. *The Eden Alternative: Renewing life in nursing homes.* Bloomington, IN: National Center on Accessibility.

National Citizens' Coalition for Nursing Home Reform. 2006. *The faces of neglect: Behind the closed doors of nursing homes.* Washington, DC: National Citizens' Coalition for Nursing Home Reform.

O'Brien, E. 2005. *Long-term care: Understanding Medicaid's role for the elderly and disabled.* Washington, DC: Kaiser Commission.

Rabig, J., Thomas, W., Kane, R. A., Cutler, L. J., & McAlilly, S. 2006. Radical redesign of nursing homes: Applying the Green House concept in Tupelo, Mississippi. *Gerontologist 46* (4), 533–39.

Rantz, M. J., Lanis, H,; Grando, V., Petroski, G. F., Madsen, R.W., Mehr, D. R., Conn, V., Zwygart-Staffacher, M., Scott, J., Flesner, M., Bostick, J., Porter, R., & Maas, M. 2004. Nursing home quality, cost, staffing, and staff mix. *Gerontologist 44* (1), 24–38.

Ronch, J. L. 2004. Changing institutional culture: Can we re-value the nursing home? *Journal of Gerontological Social Work 43* (1), 61–82.

Rosher, R. B., & Robinson, S. 2005. Impact of the Eden Alternative on family satisfaction. *Journal of American Medical Directors Association 6*(3), 189–93.

Spillman, B. C., Liu, L., & McGilliard, C. 2002. *Trends in residential long-term care.* Washington, DC: Urban Institute.

Spillman, B. C., & Lubitz, J. 2002. New estimates of lifetime nursing home use: have patterns of use changed? *Medical Care 40* (10), 965–75.

Thomas, B. 2002. Interview, "A nursing home alternative." *NewsHour with Jim Lehrer,* PBS, February 27.

Thomas, B. 2006. The Eden Alternative: Our 10 principles. http://www.edenalt .com/10.htm.

Thomas, W. H. 1996. *Life worth living: How someone you love can still enjoy life in a nursing home.* Acton, MA: VanderWyk & Burnam.

Thomas, W. H. 2004. *What are old people for? How elders will save the world.* Acton, MA: VanderWyk & Burnham.

Tornstam, L. 1998. Gertotranscendence: The contemplative dimension of aging. *Journal of Aging Studies 11*(2), 143–54.

Waidmann, T. A. 2003. *Estimates of the risk of long-term care: Assisted living and nursing home facilities.* Washington, DC: Urban Institute.

Wunderlich, G., & Kohler, P. (Eds.). 2001. *Improving the quality of long-term care.* Washington, DC: Institute of Medicine.

Zimmerman, S., Gruber-Baldini, A. L., Sloane, P. D., Eckert, J. K., Hebel, J. R., Morgan, L. A., et al. 2003. Assisted living and nursing homes: Apples and oranges. *Gerontologist 43* (special issue 2), 107–117.

Zimmerman, S., Sloane, P. D., Eckert, J. K., Gruber-Baldini, A. L., Morgan, L. A., Hebel, J. R., et al. 2005a. How good is assisted living? Findings and implications from an outcomes study. *Journal of Gerontology: Social Sciences 60* (4), S195–204.

Zimmerman, S., Sloane, P. D., Heck, E., Maslow, K., & Schulz, R. 2005b. Introduction: dementia care and quality of life in assisted living and nursing homes. *Gerontologist 45* (special issue 1), 5–7.

CHAPTER 4

The Measurement and Importance of Quality

A Collaborative Effort for Tomorrow's Assisted Living

SHERYL ZIMMERMAN, PH.D.
PHILIP D. SLOANE, M.D., M.P.H.
SUSAN K. FLETCHER, M.S.W.

Judgments about the quality of assisted living may be the single most important factor influencing how the field unfolds over the next decade. By design or default, these judgments will be based on how assisted living is defined and measured. Thus, measuring quality is not a passive exercise but, by its very questions and answers, influences what is considered important. Take nursing home care, for example, in which quality measures focus on chronic and acute illness, reflecting the fact that nursing home care has long been provided in accordance with a medical model of care. With new appreciation of the need to provide care for nursing home *residents* as opposed to treat their *illnesses,* however, critics now argue that such measures are too limited and do not include the more comprehensive components of quality of life that are central to well-being (Kane, 2003). Their concern is that by not focusing attention on domains such as enjoyment, privacy, and meaningful activities, the measures being used to determine "good" nursing home care do not reflect what is now understood to be most important to the recipients of that care. In this way, medically based criteria for measuring and regulating the quality of nursing home care not only are driving care but also may be hindering efforts to change the culture of care.

In reference to assisted living, there is as yet no widespread agreement about what constitutes quality or how it should be measured. There is, however, a valuable lesson to be learned from nursing home care: that quality is defined in accordance with underlying values, and so the criteria used to measure quality should reflect those values. That is, if the assessment of quality is to have a meaningful, positive impact on the future of assisted living, the measures employed must reflect the very substance of assisted living care. Assisted living is meant to provide room, meals, and supportive services in a way that promotes dignity, independence, privacy, autonomy, and decision making (Assisted Living Quality Coalition, 1998). Reduced to its essence, the overriding philosophy of care in assisted living is social, as opposed to medical, highlighting why measures of quality in assisted living must differ from traditional measures of nursing home quality. If quality in assisted living is measured in the same terms as quality in nursing homes, assisted living communities will come to look and feel like nursing homes. This is surely not intended to be the future of assisted living.

The critical questions, then, are *what* to measure to assess quality in assisted living and *how* best to do so. This chapter highlights key considerations in defining appropriate criteria for quality in assisted living and examines some of the challenges in measuring quality as well as implications for its future assessment.

The "What" to Measure in Quality Assessment

As will become evident, determining what to measure in quality assessment, and how to measure it, are far from straightforward and not without controversy. Fortunately, there is strong consensus that optimizing resident well-being is the outcome toward which to strive. Outcomes, of course, do not occur in a vacuum; they are conditional on the structure and process of care, as well as the care recipient's individual capacities and values. Quality of care is reflected in the relationships among the setting's capacity to provide care—structure—the manner in which care is delivered—process—and the changes in an individual that can be attributed to the provision of health care—outcomes (Donabedian, 1966). In this model, the structure of care and the processes of caregiving should be designed to optimize outcomes. This is the essence of quality care.

Figure 4.1 presents a framework to guide the comprehensive assessment of quality. It recognizes that regulatory and community factors influence the structure and process of care within assisted living and that these components of care and resident factors interact to produce outcomes. For example, in the assisted living setting an outcome such as "mobility" is the result of how federal and state regulations work to structure the local environment of care, the number and types of the residents' relationships with community volunteers and assisted living staff, and the factors unique to the residents themselves. Thus, regulation may dictate when an individual's level of impairment has progressed to the point that he or she will no longer be permitted to reside in an assisted living setting; the availability of caregivers will increase or decrease the individual's opportunities for social outings; and his or her unique genetic makeup, health habits, and recent or past experiences (e.g., trauma, injury, or obesity that resulted in osteoarthritis) all play a role in determining the outcome called "mobility." The assessment of quality must take into account these many determinants of resident outcomes. Although Figure 4.1 presents only a few examples in each area, these should be sufficient to illustrate the importance of each domain as it relates to the understanding of quality.

Regulatory Factors

In assessing the quality of assisted living, consideration must be given to the regulatory guidelines that set parameters for care. State regulations dictate such matters as admission and retention policies, licensure and training requirements, and reimbursement. For example, many states prohibit persons who need skilled nursing home care from becoming or remaining residents in assisted living, although only a few (e.g., North Carolina and Illinois) prohibit individuals who meet minimum criteria for nursing home level of care from living in assisted living (Mollica & Johnson-Lamarche, 2005). Of course, the intent of these regulations is one related to quality: to ensure that assisted living communities can meet resident needs.

Thus, quality might be considered in terms of compliance with regulatory requirements. This strategy is in large part how nursing home quality

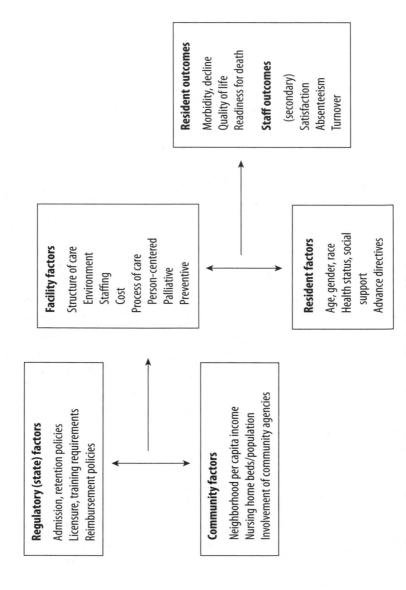

Regulatory (state) factors

Admission, retention policies
Licensure, training requirements
Reimbursement policies

Community factors

Neighborhood per capita income
Nursing home beds/population
Involvement of community agencies

Facility factors

Structure of care
Environment
Staffing
Cost
Process of care
Person-centered
Palliative
Preventive

Resident factors

Age, gender, race
Health status, social
support
Advance directives

Resident outcomes

Morbidity, decline
Quality of life
Readiness for death

Staff outcomes

(secondary)
Satisfaction
Absenteeism
Turnover

Figure 4.1. Framework for assessing quality in assisted living

is determined, but it has limited value because it sets a low standard for quality: the minimum level of care that will be considered acceptable. Another reason that regulatory compliance should not constitute the ultimate indicator of quality is that there is evidence that many of the components of care that are typically regulated do not relate to resident outcomes or do so only inconsistently and to a limited extent (Zimmerman et al., 2005).

Community Factors

Regulations are influenced by and also exert an influence on community factors. In the context of Medicaid reimbursement, for example, the very availability of assisted living beds relates to the number of nursing home beds, because both draw on the same resources. Other community factors that relate to care include what supportive resources are available locally. Such resources might include a community college that has a gerontology curriculum and brings additional expertise to residents' care, churches and civic organizations that provide social support for residents, home health care agencies that can deliver therapeutic care, and hospice for residents approaching the end of their lives.

Facility Factors: Structure and Process of Care

Both regulatory and community factors influence the structure and the process of care in assisted living. Within the category of facility factors, there are an almost unlimited number of potential determinants of quality that might be measured. For example, the structure of care can include numerous environmental indicators (e.g., home-likeness, lighting, cleanliness), staffing (e.g., experience, training, staff-to-resident ratio), and cost (e.g., whether there are multiple rate levels, whether a unit is purchased versus rented, whether the capital is surrendered when the resident dies). The process of care is similarly multifaceted and can include such components as the extent and type of person-centered, palliative, and preventive care that is available. Of course, a given assisted living setting may or may not evidence any or all of these processes of care (or others), depending on its specific mission and the values it embodies.

The structure and process of care presumably reflect the underlying values and goals of assisted living, which should be reflected in quality assessment. The efforts of two workgroups have elucidated these values

TABLE 4.1
The Goals of Assisted Living

1. Offer personalized, cost-effective, high-quality supportive services in a safe residential environment.
2. Maximize the independence of each resident.
3. Treat each resident with dignity and respect.
4. Promote the individuality of each resident.
5. Protect each resident's right to privacy.
6. Provide each resident the choice of services and lifestyles and the right to negotiate risk associated with that choice.
7. Involve residents and include family and friends in service planning and implementation when requested by a competent resident or when appropriate for incompetent residents.
8. Provide opportunity for residents to develop and maintain relationships in the broader community.
9. Minimize the need to move.
10. Involve residents in policy decisions affecting resident life.
11. Make full consumer disclosure before move-in.
12. Ensure that potential residents are fully informed regarding the setting's approach and capacity to serve individuals with cognitive or physical impairment.
13. Ensure that specialized programs (e.g., for residents with dementia) have a written statement of philosophy and mission reflecting how the setting can meet the specialized needs of the resident.
14. Ensure that residents can receive health services provided as they would be within their own home.
15. Ensure that assisted living, while health care-related, focuses primarily on a supportive environment designed to maintain an individual's ability to function independently for as long as possible.
16. Ensure that assisted living, with its residential emphasis, avoids the visual and procedural characteristics of an "institutional" setting.
17. Ensure that assisted living, with its focus on the customer, lends itself to personalized services emphasizing the particular needs of the individual and his or her choice of lifestyle. The watchwords should be "creativity," "variety," and "innovation."

Source: Adapted from Assisted Living Quality Coalition (1998).

and goals. The first is the Assisted Living Quality Coalition, which set forth the goals summarized in Table 4.1 (Assisted Living Quality Coalition, 1998). Table 4.1 suggests that the quality of assisted living might be assessed in reference to the extent to which supportive services are personalized and provided in a safe environment; processes of care promote independence, dignity, respect, individuality, privacy, choice, and involvement; family, friends, and the broader community are involved in care; consumers are informed about and understand the limits of care; independent function is allowed; and services are provided as they would be in a private home. These elements comprise the structure and process of care that presumably result in outcomes, such that, for example, *promoting* independent function will *result in* independent function.

One reason that the values reflected in the goals set out in Table 4.1 may be especially useful in assessing quality is that, to a certain extent, they embody an ideal; in fact, many communities that refer to themselves or are labeled as assisted living do not fully embrace these goals or the values on which they are founded (Zimmerman, Sloane & Eckert, 2001). To the extent, then, that the definition of quality in assisted living is taken to rest on these values, they may well differentiate those assisted living settings that are of a "good" quality from those of lesser quality.

The second source that can provide guidance with respect to identifying facility factors that are determinants of quality is the report of the Assisted Living Workgroup, *Assuring Quality in Assisted Living* (Assisted Living Workgroup, 2003). The workgroup, composed of 50 national organizations representing consumers, providers, advocates, professionals, and others, proposed criteria related to services and regulation, private units, and levels of care, that were intended to capture the underlying philosophy of assisted living to inform state and federal oversight as well as operations in assisted living settings. Like the goals articulated by the Assisted Living Quality Coalition, these criteria suggest concretely the "what" to measure in assessing quality in assisted living. Examples include the extent to which communities provide or coordinate oversight and services to meet individualized needs; whether they have 24-hour awake staff; and the extent to which they provide and oversee personal and supportive services, health-related services, social services, recreational activities, meals, housekeeping, laundry, and transportation. Also like the coalition, the Assisted Living Workgroup held that a critical indicator of quality in assisted living is the degree to which residents have the right to make choices and receive services in a way that promotes dignity, autonomy, independence, and quality of life as the residents themselves define it.

There are limitations, however, to relying on any one definition of assisted living, let alone one goal or one philosophical principle, to define quality care. For one, not all constituents agree on the importance of some of the proposed definitional components. Participants in the Assisted Living Workgroup, for example, could not agree whether assisted living should be defined in reference to privacy (i.e., units must or should be private) or whether communities should be defined in reference to specific levels of care. Another very important limitation is that, because these communities provide care to individuals with somewhat different needs and abilities, it may not be realistic or appropriate to hold all communities to a single set of policies and procedures; for example, policies related to resident control may not be appropriate across residents and facilities (Zimmerman et al., 2003). As discussed further below, differences in resident case mix present a significant challenge to assessing quality.

Resident Factors

Returning to Figure 4.1, resident factors interact with facility factors to determine outcomes. In fact, they are the strongest predictors of outcomes and are tremendously important for assessing the quality of assisted living. In the simplest of examples, older residents are likely to have worse outcomes than younger residents, and so assessment of the quality of care must allow for the effect of age. Similarly, resident preferences can influence both the process by which care is provided and the outcomes of care. Preferences are expressed through advance directives or living wills that specify what care the resident does or does not want to receive in different circumstances or through negotiated risk agreements that set forth the parameters of care that a resident desires.

Resident Outcomes

Attention can now turn to the final box in Figure 4.1, the indicator that should truly drive what is considered "quality" assisted living: outcomes. In assisted living, where it is uncommon for individuals to be in a position to markedly improve, outcomes most often refer to maintaining function or slowing decline. This is not to deny, however, that individuals may experience an increase in social involvement, positive affect, quality of life, nutrition, and other outcomes after moving into an assisted living community. As noted previously, outcomes are what should guide decisions about what to measure in the quest for quality, what services to provide, and (if necessary) what regulations to implement. Regulations, community factors, and facility factors are important to the extent that they influence resident outcomes (taking resident factors into consideration).

As was true regarding the structure and process of care, an almost limitless number of outcomes can be measured. Nursing homes, as a regulated industry, have been required to develop standardized outcome indicators, and because assisted living serves residents with similar health conditions, including cognitive impairment (Golant, 2004; Sloane, Zimmerman & Ory, 2001), many of the same outcomes may be relevant. The outcomes that have been used to assess the quality of nursing home care include worsening function, infection, inadequate pain management, pressure ulcers, daily use of physical restraints, and failure to improve and manage delirium (Fitzgerald, Shiverick, & Zimmerman, 1996). Certainly, "quality" assisted living should at least seek to avoid these negative outcomes and the care practices associated with them.

As noted previously, however, relying uncritically on nursing home quality measures carries the risk of blurring the distinction between the two care settings. Also as noted earlier, the philosophy of care in assisted living is not focused on medical status, and so more comprehensive measures of quality of life are needed when considering outcomes in the context of assisted living. There are many such measures available for this purpose, some of which assess discrete domains (e.g., depression) and some of which assess quality of life overall. Table 4.2 provides a sample of the types of measures that are available, with citations to facilitate their access. (Comprehensive lists of quality of life measures can be found in texts such as Kane & Kane, 2000.)

Staff Outcomes

Finally, the long-term care field has recently come to appreciate the importance of staff well-being as a factor in quality of care. Staff turnover, for example, can lead to poorer resident function and increased risk of resident infection and hospitalization (Spector, 1991; Zimmerman et al., 2002). The exact mechanisms through which staffing affects outcomes is unknown, but it has been suggested that turnover impedes training and supervision and reduces the familiarity between staff and residents that is integral to assessing key resident needs and detecting new events and change in resident status (Anderson et al., 1998).

The Challenge of Measuring Quality

Understanding the concept of quality and defining what should count as indicators of it in assisted living is only the first step toward actually assessing quality. The next matter is to address issues relating to how to

TABLE 4.2
Sample Measures to Assess Assisted Living Resident Outcomes

Discrete Domains of Quality of Life	Reference
Activities of Daily Living:	
Minimum Data Set Activity of Daily Living Scale (MDS-ADL)	Morris et al. (1999)
Behavior:	
Cohen-Mansfield Agitation Inventory (CMAI)	Cohen-Mansfield (1986)
Cognition:	
Mini-Mental State Exam (MMSE)	Folstein et al. (1975)
Minimum Data Set Cognition Scale (MDS-COGS)	Hartmaier et al. (1994)
Depression/Affect:	
Center for Epidemiological Studies Depression Scale (CES-D)	Radloff (1977)
Cornell Scale for Depression in Dementia (CSD-D)	Alexopoulos (1988)
Geriatric Depression Scale (GDS)	Yesavage & Brink (1983)
Older Adult Health and Mood Questionnaire (OAHMQ)	Kemp & Adams (1995)
Philadelphia Geriatric Center Affect Rating Scale (PGC-ARS)	Lawton et al. (1996)
End of Life:	
Quality of Death in Long-term Care (QOD-LTC)	Munn et al. (2007)
Life Satisfaction:	
Life Satisfaction Index (LSI-A)	Neugarten et al. (1961)
Social Function:	
Assisted Living Social Activitiy Scale (AL-SAS)	Zimmerman et al. (2003)
Resident and Staff Observation Checklist (RSOC-QOL)	Zimmerman et al. (2001)
Spiritual Well-being:	
Spiritual Experience Scale	Genia (1991)
Spiritual Well-being Scale	Ellison (1983)
Aggregate Quality of Life:	
Alzheimer's Disease Related Quality of Life (ADRQL)	Rabins et al. (2000)
Dementia Care Mapping (DCM)	Bradford Dementia Group (1997)
Dementia Quality of Life (DQoL)	Brod et al. (1999)
Quality of Life in Alzheimer's Disease (QOL-AD)	Logsdon et al. (2000)
Quality of Life in Dementia (QOL-D)	Albert et al. (1996)
Quality of Life Index (QLI)	Ferrans & Powers (1992)
Quality of Life in Nursing Homes	Kane et al. (2003)

measure quality in practice. This is not a simple matter, however, because it raises broad concerns about the place of quality assessment in assisted living and technical questions about measurement itself.

Determining the Limits of Quality Assessment

Positing quality of life as an outcome against which the quality of care in assisted living should be determined raises an important consideration: in light of the myriad factors that define quality of life for any individual, to what extent should the structure and processes of care in assisted living be held accountable for an individual's quality of life? This question might be approached in reference to the scope of human needs. Abraham Maslow (1954) outlined a hierarchy of needs ranging from (1) the most basic physical needs (such as for food, water, rest) to needs for (2) security and safety, (3) social belonging and inclusion, (4) self-esteem, recognition, autonomy, and respect, and (5) self-actualization (such as achieving a sense of purpose and realization of one's potential). Because assisted living is a social model of care and focuses on independence, dignity, respect, individuality, privacy, and choice, the assessment of quality should surely address Maslow's first four levels of human needs. Further, if it does not encompass more than the most basic needs, assisted living will come to suffer the stigma that accompanies nursing home care; however, the more we *require* assisted living to encompass, the more it will cost and the less available and accessible it will become. Arguably, then, achieving the "loftier" outcomes embedded in Maslow's fifth level of self-actualization constitutes an ideal state, but one that is beyond the responsibility of the average assisted living community.

Individualizing the Assessment of Quality

Once an outcome has been selected, it is time to turn attention to measurement. Different measures may be needed to assess the same outcome for different types of residents. Also, many measures, such as those assessing affect and cognition, have an educational and cultural bias; depression, for example, presents differently in different cultures. Further, residents who are developmentally disabled, mentally ill, or cognitively impaired may present a similar problem—such as depression—differently (Rogler, 1999). Similarly, what constitutes appropriate care may differ for different individuals; in the case of depression, this care may range from psychotherapy to medication to electroconvulsive therapy. Thus, selecting the optimal measures and determining how the resulting information should be used are not always evident.

Recognizing Differences across Facilities

Resident case mix is a reflection of the assisted living community that has implications for quality assessment. Consider the information shown in Table 4.3. These data are derived from the Collaborative Studies of Long-

TABLE 4.3

Mean Resident Impairment by Type of Assisted Living

(*N*=2,078 residents)

Impairment	Community Type		
	<16 beds	Traditional	New Model
Functional	6.1	3.0[a]	4.7[b]
Cognitive	3.2	2.1[a]	2.8[b]
Behavioral	17.5	16.6	17.0

Note: Function measured with the Minimum Data Set Activity of Daily Living Scale (Morris). Cognition measured with the Minimum Data Set Cognition Scale (Hartmaier). Behavior measured with the Cohen-Mansfield Agitation Inventory (Cohen-Mansfield). Higher scores indicate more impairment.

[a]$p<0.001$ compared to communities with <16 beds.

[b]$p<0.05$ compared to traditional communities.

Term Care (CS-LTC), a program of research into the quality of care and quality of life of residents across hundreds of assisted living communities. To ensure representation of the broad expanse of assisted living, the CS-LTC created a typology to sample facilities: smaller facilities (less than 16 beds), traditional (board-and-care style) facilities, and "new-model" facilities (Zimmerman et al., 2001). Table 4.3 shows that traditional assisted living serves a less functionally and cognitively impaired resident population than either smaller facilities or new-model facilities. Hence, their residents would be expected to be better able to achieve independence and to exercise control over care and other decisions than residents in the other types of facilities and also to have better relative outcomes. Conversely, residents in smaller facilities are less likely to be able to exercise the same degree of autonomy and control and more likely to evidence worse outcomes (regardless of the quality of care), by virtue of being more functionally and cognitively impaired. Resident case mix also relates to the structure and process of care and outcomes on a broader level. For example, facilities that serve a more Medicaid-reimbursed population tend to have a poorer environmental quality and provide less privacy, whereas those that treat more residents with cognitive and behavioral problems provide more nursing care (Park et al., 2006). For these reasons, differences in resident case mix are important to consider when assessing quality.

There is a second issue related to differences across facilities: the actual instruments that are used to measure quality. Of note, many of the measures often used to assess the structure and process of care have an institutional bias, in that that they favor larger, more complex communities. Consider the information in Figure 4.2, which illustrates components of resident control and policy choice, by facility type. Although these components do not exhaust the range of items measured, they indicate a definite bias in favor of traditional and new-model facilities. For example, traditional and new-model facilities are more likely to have a resident council and resident committees than are smaller facilities. In fact, a summary measure of control and choice using the Policy and Program Information Form of the Multiphasic Environmental Assessment Procedure (MEAP; Moos & Lemke, 1996) demonstrated the superiority of traditional and new-model facilities over small facilities (Morgan, Eckert, Gruber-Baldini & Zimmerman, 2004). On another measure developed from the MEAP relating to the flexibility of admission policies, however, traditional facilities scored lower than new-model facilities in their willingness to accept residents (Zimmerman, Eckert & Wildfire, 2001).

Thus, the assessment of quality in tomorrow's assisted living must include measures that are appropriate to all facility types, or at least are sensitive to the differences among them. For example, if resident input into decisions about the community is the outcome of interest, it must be

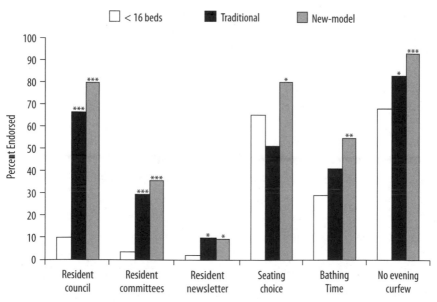

Figure 4.2. Resident control and policy choice, selected examples of difference, by type of assisted living (*N* = 193 communities). *p < 0.05 compared to communities with <16 beds; **p < 0.01 compared to communities with <16 beds; ***p < 0.001 compared to communities with <16 beds. *Source:* Measured with items from the Policy and Program Information Form of the Multiphasic Environment Assessment Procedure (MEAP; Moos & Lemke, 1996)

measured not just in terms of whether there is a formal resident council (an indicator appropriate to new-model facilities) but also in a way that can capture the extent to which residents participate in decision making in small communities that lack formal mechanisms for resident input.

Recognizing the Perspective of the Assessor

A fourth consideration relates to the vantage point of whoever is conducting the evaluation. This is an important matter for two reasons. First, different raters may value different things, such as a daughter who wants her mother to live in a hotel-type setting while the mother prefers something more homelike. Second, even when they agree on the focus of assessment, there is often disagreement about its rating—as a case in point, there is little to no agreement between resident and care provider ratings regarding quality of life (Sloane et al., 2005). Different ratings should not be taken to imply that one rater is right and the other wrong; rather, each is assessing the feature somewhat differently from the other. Recognizing this, and in light of the notable proportion of residents who have cognitive impairment, it is advisable to include ratings from others when assessing quality. Whenever possible, however, assessment should always include the resident's perspective.

Weighing Sensitivity and Significance

The measurement of quality is further complicated by the metric used. A gross scale that allows an assessor to rate quality of life only as "bad" or "good" is unlikely to show change. In contrast, a 10-point scale, with anchors of 0 representing bad and 10 representing good, *is* likely to show change, in part because there are more options but also because random error is more likely when choosing between any two points on this more discrete scale. Thus, the former scale is insensitive to small change, whereas the latter is overly sensitive to change, and to error. Any change seen on the former scale is likely to be meaningful, whereas change from one point to another on the latter may not indicate a true difference. The solution is to use established scales with known ability to discriminate important differences.

Appreciating the Complexity of Quality Assessment

As the foregoing has shown, measuring quality in tomorrow's assisted living should consider factors ranging from regulation to resident outcomes. Appropriate measures must be selected with an understanding of the philosophy and variability of assisted living, the challenges of quality measurement, and how these measurement issues can and will affect the resultant findings and recommendations. Beyond the challenges of identifying appropriate measures, further challenges arise when quality assessment must take into account multiple influential factors in the complex world of caregiving and those encountered when putting the findings of quality assessment into practice.

The Multifactorial Nature of Quality

One of these further challenges is the complexity of determining quality when there are multiple factors potentially influencing any one outcome and when the same factor can influence different outcomes in different ways. Figure 4.3 illustrates some of these complex relationships.

A Single Component of Care Might Have Both Bad and
Good Care Correlates

A multitude of structure and process components of care could rightfully be included in quality assessment. The structure of care could assess room type and size, toilet access, the availability and attractiveness of outdoor space, or the number of amenities, for example. The process could refer to care planning, service provision, whether or not there is a resident council, the degree of resident autonomy, and the like. In Figure 4.3, three components of care have been selected for illustration: facility size, the provision of informal activities, and the number of safety features that are available. Panel A1 illustrates the relationship between facility size and informal activities and shows that as facility size increases, the number of informal activities decreases. A proponent of informal activities would favor a smaller community. Panel A2, however, shows that, as facility size increases, so too does ability to provide more safety features—call bells, perhaps. A proponent of safety would favor a larger community.

A Single Component of Care Might Relate to Both Bad and Good Outcomes

Of course, whether a certain component of the structure or process of care is important depends on how it relates to resident well-being, so it is necessary to bring resident outcomes into the picture. Once again, there are many from which to choose, and unfortunately, optimizing one outcome might require that another, also important state of being, be downplayed or ignored—for example, autonomy versus safety, social involve-

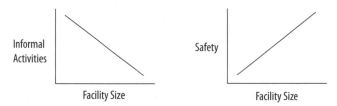

A1-2. **One Component of Care Might Have Both Bad and Good Care Correlates.**
Relationship between one facility characteristic (size) and two other facility characteristics.

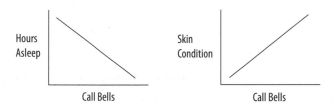

B1-2. **One Component of Care Might Relate to Both Bad and Good Outcomes.**
Relationship between one facility characteristic (bells) and two different resident outcomes.

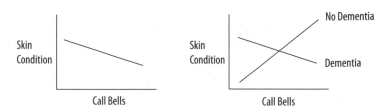

C1-2. **One Component of Care Might Act Differently for Different Residents.**
Relationship between one facility characteristic (bells) and one resident outcome, for residents without dementia (B2), with dementia (C1), and displayed together (C2).

Figure 4.3. Relationships among the structure, process, and outcomes of care

ment versus privacy, or services versus cost. These types of tradeoff are reflected in negotiated risk agreements between residents and providers, which expressly state that the resident chooses to accept certain risks associated with care in order to maximize preferences (e.g., the choice not to adhere to dietary restrictions in favor of following a preferred diet). There is some concern that allowing such choice might lower the standard of care and absolve communities from responsibility for bad outcomes (National Senior Citizens Law Center, 2000). Thus, even the matter of allowing residents to choose outcomes based on personal values is not without controversy.

Panels B1 and B2 relate two resident outcomes—sleep and skin condition—to one component of care: call bells. As panel B1 indicates, if call bell use is high at night, resident sleep could well be disrupted; however, as panel B2 indicates, if the call bells are being used to obtain help with toileting during the night, having call bells available at night might help improve skin condition. Thus, depending on the outcome of interest, call bells could be considered bad or good. In reality, of course, sleep and skin condition relate to many more components of care than just call bells, and so these panels could conceivably be repeated for facility temperature and staffing, among others.

A Single Component of Care Might Act Differently for Different Residents

Panels C1 and C2 take the posited relationship between call bells and skin condition a step further. If the positive relationship between call bells and skin condition holds true only for those residents who are able to use the bells when needed (e.g., residents who do not have dementia), it is conceivable that residents who are not able to use the bells (e.g., those who *do* have dementia) might actually receive less care, and might in fact develop more skin breakdown, because staff are attending more often to the residents who are ringing their call bells. That is, there could be a negative relationship between these variables, such that, as the use of call bells increases, skin condition actually worsens for residents with dementia. Panel C2 demonstrates this more complex relationship among this single component of care, this single outcome, and the resident's cognitive status. Of course, care and outcomes in assisted living can never really be reduced to components as simple as these, and so the complexity of quality assessment must by now be evident. Adding to the challenge is the fact that neither consumer need and nor care provision is stable; assessment of quality must also take into account changing need and the ability of care to respond to change over time. The measurement of quality is challenging indeed.

The Matter of Causality

There is an additional matter to consider when drawing conclusions about care related to outcomes: whether there is a causal relationship between the components under study. It is logical to assume that how satisfied assisted living residents are with the quality of their lives (an outcome) is influenced by life within the community (the structure and process of care), but one study found that it was associated with their relationship with their family members (National Investment Conference, 1998). Findings such as this, and others that use a cross-sectional design wherein care and outcomes are assessed and compared at a single point in time, make it impossible to determine cause and effect. An additional limitation of cross-sectional assessment is that, if the structure and process of care do have a causal relationship to outcomes, the outcome has typically already occurred by the time assisted living providers, regulators, and researchers tend to measure it. Thus, it is not typically the case that quality assessment provides certainty that care *caused* the outcome.

Because of these limitations, the optimal design with which to assess quality is a longitudinal study of newly admitted residents. In addition, if two treatment approaches were being compared, random assignment of residents would be necessary to be certain that it was the treatment (and not some other difference between the groups) that was the causal agent. Unfortunately, it is virtually impossible to conduct such assessments in a reasonable period of time and without an extremely and often prohibitively large number of participating assisted living communities. Thus, hopes for what can be learned in the measurement of quality in tomorrow's assisted living must be tempered by the realities of resources and time.

Quality Assessment, Quality Improvement, and the Realities of Providing Care

There are also some potentially unfounded assumptions underlying the very rationale of quality assessment. One is that outcomes are modifiable;

another is that assisted living's social model of care influences outcomes in a predictable manner. As noted earlier, these assumptions must recognize that residents' health status has the strongest relationship to outcomes of care. Other important considerations are that countless human differences characterize both the care provider and the care recipient; that residents' needs and the care they receive change over time; and that the care provided to assisted living residents consumes only a small fraction of their day (e.g., in smaller assisted living communities, where more time is devoted to actual caregiving than in any other assisted living setting, any one resident receives approximately 1.5 hours of personal care assistance per day) (Stearns & Morgan, 2001). Thus, it is almost foolhardy to expect that care can affect outcomes in predictable ways.

Two other potentially false assumptions are that providers have the knowledge and the ability to modify care once armed with the information that there is reason to do so. For example, knowing that some residents with dementia become agitated during bathing implies neither that a better technique is available nor that the organizational structure of an assisted living setting will support a suggested change in care practices. In fact, one recent randomized trial of an effort to improve the bathing experience cost millions of dollars to develop and evaluate and demonstrated the value of the new practice, but adoption of it has been incomplete (Sloane et al., 2004). Of course, quality improvement does not require that evidence for change be based on the gold standard of a randomized, controlled trial. In most cases, however, it does require a change in care practices, and, in some cases, it requires additional resources or a reallocation of existing resources. In these latter instances, it may well be necessary to consider whether the benefits of change are likely to be worth the cost. There is good reason, then, to reflect on whether findings can feasibly be implemented—or what it will take to implement them successfully—before undertaking quality assessment.

Conclusions and Implications for the Future

The foregoing discussion has pointed out only some of the more significant challenges to measuring quality in assisted living. It was not intended to be exhaustive, and many pressing concerns remain—for example, the validity of quality assessment (i.e., whether it captures what it intends to) or whether there are measures for what is considered important in assisted living. The wise policy maker, provider, or researcher will recognize the need for thorough analyses before making broad claims about quality assessment in assisted living.

One claim that can safely be made, however, is that the measurement of quality must be pragmatic, undertaken with a clear understanding of its purpose and limitations. In light of the considerations reviewed in this chapter, one strategy seems optimal: the measurement of quality should be a collaborative effort among providers, policy makers, and researchers. Neither providers nor policy makers alone can or should be expected to have the expertise to deal successfully with the myriad challenges of valid, meaningful quality assessment. Similarly, it is not to be expected that researchers can or do have their finger on the pulse of the field, or understand which issues are of most concern to the practice and policy community. This suggests a model of multidisciplinary, community-based, participatory research—in which providers, residents, and other stakeholders work with researchers to define a problem, obtain information to assess it, and use the findings to modify care—is most appropriate. The benefit of such an approach, because it is grounded in actual practice, is that it addresses concretely identified needs and is more likely to result in sustainable change in practice than other strategies (Altman, 1995).

As the measurement of the quality in assisted living proceeds in this collaborative model, it will be wise to focus on multiple components of the structure, process, and outcomes of care to understand not only the tradeoffs among, but also the consistency of, quality indicators. To the extent that nursing home measures of quality are appropriate, they should be used, or adapted; however, nursing home measures are insufficient, because they do not reflect the distinctive philosophy, structure, and caregiving processes that are central to assisted living or the quality-of-life outcomes that are the objective of care. Also, careful consideration should be given to identifying who is the best source of quality information, keeping in mind two prime considerations: that the consumer's voice be included whenever possible and that data collection not become the tail that wags the dog. In tomorrow's assisted living, the effort to collect information should be reasonable and should be monitored to ensure that it is being used to improve care.

ACKNOWLEDGMENTS

The work on this manuscript was supported by a grant from the National Institute on Aging (K02 AG00970).

REFERENCES

Albert, S. M., Del Castillo-Castaneda, C., Sano, M., Jacobs, D. M., Marder, K., Bell, K., Bylsma, F., Lafleche, G., Brandt, J., Albert, M., & Stern, Y. 1996. Quality of life in patients with Alzheimer's disease as reported by patient proxies. *Journal of the American Geriatrics Society 44,* 1342–1347.

Alexopoulos, G. S., Abrams, R. C., Young, R. C., & Shamoian, C. A. 1988. Cornell scale for depression in dementia. *Biological Psychiatry 23,* 271–284.

Altman, D. G. 1995. Sustaining interventions in community systems: on the relationship between researchers and communities. *Health Psychology 14* (6), 526–536.

Anderson, R. A., Hsieh, P. C., & Su, H. F. 1998. Resource allocation and resident outcomes in nursing homes: comparisons between the best and worst. *Research in Nursing and Health 2* (4), 297–313.

Assisted Living Quality Coalition. 1998. *Assisted living quality initiative: Building a structure that promotes quality.* Washington, DC: Public Policy Institute, American Association of Retired Persons.

Assisted Living Workgroup. 2003. *Assuring quality in assisted living: guidelines for federal and state policy, state regulation, and operations: A report to the U.S. Senate Special Committee on Aging.* Washington, DC: Government Printing Office.

Bradford Dementia Group. 1997. *Evaluating Dementia Care: The DCM Method.* 7th ed. Bradford, England: Bradford Dementia Group.

Brod, M., Stewart, A. L., Sands, L., & Walton, P. 1999. Conceptualization and measurement of quality of life in dementia: The Dementia Quality of Life instrument (DQoL). *Gerontologist 39,* 25–35.

Cohen-Mansfield, J. 1986. Agitated behaviors in the elderly. II. Preliminary results in the cognitively deteriorated. *Journal of the American Geriatrics Society 34,* 722–727.

Donabedian, A. 1966. Evaluating the quality of medical care. *Milbank Memorial Fund Quarterly 44* (3) supplement, 166–206.

Ellison, C. W. 1983. Spiritual well-being: Conceptualization and measurement. *Journal of Psychology and Theology 11* (4), 330–338.

Ferrans, C. E., & Powers, M. J. 1992. Psychometric assessment of the quality of life index. *Research in Nursing Health 15* (1), 29–38.

Fitzgerald, R. P., Shiverick, B. N., & Zimmerman, D. 1996. Applying performance measures to long-term care. *Joint Commission Journal of Quality Improvement 22* (7), 505–517.

Folstein, M. F., Folstein, S. E., & McHugh, P. R. 1975. "Mini-Mental State": A practical method for grading the cognitive state of patients for the clinician. *Journal of Psychiatric Research 12,* 189–198.

Genia, V. 1991. The Spiritual Experience Index: A measure of spiritual maturity. *Journal of Religion and Health 30* (4), 337–347.

Golant, S. M. 2004. Do impaired older persons with health care needs occupy U.S. assisted living facilities? An analysis of six national studies. *Journal of Gerontology: Social Sciences 59B,* S68–79.

Hartmaier, S., Sloane, P. D., Guess, H., & Koch, G. 1994. The MDS cognition scale: A valid instrument for identifying and staging nursing home residents with dementia using the Minimum Data Set. *Journal of the American Geriatrics Society 42,* 1173–1179.

Kane, R. L., & Kane, R. A. 2000. *Assessing older persons: Measures, meaning and practical applications.* New York: Oxford University Press.

Kane, R. A., Kling, K. C., Bershadsky, B., Kane, R. L., Giles, K., Degenholtz, H. B., Liu, J., & Cutler, L. J. 2003. Quality of life measures for nursing home residents. *Journal of Gerontology: Medical Sciences 58A,* 240–248.

Kemp, B., & Adams, B. 1995. The Older Adult Health and Mood Questionnaire: A measure of geriatric depressive disorder. *Journal of Geriatric Psychiatry and Neurology 8,* 162–167.

Lawton, M. P., Van Haitsma, K., & Klapper, J. 1996. Observed affect in nursing home residents with Alzheimer's disease. *Journal of Gerontology B: Psychological Sciences and Social Sciences 51,* P3–14.

Logsdon, R. G., Gibbons, L. E., McCurry, S. M., & Teri, L. 2000. Quality of life in Alzheimer's disease: Patient and caregiver reports. In S. M. Albert & R. G. Logsdon (Eds.), *Assessing quality of life in Alzheimer's disease* (pp. 17–30). New York: Springer.

Maslow, A. 1954. *Motivation and personality.* New York: Harper

Mollica, R., & Johnson-Lamarche, H. 2005. State residential care and assisted living policy, 2004. http://aspe.hhs.gov/daltcp/reports/04alcom.htm.

Moos, R. H., & Lemke, S. (Eds.). 1996. *Evaluating residential facilities: The Multiphasic Environmental Assessment Procedure.* Thousand Oaks, CA: Sage.

Morgan, L. A., Eckert, J. K, Gruber-Baldini, A. L., & Zimmerman, S. 2004. Policy and research issues for small assisted living facilities. *Journal of Aging and Social Policy 16,* 1–16.

Morris, J. N., Fries, B. E., & Morris, S. 1999. Scaling ADLs within the MDS. *Journal of Gerontology: Medical Sciences 54,* M546–553.

Munn, J. C., Zimmerman, S., Hanson, L., Sloane, P. D., Clipp, E. C., Tulsky, J. A., & Steinhauser, K. E. 2007. Measuring the quality of dying in long-term care. *Journal of the American Geriatrics Society 55,* 1371–1379.

National Investment Conference. 1998. *National survey of assisted living residents: who is the customer?* Annapolis, MD: National Investment Conference.

National Senior Citizens Law Center. 2000. Assisted living. www.nsclc.org/news/04/april/expect_management.htm.

Neugarten, B. L., Havighurst, R. J., & Tobin, S. S. 1961. The measurement of life satisfaction. *Journal of Gerontology 16,* 134–143.

Park, N. S., Zimmerman, S., Sloane, P. D., Gruber-Baldini, A. L., & Eckert, J. K. 2006. An empirical typology of residential care/assisted living based on a four state study. *Gerontologist 46,* 238–248.

Rabins, P. V., Kasper, J. D., Kleinman, L., Black, B. S., & Patrick, D. L. 2000. Concepts and methods in the development of the ADRQL: An instrument for assessing health-related quality of life in persons with Alzheimer's disease. In S. M. Albert & R. G. Logsdon (Eds.), *Assessing quality of life in Alzheimer's disease* (pp. 51–68). New York: Springer.

Radloff, L. S. 1977. The Center for Epidemiological Studies-Depression Scale: A self-report depression scale for research in the general population. *Applied Psychological Measurements 3,* 385–401.

Rogler, L. H. 1999. Methodological sources of cultural insensitivity in mental health research. *American Psychologist 54,* 424–433.

Sloane, P. D., Hoeffer, B., Mitchell, C. M., McKenzie, D. A., Barrick, A. L., Rader, J., Stewart, B. J., Talerico, D. A., Rasin, H. H, Zink, R. C., & Koch, G. G. 2004. Effect of person-centered showering and the towel bath on bathing-associated aggression, agitation, and discomfort in nursing home residents with dementia: a randomized, controlled trial. *Journal of American Geriatric Society 52* (11), 1795–1804.

Sloane, P. D., Zimmerman, S., & Ory, M. 2001. Care for persons with dementia. In S. Zimmerman, P. D. Sloane, & J. K. Eckert (Eds.), *Assisted living: Needs, practices and policies in residential care for the elderly* (pp. 242–270). Baltimore: Johns Hopkins University Press.

Sloane, P. D., Zimmerman, S., Williams, C. S., Reed, P. S., Gill, K. S., & Preisser, J. S. 2005. Evaluating the quality of life of long-term residents with dementia. *Gerontologist 45,* special issue 1, 37–49.

Spector, W. D., & Takada, H. A. 1991. Characteristics of nursing homes that affect resident outcomes. *Journal of Aging Health 3* (4), 427–454.

Stearns, S., & Morgan, L. A. 2001. Economics and financing. In S. Zimmerman, P. D. Sloane, & J. K. Eckert (Eds.), *Assisted living: needs, practices and policies in residential care for the elderly* (pp. 271–291). Baltimore: Johns Hopkins University Press.

Yesavage, J. A., & Brink, T. L. 1983. Development and validation of a geriatric depression screening scale: A preliminary report. *Journal of Psychiatric Research 17* (1), 37–49.

Zimmerman, S., Eckert, J. K., & Wildire, J. 2001. The process of care. In S. Zimmerman, P. D. Sloane, & J. K. Eckert (Eds.), *Assisted living: Needs, practices and policies in residential care for the elderly* (pp. 198–223). Baltimore: Johns Hopkins University Press.

Zimmerman, S., Gruber-Baldini, A. L., Hebel, J. R., Sloane, P. D., & Magaziner, J. 2002. Nursing home facility risk factors for infection and hospitalization: Importance of RN turnover, administration and social factors. *Journal of the American Geriatrics Society 50,* 1987–1995.

Zimmerman, S., Gruber-Baldini, A. L., Sloane, P. D., Eckert, J. K., Hebel, J. R. Morgan, L. A., Stearns, S. C., Wildfire, J., Magaziner, J., & Chen, C. 2003. Assisted living and nursing homes: Apples and oranges? *Gerontologist 43,* 107–117.

Zimmerman, S., Scott, A. C., Park, N. S., Hall, S. A., Wetherby, M. M., Gruber-Baldini, A. L., & Morgan, L. A. 2003. Social engagement and its relationship to service provision in residential care/assisted living. *Social Work Research 27,* 6–18.

Zimmerman, S. I., Sloane, P. D., & Eckert, J. K. 2001. The state and quality of assisted living. In L. S. Noelker & Z. Harel (Eds.), *Linking quality of long-term care and quality of life* (pp. 117–135). New York: Springer.

Zimmerman, S., Sloane, P. D., Eckert, J. K., Buie, V. C., Walsh, J., Hebel, J. R., & Koch, G. 2001. An overview of the collaborative studies of long-term care. In S. Zimmerman, P. D. Sloane, & J. K. Eckert (Eds.), *Assisted living: Needs, practices and policies in residential care for the elderly* (pp. 117–143). Baltimore: Johns Hopkins University Press.

Zimmerman, S., Sloane, P. D., Eckert, J. K., Gruber-Baldini, A. L., Morgan, L. A., Hebel, J. R., Magaziner, J., Stearns, S. C., & Chen, C. K. 2005. How good is assisted living? Findings and implications from an outcomes study. *Journal of Gerontology: Social Sciences 60B,* 195–204.

CHAPTER 5

Small Board-and-Care Homes

A Fragile Future

PAULA C. CARDER, PH.D.
LESLIE A. MORGAN, PH.D.
J. KEVIN ECKERT, PH.D.

One of the great secrets in the era of new, corporate-built assisted living properties is the presence of a large number of quiet, anonymous, small board-and-care homes that offer housing and long-term care services to older adults who require a supportive environment. These small homes care for substantial numbers of moderately to seriously impaired people at relatively low cost in neighborhoods all around the country.

In examining the future of small homes, we recognize that many terms have been used to refer to them, including "adult foster care," "family care," "rest home," "domiciliary care home," and "adult care home." More recently, with the growing popularity of assisted living, small homes have sometimes taken (or have been given) that title (Mollica, 2002). In keeping with studies during the past 10 years (Morgan, Eckert, Gruber-Baldini, & Zimmerman, 2004; Morgan, Eckert, & Lyon, 1995), we use the phrase "small board and care." More important than what they are called is understanding the essential role that these small-group residences continue to play for frail older persons.

Rationale for the Focus on Board and Care

Why a chapter on small board-and-care homes in a book about assisted living? First, these homes are a part of the dynamic "housing with services" sector, of which assisted living has become so prominent a part. As one of the diverse array of providers and models of care, the fates of small board-and-care homes are necessarily connected to the future of the sector as a whole. Second, some states have chosen to include board and care under the same regulatory umbrella as assisted living, building an even more explicit connection between the two clusters of housing/care environments. As we shall discuss below, these two broad categories share many elements, thus supporting unified regulation; at the same time, many distinguishing traits argue against common regulation. Third, although assisted living is the "new thing" in senior housing with services, it is not the only thing, nor do we expect it to fully replace long-standing models, such as board and care. Small board-and-care homes serve as a signpost of significant challenges that face the assisted living sector overall.

In this chapter, we summarize what is known (and not known) about the number of small board-and-care homes and the clients they serve; describe some challenges they share with the long-term care market overall; profile two such homes from an ongoing ethnographic study of assisted living (Mead, Eckert, Zimmerman, & Schumacher, 2005; Schumacher et al., 2005); and summarize five key challenges facing the fragile small board-and-care home sector, including competition, financial pressures, staffing concerns, regulatory pressures, and uncertainty over public financing. These challenges represent significant threats to the future of small homes in the current, shifting contexts of long-term care and, most especially, the growth of assisted living.

The Variety of Small Board-and-Care Homes

Current knowledge about the number of small board-and-care homes and the numbers and characteristics of their residents is imprecise at best. In light of the varied names by which they are known, categories under which they are regulated, constituencies they serve (elderly, developmentally disabled, and mentally ill, among others), and varying definitions used for research purposes (e.g., based on size, licensure category, client mix), estimates of the number of homes of interest vary considerably. There are few recent studies on the numbers, sizes, and resident profiles to permit us to compare small board-and-care homes to larger assisted living buildings or nursing homes.

In the early 1990s, estimates of the number of licensed board-and-care homes ranged from 31,942 nationwide occupied by 504,750 residents (Hawes, Wildfire, Lux, & Clemmer, 1993) to 34,090 homes occupied by 613,483 persons (Clark, Turek-Brezina, Chu, & Hawes, 1994). Most had a capacity for 2–10 residents. (This upper limit was sometimes an artifact of how "small" residences were defined by different studies.) In the same period, there were estimated to be an additional 28,000 unlicensed board-and-care homes in the United States (Clark et al., 1994). No studies since then have provided national estimates, but, based on anecdotal information, we contend that small homes continue to house and care for a large number of older adults nationally. For example, in the fall of 2005, there were 1,579 licensed assisted living residences in Maryland, of which 963 (61 percent) had a capacity for 5 or fewer residents, and another 463 (29 percent) were licensed for 6–16 residents (Office of Health Care Quality, 2005a).

Data are similarly limited with respect to how the characteristics of residents in small homes differ from occupants of other types of residential care. One distinction is that small board-and-care homes are more diverse in terms of their resident populations than assisted living. Thus, some small homes accommodate younger disabled people, the chronically mentally ill, and older frail adults or dementia sufferers in the same residential setting (Clark et al., 1994; Folkemer et al., 1996; Sherman & Newman, 1988), whereas others house only persons with dementia, only women, or only individuals with physical disabilities. Further, in light of the limited shared living and eating spaces of small homes, resident diversity presents added challenges to these care providers (Ball et al., 2005; Morgan et al., 1995).

In the 1990s, data from two large studies (Phillips et al., 1995; Morgan, Gruber-Baldini, & Magaziner, 2001; Zimmerman et al., 2001) indicated that compared to larger and newer assisted living properties, small board-and-care residences were likely to house older persons with more cognitive impairments, chronic health conditions, and impairments in activities of daily living who rely more on mobility devices like walkers and wheelchairs. Somewhat more recent studies have suggested that residents in small homes are more often members of minorities, especially African Americans (Howard et al., 2002); have lower educational levels (Morgan et al., 2001); and are more likely to rely on public assistance (Stearns & Morgan, 2001). Studies in Georgia (Ball et al., 2005; Quinn et al., 1999), Maryland (Morgan et al., 1995), Oregon (Kane et al., 1991), and Washington (Curtis, Kiyak, & Hedrick, 2000), confirm this picture of the frailty and limited economic resources of small board-and-care residents.

Research that compares settings by number of residents offers an interesting, but not always clear, picture of the differences between smaller and larger residences. For example, in a four-state study, small residences scored lower on topics such as environmental quality, privacy, resident choice, administrative tolerance for problematic behaviors, and services (Morgan et al., 2004). These findings do not imply that small homes are "bad." Rather, the authors note that the surveys used to collect information sometimes give credit to larger buildings that have the economies of scale to offer in-house services such as an on-site bank or adult day care. Similarly, the survey questions failed to account for the homelike and personal nature of care provided by smaller homes (Morgan et al., 2004). Analyses of the medical outcomes and functional decline of residents found that those living in smaller homes either fared the same or better when compared to residents of newer and larger assisted living residences (Zimmerman et al., 2005). These findings suggest that something other than size accounts for the quality-of-life and care differences between large and small settings.

Finally, policy and regulation governing small homes reflect their ambiguous position among new, corporate-built assisted living and numerous older categories of housing and care institutions. In the 1990s, states moved rapidly to regulate the growing assisted living sector (Mollica, 2002; Mollica & Johnson-Lamarche, 2005). An ongoing question in many states has been whether to include small board-and-care homes within the scope of newly developed assisted living regulations and whether to regulate small homes separately or to leave them either minimally regulated or even unregulated (Mollica & Johnson-Lamarche, 2005).

Board and Care versus Assisted Living: Similarities and Differences

Depending on your perspective, there is either no difference between board-and-care homes and assisted living residences, or there are almost no similarities. The crux of the problem is definitional. "Assisted living" is sometimes used to refer to only settings with apartment-style units and a social model of care that emphasizes noninstitutional architectural design and respect for consumer-oriented demands like the right to make decisions that could result in negative outcomes (Carder & Hernandez, 2004). Others define assisted living as any setting or program of personal care and housing short of a facility that is licensed to provide skilled nursing care (Kane & Wilson, 2001). Size, services provided, living environment, staffing, philosophy of care, and consumer demand delineate this admittedly gray area.

Residence Size

State regulations rely on different number (of residents or beds) thresholds to define where assisted living begins and any other category of housing with care ends (Mollica & Johnson-Lamarche, 2005). Yet in some states, "assisted living" means any residence with two or more unrelated occupants who receive supportive services. Research has also ambiguously used size to define "small board-and-care home"—e.g., 10 or fewer residents (Phillips et al., 1995) versus 16 or fewer (Zimmerman et al., 2001).

Services

The type and level of services offered in both settings are partly a product of state regulatory requirements and partly a product of organizational decisions and staff capabilities. Although some board-and-care settings offer only minimal assistance with personal care, the same can be said of some assisted living residences. Either type may provide end-of-life care, but such care is not universal in either. Thus, as with size, type and level of services is not a definitive method of distinguishing board and care from assisted living.

Living Environment

Small board-and-care homes are highly variable in appearance. Some are renovated single-family homes and may not be immediately recognizable as senior housing. Many feature shared living environments paired with either private or shared bedrooms. Others are somewhat more institutional in look and feel, but seldom do they offer apartment-style accommodations. In contrast, when most of us think of assisted living, we envision larger, corporate-built properties with an array of public and private spaces that are recognizable as congregate living environments. Public eating and social spaces are paired with apartment-style residential spaces. A small number of states require assisted living to provide a private accommodation with bathroom and kitchenette, and there is consumer preference for such units (Reinardy & Kane, 2003). Again, however, the distinctions are neither clear-cut nor consistent.

Staffing

Both board and care and assisted living rely predominantly on unlicensed personnel to provide services, including personal care, housekeeping, meals, and activities. Larger establishments require a larger staff and typically a more hierarchical and shift-based staffing structure, which may or may not include medical care providers. Few small board-and-care homes offer on-site medical services. Some states require larger assisted living residences to have licensed nurses on staff or permit licensed nurses to delegate specific tasks to unlicensed staff. If small homes are regulated as assisted living, such policies include them. Smaller homes have relatively small staffs; typically they have at least one live-in staff member— either the owner or a paid employee—and a small number of employees who work on a rotating shift basis (Zimmerman et al., 2001).

Philosophy of Care

Perhaps the most talked about aspect of housing with care is its "philosophy of care" (Kane & Wilson, 2001). Our research suggests that for small board-and-care homes as well as assisted living residences the model of care includes respect for resident privacy, choice, and independence, though the rhetoric of philosophy of care is more typical of assisted living. At least 29 states include these values when defining assisted living (Mollica & Johnson-Lamarche, 2005), though the degree to which they are actually embodied in practice remains largely unstudied. We lack clear research on the extent to which this model has penetrated across the housing-with-services sector.

Consumer Demand

Finally, consumer demand plays a different role in board and care from assisted living, reflected in differing emphasis on individual entrepreneurship and corporate development. There is no board-and-care "industry" comparable to what has been described as a consumer-driven industry of assisted living (Carder & Hernandez, 2004; Kane & Wilson, 2001), though in some states consumers have shown interest in small board-and-care homes as an alternative to nursing homes (Kane et al., 1991). In contrast, assisted living developers at both the local and national levels offer a style of shelter and care that includes private apartments, personal care assistance, electronic monitoring systems, and social activities, as well as a range of on-site amenities designed for consumer appeal.

Small homes share many of the key challenges facing the overall housing-with-services sector. First, along with other residences, small homes must compete in an ever-changing market in which new buildings open while existing ones change hands or close and the array of services, prices, and players changes constantly. Second, small board-and-care homes share the challenge of operating in a sector in which getting and keeping high-quality workers remains a widespread concern. A third common challenge is the everyday balancing act—keeping prices competitive in the face of rising costs, especially liability insurance, and balancing the demands of residents who want to maintain independent while at the same time protecting them from potential harm. Fourth, small homes are part of a growing and diverse senior housing market that remains ill defined and confusing to consumers. Finally, small board-and-care homes share with larger assisted living buildings the challenge of helping residents age in place (see chapter 2), given constraints of state regulations, staffing, and building design. For example, allowing a resident who has suffered a debilitating stroke to remain in the residence might conflict with limits placed by state regulations, the abilities of current staff to meet the resident's specific needs, or the physical characteristics of the building (e.g., handicapped accessibility).

Challenges and Benefits of Small Homes
Two Small Homes: Quasi-familial and Connected

Despite similarities, small homes differ in important ways from the larger, assisted living environments. These differences relate to the often quasi-familial, interpersonal bonds that form between caregivers and residents and the environment of interpersonal connectedness that characterize many of the small board-and-care settings we have studied. Two small residences in Maryland that have been sites for ethnographic research in assisted living (Mead et al., 2005; Morgan, Eckert, Piggee, & Frankowski, 2006; Zimmerman et al., 2001) illustrate this feature of small board-and-care homes.

These homes, which we will call Valley Glen Home and Franciscan House, have much in common: both are owned and operated by immigrant families, both occupy renovated single-family homes located in suburban neighborhoods, and both are licensed to accommodate as many as 8 residents. They both participate in Maryland's home- and community-based waiver program for Medicaid-eligible clients, and Franciscan House has occasionally taken residents subsidized by the county, who rely on the Supplemental Security Income (SSI) program. Valley Glen Home is licensed to care for individuals with the highest level of needs (e.g., physical and/or cognitive impairment) permitted under state rules, while Franciscan House is at an intermediate level.

Rani opened Valley Glen Home in 1995 after moving to the United States from Southeast Asia with her son and mother. Rani's sister, who immigrated 15 years prior, suggested the idea of operating a group home. Maria Agbuya and her husband opened Franciscan Home in 1989. Originally from the Philippines, they moved to the United States with the hope that their teenage children would get a better education and to be closer to Mr. Agbuya's sister, who suggested that operating a group home would provide a good source of income.

In both settings the majority of residents have impaired memory and/ or dementia, as well as other common chronic conditions associated with advanced age. As Rani explained, "In group homes, the kind of people who come are not the ones who can decide things for themselves. Many of them have dementia or forgetfulness to some extent." Five of the 7 residents at Valley Glen have some degree of dementia; 2 are so frail that they cannot feed themselves; all are women ranging in age from 78 to 90 years (average age, 85 years). These elderly women have lived at Valley Glen from a few weeks to 3 years, with an average of 2 years. Residents at Franciscan Home are less physically impaired, but all 7 have some level of cognitive impairment. The 6 women and one man range in age from 75 to 87 (average age, 83) and had lived at the home from 2 months to 4 years (average, 2 years). Franciscan House is a two-story house, so all but two residents, whose rooms are on the main floor, must be able to negotiate stairs.

Rani and her family live with the residents and she considers these seven older persons members of her extended family. This quasi-familial approach to operating a group home has been described as "fully integrated" and represents the most connected and personal approach to operating a group home (Eckert, Cox, & Morgan, 1999). Rani extends her welcome to family members of the residents, who are highly engaged in the life of the home and in meeting the ongoing needs of their resident kin. When asked to describe one thing that she would most want others to know about small group homes, Rani said, "We are different, mainly because we interact with the residents so much more [closely]. In time to come we feel they are a part of us. We are a big family. That's how we feel, as time goes on."

Maria, whose deep Catholic faith guides her, explained that "it's a calling . . . the principle that guides me is, what I want others to do unto me, I do unto them, basically. So I hope somebody will take care of me when I get old." Maria's philosophy of care is best described as a "nonintegrated" approach because she clearly separates her own family life from the life of the residence, living in a home several miles from Franciscan House (Eckert et al., 1999). Maria focuses on meeting health needs, a priority well served by her husband, who is the registered nurse serving her residents.

During several interviews over the course of a year, Rani and Maria each explained how they provide personalized care to very frail individuals, draw on their long experience with them to identify the needs of those who can no longer speak, coordinate various activities with residents' family members (e.g., medical appointments, purchasing clothing and other supplies, paying bills), and communicate with residents' physicians. We observed as Rani helped two new residents adjust to life in assisted living, one who bitterly resented it and another who daily asked why she was there. Maria explained her frustration in balancing regulatory demands with keeping her residents healthy and stable. Each woman described her work as difficult, yet worthwhile.

Five Challenges to Small Homes

Our experience studying these and other small homes in a total of five states (Morgan et al., 1995; Zimmerman et al., 2001) has led us to identify five major challenges facing small board-and-care homes: competition, financing, staffing, regulation, and public subsidies for housing with services.

The Competitive Challenge

With the increase in numbers of corporate-built assisted living settings, small board-and-care homes face growing competition. When consumers (often adult children) seek a care environment, their search is typically rushed, the need to move to housing with services precipitated by some specific event (Frank, 2002). In these circumstances, potential customers may be more aware of the larger settings that they see routinely as they travel through their communities than of small neighborhood homes; they may be impressed by attractive environments, offering so-called care with a chandelier.

Small board-and-care homes suffer from low visibility. For example, neither Valley Glen Home nor Franciscan House looked different in any way from neighboring houses, because they have no signs or other markers indicating that they provide housing with services. For many small board-and-care homes, which are typically located in residential neighborhoods, local zoning codes prohibit posting commercial signs or other advertising on their property. Limited budgets and time also mean they make essentially no effort to market themselves. Their capacity to attract residents may be limited to word-of-mouth, lists kept by private housing placement consultants, referrals from public agencies and hospitals, or information provided through local community venues such as churches or senior centers. Neither Rani nor Maria used glossy marketing materials like those commonly used by the newer and larger assisted living settings.

In addition, most small homes offer fewer amenities and provide a narrower range of extra services than larger, corporate-built assisted living—small homes aren't the places to look for fitness centers, organized activities, beauty salons, or on-site health clinics, for example. Comparing small board-and-care homes with newer and professionally managed assisted living settings is doubtless challenging for any consumer. People may especially be attracted to their apartment-style environments, which promise privacy and autonomy to worried kin seeking to balance safety with care for their family member. The daughter of a Valley Glen resident described one of the senior housing communities her mother lived in before moving to Valley Glen: "It kind of looks like one of the Disney hotels, you know . . . like the one on the beach in Orlando. . . . It's very pleasant. I think it is a decent facility for people who don't need much [care]."

In contrast, Valley Glen and Franciscan House are typical examples of 1970s suburban homes, with a "family-sized" living and dining room, a residential kitchen, and bedrooms of varying sizes. The unmatched furniture shows physical wear. On a typical day in Valley Glen, many residents would be found in the living room, with a television on and a staff member in attendance to monitor and address their needs for mobility, toileting, comfort, and so forth. The aesthetic surroundings, privacy, and typically broader range and flexibility of services offered in larger environments may win the competition, at least for an older person's first move from home to senior housing. As the daughter above subsequently explained, however, three larger assisted living residences could not accommodate her mother's declining cognitive ability. It was only at Valley Glen that she found the housing and care combination that best suited her mother's needs.

Issues of resident retention and aging in place are also part of the competitive challenge for small homes. For larger residences that have waiting lists, there is relatively little lost revenue when residents with growing dependency relocate to a dementia unit or nursing home. For small residences, however, the loss of one resident can have significant social and financial impact. For a small board-and-care home, filling a vacancy requires effort and means lost income until a new resident is located. Although our research has not revealed cases of inappropriate care, the greater impact of losing one resident, as well as the strong interpersonal connections in small homes, could create pressure to keep residents in place even when they need more care than the homes are licensed to provide or their staffs are able to render. Small homes may also feel pressured to admit residents with behavioral problems or high care needs to fill vacancies. As summarized above, we know that small homes care for a more impaired population; whether this reflects lengthier aging in place, acceptance/retention of more impaired residents, or some combination of both is not clear.

Although some critics worry that small homes lack the capacity to care for individuals with complex needs, some states grant case-based waivers to operators who demonstrate ability to provide a higher level of care to specific individuals. This option may allow a resident with special needs to delay or avoid institutionalization and at the same time permits greater oversight of the individual at risk. Small homes with a proven track record in caring for such individuals might have a competitive edge, if consumers can find them.

The Financial Challenge

Most senior housing and service settings face financial pressures of various types: setting rates high enough to cover operating expenses but still low enough to remain competitive with other providers; offering wages that allow them to attract and retain staff; and, for small home operators, balancing the responsibilities of being a financial manager while simultaneously being a primary care provider. They differ from the new industry of assisted living providers that is largely for-profit and caters to a private-pay market of older consumers who are willing to spend an average of almost $3,000 per month—although rates vary by region and the amenities or services offered (MetLife, 2005). Only a few "upscale" small homes have pricing structures and financial operations more like their larger counterparts in assisted living (Morgan et al., 1995). Although small board-and-care homes are also predominantly private-pay and for-profit, they typically charge lower fees (Stearns & Morgan, 2001).

Small homes face many of the same kinds of costs as larger residences, but they do not benefit from the economies of scale that are possible for larger settings or chains (see chapter 1). In many small homes housing low-income elders, we found that operators essentially pooled income from residents and from any other sources (e.g., spouse wages, pensions) and used these funds to meet the combined needs of all in the household (Morgan et al., 1995). Incontinence supplies, food for family-style meals, and toiletries for family and residents alike might be purchased together at a grocery store, without subsequently itemizing "charges" to residents. The operators of many of these homes did not take a regular salary, instead benefiting from profits—if and when there were any (Morgan et al., 1995). At best, operating a small home might be marginally profitable (Morgan et al., 1995; Stearns & Morgan, 2001), because such homes are often a matter of poor people caring for other low-income individuals (Perkins, Ball, Wittington, & Combs, 2004).

As examples of the modest fees such homes charge, Maria's normal rate at Franciscan House was $1,600 per month for basic services, typically including rent, meals, housekeeping, and laundry. (She explained that she had had to raise her rates because of increases in her liability insurance premium.) Rani charged $1,600–$1,800 for basic services, with her highest monthly fee totaling $2,500 for a person who was dependent in all personal care tasks, including eating. Although this approaches the national average of $2,905 for assisted living, as a "base rate" that figure may not include all personal care services and ancillary fees. But these figures do not tell us what people believe they are "getting" for their money or how services, amenities, and such intangible qualities as a "homelike" environment factor into an individual's choice of one setting over another. Absolute costs cannot be compared between board and care and assisted living because detailed information about the total cost of care—including room, board, all services, fees, and ancillary costs such as medication administration, transportation, personal needs—has not been reported for either housing type.

Other researchers have found that operators who cater to low-income individuals must find ways to save money. One small home provider conserved water and other household utilities, relied on free community resources, and even flirted with questionable, even potentially illegal, strategies, such as asking capable residents to help with chores in exchange for lower fees, hiring staff with "dubious" backgrounds, and even "shifting" (or moving) residents between a licensed and an unlicensed setting (Perkins et al., 2004). Such actions make clear the financial distress that some small homes experience in serving very low-income individuals.

The Staffing Challenge

Settings that provide housing with services to older adults compete to attract, train, and retain staff from a common, limited pool of potential employees. Small board-and-care homes face challenges in recruiting staff akin to those in recruiting residents: their relative invisibility and absence of formal mechanisms for referral. While some individuals might enjoy working in a small board-and-care home, preferring the personalized and broader level of contact permitted by this setting, larger homes often provide more tangible rewards in terms of benefits, training, and opportunities for career advancement. For small homes, by contrast, finding the right kind of person is a challenge sometimes undertaken through informal networks. Rani, for example, prefers to locate individuals privately as opposed to hiring through agencies that charge an hourly rate she finds difficult to meet; she relies on agencies only when she cannot locate available workers through newspaper ads or by word of mouth (see chapter 2).

Training the staff who provide hands-on care presents a different kind of challenge for a home with few employees who are not available to "cover" for one another when staff or operators need to be trained in new regulatory procedures or to expand technical skills such as medication management or life safety training. Care providers in small board-and-care homes are typically trained by the operator, as exemplified by Rani, who likes to teach individuals her own way of doing things. She explained, "Initially I have to get myself involved a lot. In fact, every moment I am with them [the new employee] in the beginning. But if they are here, for the next six months, say, then they get settled. They get to know the person [resident] and so they know how each one will react and what they require and so on." Maria echoed the amount of time and effort required to train a new staff member, explaining that, "It's a process of training. It takes a long time. So every day I try to . . . whatever she can do, I let her do. If she misses something, I will do it for the meantime until she gets used to something and when she can absorb it."

Rani and Maria both provide hands-on training tailored for each specific resident; and both prefer to hire live-in staff. Rani explains that it is best to hire someone who sees the job as a career rather than someone who just wants to make extra money. Finding such individuals, however, is a matter of trial and error. The time and effort dedicated to training just one employee translates into significant costs, both financial and emotional, for these operators, who typically are also providing direct care for residents themselves. These two operators and others have described staff continuity as critical to providing quality care to older persons, especially those with cognitive impairment.

As organizations, small board-and-care homes are relatively "flat," with an operator (often the owner) and a relatively small staff of care providers. Thus, being an employer and employee in the smaller homes is substantially different than in large, hierarchically organized settings that provide 24-hour care in shifts. First, there is relatively little specialization. Everyone does the work of maintaining the space (e.g., cleaning, emptying trash), making meals, and responding to residents' ongoing care needs. A second consequence of this flat structure is few opportunities for advancement. For example, Rani hired several nursing students, knowing she would likely lose them because she would not be able to pay registered nurse salaries once they completed their educations. We lack data on whether turnover of staff is higher or lower in small board-and-care homes than in larger residences, but the loss of a staff member could arguably have a greater impact, given that a small home may employ only three or four individuals at any given time. Also, smaller homes lack a pool of employees to draw on when one calls in sick. Thus, although both smaller and larger assisted living settings face workforce issues, the impact may be greater in smaller homes. The operator is responsible not only for hiring staff but also for training them, paying them, and picking up the slack if they do not measure up to expected standards.

The Regulatory Challenge

The board-and-care debate over the past 30 years has centered on whether to regulate and if so, how strictly and on what aspects of the physical environment, services, staffing, and oversight provided (Dobkin, 1989). As discussed in chapter 13, some states use a one-size-fits-all approach in which small homes must meet the same standards as larger assisted living buildings. Other states treat small homes as a distinct class, recognizing that care occurs in family homes on a very small and personal scale (Carder, Morgan, & Eckert, 2006). Opponents of regulating small homes argue that government oversight favors the kind of standardized, bureaucratic, institutional approaches to care evident in skilled nursing homes, in contrast to the personalized, homelike care that small settings characteristically offer (see chapter 13). Those who argue for regulating small homes, in turn, point to the need to monitor and improve quality, safety, and accountability (Hawes, 1997; Phillips et al., 1995).

Maryland's experience exemplifies the dilemma of regulation. In 1999 Maryland moved from a largely unregulated system of small board-and-care homes to a regulatory system that included even the smallest homes under the assisted living umbrella. This one-size-fits-all approach remains controversial among operators and regulators today. Rani's home, where 7 older persons live and receive daily assistance, must meet the same standards as an assisted living owned by a national corporation that has 150 residents and 70 employees organized into departments, levels, and three rotating shifts. This regulatory approach makes sense in reference to providing direct personal assistance—an individual moving into Rani's home should expect the same quality of care as she would receive from a corporate chain (and vice versa).

Both Rani and Maria, however, expressed frustrations related to the current assisted living regulations. They faced uncertainties about how to meet these requirements and found the assessment and care planning process, as well as other paperwork demands (like posting menus and activity calendars), overwhelming at times. Maria explained,

> Before the year 2000, the rules were not as strict, okay, like they didn't ask for too many things. Now we have so many paperworks [sic]. We have to send this to the doctor. We have to do our own assessment. We didn't have that before. We have to have a 45-day nursing assessment and then we have so many reports like everything has to be documented just for the record, maybe because of so many lawsuits, I don't know. It's just that we are swamped with paperworks [sic]; that's it. Every little thing we have to like write it down and send it to this form and send that form over there. It's too much. . . . We're not machine, you know, and everybody needs to rest and take off and take a break.

Maria's frustration was echoed by other small home operators who attended public meetings organized by the state licensing agency (Office of Health Care Quality, 2005b).

Even in states that have separate oversight or regulation for small homes, the relative burden of responding to regulatory requirements weighs more heavily on small homes, which have so few staff members. Although regulation is well intentioned, the time and paperwork demands create a greater challenge for small board-and-care homes to conform to all requirements in a responsible fashion while simultaneously meeting needs for care, than is the case for their larger counterparts (see chapter 1).

Such differences in scale between small and larger providers have led to debate among providers, public agency staff, medical providers, and consumers. A recent Maryland report suggested that policy be changed to reclassify homes that care for one to four individuals in a category distinct from assisted living (Office of Health Care Quality, 2005b). In keeping with the goal of offering "family-like" care, under this proposed policy owners of small homes would not be permitted to have financial interest in more than one home. Other states are also questioning whether multiple ownership, or "chains," threatens the personalized qualities of small homes (Folkemer et al., 1996). Such a business arrangement, however, might strengthen the financial viability of some small homes. For example, owning more than one home, especially if the buildings were situated adjacent to each other, might help create economies of scale in terms of purchasing food and household supplies, hiring or contracting with service providers, such as medical professionals and home and lawn maintenance, and sharing other operating expenses.

The Public Subsidy Challenge

Given the sizable concentrations of lower-income individuals in the smaller homes, more residents of small board-and-care homes receive some sort of public subsidy than do residents of larger or newer assisted living residences. For example, in Maryland, 49 percent of the homes licensed for 16 or fewer residents are certified to accept Medicaid waiver clients, as compared to only 29 percent of settings with 17 or more residents. Primary among public finance sources are SSI and Medicaid (Morgan et al. 1995; Phillips et al., 1995).

Forty-one states now use Medicaid to pay for services provided in residential settings, such as board-and-care homes, and other states use general revenues to subsidize some portion of this care (Mollica & Johnson-Lamarche, 2005). Public payments for board and care are limited to individuals who qualify both financially and medically. States are increasingly looking to reduce their Medicaid expenses by subsidizing the cost of assisted living for eligible individuals who might otherwise enter a higher cost nursing home (Justice & Heestand, 2003; National Governors Association, 2000). States, however, have taken different approaches to determining who qualifies, what scope of services should be covered, and what level of reimbursement should be provided (for a fuller discussion of this issue, see chapters 11 and 14). Providers often argue that Medicaid reimbursement rates do not cover their operational costs and that when states place caps on the number of Medicaid "slots" available providers are left uncertain whether residents who spend down will qualify. Many providers opt not to accept Medicaid because of such uncertainties. At a 2003 meeting to discuss issues faced by operators of small homes, one Maryland operator reported that only 31 of 155 small board-and-care providers in the county accepted subsidy clients, down from 55 in the prior year. He attributed this decline to increased liability insurance rates that made it too expensive to care for very low-income individuals.

Deciding whether to accept individuals with public subsidies can be a particular challenge for operators of small homes. When the individual's public funding (e.g., a monthly SSI payment) fails to cover the actual cost of housing and services fully, an operator must decide which is worse: letting a bed remain empty for a month or more or accepting a very poor resident who may remain for a long time. This sort of pressure may not affect larger residences, for which the addition of one or two residents whose costs are not fully covered may have less impact on the overall income, social dynamics, and staffing needs. Providers' decision making is further compounded by the fact that rapidly rising health care costs threaten the future availability of Medicaid funding (Coleman, Fox-Grage, & Folkemer, 2003).

Future Prospects for Small Homes

Clearly, although they are not entirely distinct from the larger housing with services sector that includes assisted living, small board-and-care homes face a number of challenges to survival that are specific to their smaller size and less visible place in ongoing national discussions. With the rapid growth of larger, corporate-developed assisted living during the past 15–20 years, many people have largely lost sight of the small homes, which continue to provide care to older adults in substantial numbers across the country. In some instances, the fates of the two sectors are intertwined. For example, many of the challenges related to staffing and competition are shared by residences of all sizes. Solutions to these problems, if they appear, will benefit both small and large-scale providers of housing with services, but other challenges are unique to small homes.

What is the likely future for small board-and-care homes? Significant anecdotal evidence suggests high rates of turnover among homes in this sector, from a rash of closings to the conglomeration of small homes into minichains. Some of the small operators in our research describe feeling pushed toward a decision to sell or cease operation. Such a shakeout could be viewed simply as the market operating to remove less viable businesses in favor of the more viable, larger scale operations. This outcome, however, overlooks important questions about the value of small homes among the array of housing with services and whether this alternative should remain available in the marketplace.

Small homes broaden the array of alternatives for meeting the needs of a highly diverse pool of residents. Some consumers prefer smaller settings, and such homes may be especially appropriate for individuals who have cognitive impairments. If smaller homes are to remain competitive, they must capitalize on their unique, family-like environment by forming coalitions and cultivating advocates. Operators of small board-and-care residences might follow the successful model of the assisted living movement by being proactive and educating consumers and public officials about their distinctive "product." Moreover, the survival of the small-scale housing and care environments could be enhanced if older adults who qualify for public subsidies were empowered to select among the broadest range of alternatives to meet their needs, as do private-pay consumers.

Just how regulation evolves will make an important difference. Clearly one-size-fits-all regulation creates differential impacts based on size, and the pressure to increase regulatory oversight, staffing, and training requirements may create greater pressure on small homes than on larger ones. Nevertheless, we recognize that size alone is not the most important factor in defining and regulating housing with services. For example, although the difference between a 6-unit and an 80-unit building might be obvious, the distinction between a 6-unit and an 11- or 12-unit home is not. To be meaningful, regulation must focus on level and type of services provided.

As residents in all types of nonmedical housing with services age in place and manifest greater physical and cognitive limitations, states are considering "upping the ante" with regard to nursing staff, credentialing of operators, and related changes that might result in assisted living settings coming to resemble nursing homes. Policies that require licensed nurses across the sector, even in the smallest of board-and-care homes, would fundamentally change the nature of care provided toward a more "medicalized" approach, and would increase staffing costs. By contrast, if states develop alternative regulation and oversight for small residences that are geared to their unique circumstances and needs (e.g., adjusted staffing and record-keeping requirements), small providers will be better able to meet standards and afford to continue their businesses, while also preserving their special character of care.

Public policies that support community-based settings create a market for small homes. Some states, including Oregon and Washington, have created a regulatory infrastructure that addresses the characteristics of small settings by providing case management to residents, specialized training for staff, and ongoing quality monitoring of all licensed homes. With support from a Real Choice Systems Change grant from the Centers for Medicare and Medicaid Services, Arkansas is currently preparing adult foster care regulations. When implemented, these regulations will allow for the development of licensed adult foster homes.

In addition to providing less medicalized care, small homes currently house a higher percentage of lower-income and minority individuals, including more persons who rely on SSI, Medicaid home- and community-based waivers, and other publicly funded programs, than do other housing with care settings. Should small homes disappear from the market, a significantly greater number of older adults would require placement in alternative settings that accept their lower fee-reimbursement rates. Barring expansion of alternative housing options offering more affordable care (see chapter 12) or greater acceptance of public reimbursement among other assisted living settings, the only option for such individuals would be relocation to Medicaid-funded nursing home beds. This would be an extremely unwelcome irony in an era when policy makers are seeking community-based alternatives for care, both because of their lower cost and because of consumer preferences to avoid nursing homes.

Finally, small board-and-care homes face unique challenges in terms of advocating for their specific business and resident needs. Operators of small homes with few employees have little time to attend meetings, organize, or lobby legislators to keep their issues in mind as laws and regulations are developed. In our research, operators of small homes reported difficulty getting away for any reason, and few were involved with organizations or political activities that might have increased the visibility of the smallest homes. As a result, regulations often mirror the realities only of the larger, corporate-built assisted living settings. Getting more information about the needs of small homes and their residents into the hands of those contemplating creating or altering public policies would help to redress this imbalance.

Conclusions and Implications for the Future

We are in a formative period for policy regarding housing with services. To avoid making decisions in a void, or reacting only to sensational reports of egregious abuse and neglect, policy makers and regulators need accurate information about the number of small board-and-care homes, the people they serve, and the people who operate and work in them. To date, much of the research conducted in assisted living (of all sizes) has used measures that favor the characteristics of larger residences; thus, valid and reliable measures are needed to guide future research in small settings (Morgan et al., 2004). Generating up-to-date data on these small board-and-care homes and the significant role that they continue to play in the housing with services sector will help assure a true picture of where care is provided as we approach key decisions influencing the future of this fragile segment of the market.

In future decades we will face critical choices that will determine the viability of small homes, which have been a bulwark of caring for frail elders for many decades. Beyond accurate data, advocacy is needed to support small homes, whose resources do not promote lobbying or the creation of state- or national-level organizations to call policy makers' attention to their needs. The decidedly marginal place of small board-and-care homes in policy discussions means that public programs to ensure safety and improve services may miss the specialized needs of small homes and their residents, as well as the potential to support these different environments. The quasi-familial and connected environment that typifies the best of small homes is a good fit for many older adults requiring a supportive housing and care environment. Sustaining this distinctiveness through policies that support, as well as regulate, may enable small homes to survive some of their unique challenges. The imbalance between the organizational and advocacy base of the larger, for-profit and chain-based assisted living sector and the small providers is a noteworthy issue as we look forward. Without broader awareness of the critical role small homes play, their future remains clouded.

REFERENCES

Ball, M. M., Perkins, M. M., Whittington, F. J., Hollingsworth, C., King, S. V., & Combs, B. 2005. *Communities of care: Assisted living for African American elders*. Baltimore: Johns Hopkins University Press.

Carder, P. C., & Hernandez, M. 2004. Consumer discourse in assisted living. *Journals of Gerontology: Social Sciences 59B,* S58–67.

Carder, P. C., Morgan, L. A., & Eckert, J. K. 2006. Small board-and-care homes in the age of assisted living. *Generations 29* (4), 24–31.

Clark, R. F., Turek-Breznin, J., Chu, C.W., & Hawes, C. 1994. *Licensed board-and-care homes: Preliminary findings from the 1991 National Health Provider Inventory.* Washington, DC: U.S. Department of Health and Human Services. www.aspe.hhs.gov/daltcp/reports/rn06.htm.

Coleman, B., Fox-Grage, W., & Folkemer, D. 2003. *State long-term care: Recent developments and policy directions*. Washington, DC: National Council of State Legislatures.

Curtis, M., Kiyak, A., & Hedrick, S. 2000. Resident and facility characteristics of adult family homes, adult residential care, and assisted living settings in Washington State. *Journal of Gerontological Social Work 34,* 25–41.

Dobkin, L. 1989. *The board and care system: A regulatory jungle*. Washington, DC: American Association of Retired Persons.

Eckert, J.K., Cox, D., & Morgan, L.A. 1999. The meaning of family-like care among operators of small board and care homes. *Journal of Aging Studies 13*(3), 333–347.

Folkemer, D., Jensen, A., Lipson, L., Stauffer, M., & Fox-Grage, W. 1996. *Adult foster care for the elderly: A review of state regulatory and funding strategies (report #9604A)*. Washington, DC: American Association of Retired Persons.

Frank, J. B. 2002. *Paradox of aging in place in assisted living*. Westport, CT: Bergin & Garvey.

Hawes, C. 1997. Regulation and the politics of long-term care. *Generations 21 (4),* 5.

Hawes, C., Wildfire, J. B., Lux, L. J., & Clemmer, E. 2000. *Regulation of board and care homes: results of a survey in the 50 states and the District of Columbia.* Washington, DC: American Association of Retired Persons.

Howard, D. L., Sloane, P. D., Zimmerman, S., Eckert, J. K., Walsh, J. F., Buie, V. C., Taylor, P. J., & Koch, G. G. 2002. Distribution of African Americans in residential care/assisted living and nursing homes: More evidence of racial disparity? *American Journal of Public Health 92* (8), 1272–1277.

Justice, D., & Heestand, A. 2003. *Promising practices in long-term care systems reform: Oregon's home and community based services system*. Washington, DC: Medstat. www.cms.hhs.gov/promisingpractices/mfp92903.pdf.

Kane, R. A., Kane, R. L., Illston, L. H., Nyman, J. A., & Finch, M. D. 1991. Adult foster care for the elderly in Oregon: A mainstream alternative to nursing homes? *American Journal of Public Health 91* (9), 1113–1120.

Kane, R. A., & Wilson, K. B. 2001. *Assisted living at the crossroads: Principles for its future.* Portland, OR: Jessie F. Richardson Foundation.

Mead, L. C., Eckert, J. K., Zimmerman, S., & Schumacher, J. G. 2005. Sociocultural aspects of transitions from assisted living for residents with dementia. *Gerontologist 45 (special issue),* 115–123.

MetLife. 2005. *The 2005 MetLife market survey of assisted living costs.* Westport, CT: MetLife Mature Market Institute. www.metlife.com.

Mollica, R. 2002. *State assisted living practices and options: A guide for state policy makers.* Portland, ME: National Academy for State Health Policy.

Mollica, R., & Johnson-Lamarche, H. 2005. *State residential and assisted living policy, 2004.* Portland, ME: National Academy for State Health Policy.

Morgan, L. A., Eckert, J. K., Gruber-Baldini, A.L., & Zimmerman, S. 2004. Policy and research for small assisted living facilities. *Journal of Aging and Social Policy 16* (4), 1–16.

Morgan, L. A., Eckert, J. K., & Lyon, S. L. 1995. *Small board-and-care homes: Residential care in transition.* Baltimore: Johns Hopkins University Press.

Morgan, L. A., Eckert, J. K., Piggee, T., & Frankowski, A. C. 2006. Two lives in transition: Agency and context for assisted living residents. *Journal of Aging Studies, 201* (1), 123–132.

Morgan, L. A., Gruber-Baldini, A. L. & Magaziner, J. 2001. Resident characteristics. In S. I. Zimmerman, P. D. Sloane, & J. K. Eckert (Eds.), *Assisted living: needs, practice, and policies in residential care for the elderly* (pp. 144–172). Baltimore: Johns Hopkins University Press.

National Governors Association. 2000. *Challenges and opportunities for states in providing long-term care for the elderly.* Washington, DC: National Governors Association.

Office of Health Care Quality. 2005a. *Assisted living program licensee directory.* www.dhmh.state.md.us/ohcq/licensee_directory/licensee_directory.htm.

Office of Health Care Quality. 2005b. *Maryland assisted living program 2004 evaluation.* Baltimore: Department of Health and Mental Hygiene, Office of Health Care Quality. www.dhmh.state.md.us/ohcq/alforum/2004_alp_rpt.pdf.

Perkins, M. M., Ball, M. M., Whittington, F. J., & Combs, B. L. 2004. Managing the care needs of low-income board-and-care home residents: A process of negotiating risks. *Qualitative Health Research 14* (4), 478–495.

Phillips, C., Lux, L., Wildfire, J., Greene, A., Hawes, C., et al. 1995. *Report on the effects of regulation on quality of care: Analysis of the effect of regulation on the quality of care in board and care homes.* Washington, DC: U.S. Department of Health and Human Services, Assistant Secretary for Planning and Evaluation.

Quinn, M. E., Johnson, M. A., Andress, E., McGinnis, P., & Remesh, M. 1999. Health characteristics of elderly personal care home residents. *Journal of Advanced Nursing 30* (2), 410–417.

Reinardy, J. R., & Kane, R. A. 2003. Anatomy of a choice: Deciding on assisted living or nursing home care in Oregon. *Journal of Applied Gerontology 22* (1), 152–173.

Schumacher, J. G., Eckert, K., Zimmerman, S., Carder, P. & Wright, A. 2005. Physician care in assisted living: A qualitative study. *Journal of the American Medical Directors Association 6*, 34–45.

Sherman, S., & Newman, E. 1988. *Foster families for adults: A community alternative in long-term care.* New York: Columbia University Press.

Stearns, S. C., & Morgan, L. A. 2001. Economics and financing. In S. I., Zimmerman, P. D. Sloane, & J. K. Eckert (Eds.), *Assisted living: Needs, practices, and policies in residential care for the elderly* (pp. 271–191). Baltimore: Johns Hopkins University Press.

Zimmerman, S. I., Sloane, P. D., Eckert, J. K., Buie, V. C., Walsh, J. F., Koch, G. G., & Hebel. J. R. 2001. An overview of the collaborative studies of long-term care. In S. I. Zimmerman, P. D. Sloane, & J. K. Eckert (eds), *Assisted living: Needs, practices, and policies in residential care for the elderly* (pp. 117–143). Baltimore: Johns Hopkins University Press.

Zimmerman, S., Soane, P. D., Eckert, J. K., Gruber-Baldini, A., Morgan, A. L., Hebel, J. R., Magaziner, J., Stearns, S. C., & Chen, C. K. 2005. How good is assisted living? Findings and implications from an outcomes study. *Journal of Gerontology: Social Sciences 60B* (4), S195–204.

PART II

PRIVATE-SECTOR INFLUENCES ON TOMORROW'S ASSISTED LIVING RESIDENCES

CHAPTER 6

The Future of Assisted Living

Residents' Perspectives, 2006–2026

MARGARET A. WYLDE, PH.D.

Were this chapter being written "by the book," it would begin with a discussion of the likely *old, older, senior,* or *elder* assisted living consumer during the next 20 years. To be sure, the chapter will describe that consumer, but the primary intent here is to approach assisted living from the consumer's perspective. And the last thing today's and tomorrow's consumer wants is to be classified, categorized, enumerated, or called *old, older, senior, elder,* or anything else that negates everything about them except their age.

Any discussion of consumer preferences for assisted living must also begin by recognizing a well-publicized finding. The American Association of Retired Persons (AARP) has shown repeatedly that "What I really want is to stay in my current residence as long as possible" (AARP, 2005). Other surveys have shown much the same (e.g., 84 percent of the 50-plus population surveyed by Roper Public Affairs agreed with this statement; see Figure 6.1). Concomitantly, the proportion that own their homes has continued to increase significantly among 75-plus households (Figure 6.2), from 70 percent in 1998 to 78 percent in 2002 (U.S. Department of Commerce,

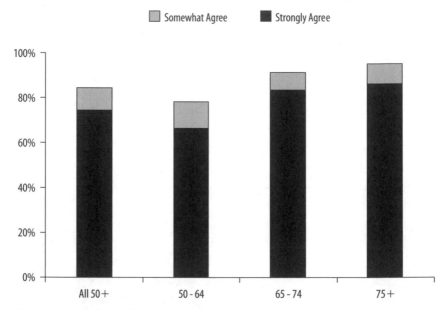

Figure 6.1. Proportion who strongly agree or agree that they want to remain in their current residence for as long as possible

2002). To be successful, assisted living providers must look for ways to counter these preferences.

A third critical insight, when one considers the studies focused on the care needs of consumers, is that the assisted living alternatives have at times lost sight of the person. By boiling people down to an average age (a faceless, useless group called "old"), the number of activities of daily living (ADLs) with which they need assistance, and the type of community in which they live, the alternatives fail to see who these people are and were and who they may still become.

The result is that many of the prognostications made about tomorrow's consumers of assisted living are antithetical to *consumer* trends and preferences. Well-meaning stakeholders may advocate for more regulations, the government may issue them, and some developers will adhere to them, but other developers, who are in tune with consumers' wants, will invent the next metamorphosis of the assisted living/nursing care product, aspiring once again to provide what consumers want.

Resident, Consumer, or Customer?

A few years ago, the term *mass customization* received focus as retailers began to take advantage of online communication and computer-controlled manufacturing. Consumers enjoy being able to enter their measurements and preferences into a short online questionnaire and place their order for the "custom-made" jeans, dress suits, and swimming suits. Some shoe manufacturers send you a kit to make molds of your feet, all to deliver you a better product custom fit to you.

In this period, even as assisted living providers were developing individual care plans for residents, they were also being accused of "warehousing" elderly people. The charge of warehousing was a result of many industry blights that have been evident in the past decade. It was manifested by the rapid construction of thousands of assisted living residences with "shoe box"–size and –style apartments, the paucity of interesting and beneficial educational and recreational programs for customers, the scarcity of staff on weekends, ready-made, processed food that could be elegantly overcooked by anyone, and dining schedules that had residents lining up for the evening meal by 4:00 p.m., being served at 4:30, and being finished by 4:45 so that the staff could clear the tables and be off by 5:00. The lucid, engaged assisted living resident who had enjoyed decades of fine dining, stimulating conversations, engaging friends and acquaintances, and at least modest command of the world around her was now

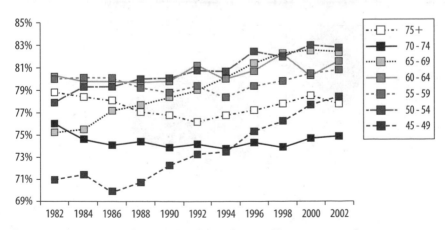

Figure 6.2. Proportion who own their home, by age of homeowner and year

relegated to bingo, keeping-the-beach-ball-in-the-air exercises, lukewarm processed dinners served in the middle of the afternoon, and spirited discussion of someone's latest trip to the podiatrist.

As an industry, we have focused on providing individual care of high technical quality, but to a great extent we have lost the person. When you move to an assisted living residence, you are no longer an individual; you become "one of our residents." Indeed, despite the fact that you pay for your apartment, services, and dining room fare you are not even one of our "customers," you are simply one of the residents to whom we provide high-quality care. There is a huge difference between being a customer with preferences and purchasing power and being a resident.

Given that the assisted living customer is not sick and does not require medical attention, the customer's multifaceted journey in the assisted living residence combines a transaction for use of real estate, a contract for services, and pursuit of enjoyment of life. The customer focuses not on the care received, but on the life to be lived.

It is a stark comeuppance when you realize you need someone to help you bathe. You, who have jumped from rocks into rivers, jack-knifed from

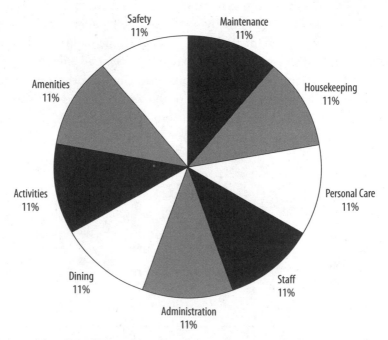

Figure 6.3. The effect of assisted living services on overall sense of quality if all services affect quality of life equally

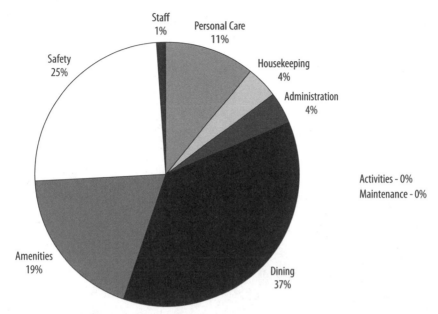

Figure 6.4. Results of satisfaction surveys of assisted living customers (residents) and the extent to which each service area correlated with "overall sense of satisfaction"

the high dive, and spent Sunday mornings in the hot tub, are now expected to sit there while a stranger gives you a bath. As one resident said recently after a trip to the "shower" room, "I felt like I was being hosed down like a dog." But, you can tolerate the mechanics of care, as long as they are done well and efficiently and you're able to get on with your day—if it offers something new, different, fun, educational, interactive, challenging, of use to others, and perhaps a good "belly laugh."

Ay, there's the rub. The assisted living residence invests predominantly in providing care and sparingly in enhancing life. For the assisted living customer, it is not the quality of personal care assistance that correlates with her overall satisfaction or willingness to recommend your place to friends; it is how she spends her day. The fact that she is bathed, her meals and snacks are prepared, her bed is made, and her apartment is cleaned is not the focus of her existence. Those things are appreciated because they are needed, but they play minimally into her assessment of the quality of her life.

The importance of everyday life to assisted living customers is evident from satisfaction surveys. Figures 6.3, 6.4, and 6.5 reveal the relative contribution each of nine service areas made to customers' satisfaction with

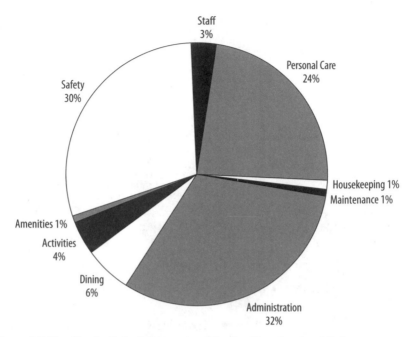

Figure 6.5. Results of satisfaction surveys of the families of assisted living customers (residents) and the extent to which each service area correlated with "overall sense of satisfaction"

their assisted living residence. (The results indicate only relative importance from the customers' perspectives, not whether the individual services were judged to be satisfactory or unsatisfactory.)

If each of the services areas traditionally measured in satisfaction surveys of assisted living—staff performance, personal care, housekeeping, maintenance, administration, dining, activities, amenities, and safety— were equally important to customers, we could represent the relative contribution of each as shown in Figure 6.3—that is, as a pie chart with nine identical slices. But surveys show that these service areas in fact *do not* contribute equally to customers' satisfaction with assisted living. Consumers rather slice their pie of priorities into larger and smaller pieces. For example, Figure 6.4 shows data from one assisted living company indicating clearly that customers (residents) felt some service areas were more important than others. For these customers, dining (37 percent), safety (25 percent), and amenities (19 percent) contributed a good deal more to their satisfaction with the assisted living residence than did personal care (11 percent) or other service areas.

The family members of assisted living customers who play key roles in the decisions older people make about their care decisions in turn value differently the attributes of the assisted living residence. Figure 6.5 graphs family members' rating of the relative contributions of different service areas. Although family members, like customers, felt that residents' safety was an important contributor to overall satisfaction (30 percent), they had a different perspective on other service areas. Thus, personal care counted far more among family members (24 percent) than among residents, whereas administration topped the list (32 percent) and was considered much more important than it was by customers (4 percent). The message is clear. Assisted living customers want to enjoy their days, some may want to do something useful, and others would like a mental challenge and the opportunity to "exercise their brain." Families, by contrast, want to be sure their loved ones are safe and that their personal care needs are met. They also want to have "hassle-free" dealings with the operators of the facility.

Assisted Living Customers: The Next 20 Years

The characteristics of the next generation of assisted living customers will help shape their purchase decisions and satisfaction. During the next 20 years, the last members of the "Greatest Generation" (those born in 1924 or earlier) will be cycling out of assisted living and members of the "Silent Generation" (those born between 1925 and 1942) will become assisted living's principal customers. With the average age of entry into assisted living today being 83, the Silent Generation—whose oldest members are this age at the time of this writing—are just beginning to cross the thresholds of assisted living residences. In 20 years, their youngest members will be 86 years of age.

About 95 percent of members of the Silent Generation are retired today. This group has been labeled conformist, believers in the status quo, adapters, people who went along and got along. Members of the Silent Generation have not been seen as risk takers—for example, only 2 percent took the risk to be self-employed, whereas the majority included long-term employees of companies that provided them a good living, good benefits, and retirement pensions.

The Silent Generation, however, may mistakenly be perceived as a group unlikely to clamor for change, and the assisted living industry should not be too complacent. The Silent Generation *has* taken a stand on some issues.

It legitimized divorce, for example. After marrying at an average age of 23 years for men and 20 for women, the "divorce epidemic" was started among men and women born between 1930 and 1940, who showed the biggest age-bracket jump in divorce rate in history. And the Silent Generation can claim kinship with one of the greatest leaders for social change in American history, Dr. Martin Luther King, Jr., who was born in 1929.

The growth of assisted living during the next 20 years will depend on how the next generation of consumers views this long-term care alternative. Several factors will be influential: their level of family support, economic resources, health status, and the availability of technology.

Family Support

Many among the next generation of assisted living customers have adult children. Ninety-four percent of women in the Silent Generation became mothers and stayed at home, where they raised an average of 3.3 children. So unlike many of their daughters, women of the Silent Generation may have children to support them when they need help. And, although not all adult children will behave the same, many will want the same independence for their parents as they will want for themselves.

Economic Outlook

Tomorrow's assisted living consumers may be reluctant to spend money unless they see clear benefit and value from the products and services they purchase. Children of the Great Depression and the upheavals of World War II, the Silent Generation is not inclined to take on debt or financial risk. This group has learned to hunker down with their families and weather the storm. They may be particularly averse to taking risks in uncertain times of increasing threats of terrorism worldwide and escalating oil prices.

Although a majority of the upcoming generation of potential assisted living customers own their homes (Figure 6.2), their annual household income has stagnated—there has not been a net real increase in family incomes among age 50 and older households since 1999 (AARP, 2006). The estimated median annual household incomes of the target market sector, 75-plus years of age, are expected to increase only 2.5 percent during the next five years—for example, from $29,312 in 2006 to $33,028 in 2011 for

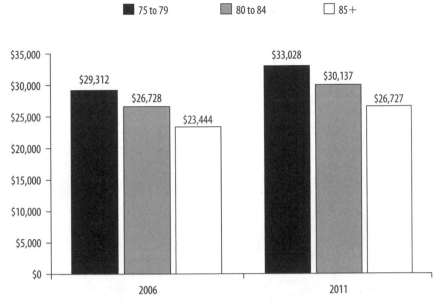

Figure 6.6. Estimated median annual household incomes, by age of head of household, 2006 and 2011

the 75–79 age group (Figure 6.6). At best, this increase will only keep pace with inflation.

If the price of assisted living charged to customers keeps pace with inflation, the proportion of consumers with sufficient funds to afford out-of-pocket payments is likely to shrink. On the positive side, the proportion of households who rely for more than half of their income from Social Security (Figure 6.7) has also been shrinking, albeit slowly (AARP, 2006).

Health Status

Health trends among the target market sector for assisted living have begun to turn downward. The proportion of individuals at least 75 years of age who report that their health is "excellent" or "very good" dropped from 35 percent to 31 percent between 1994 and 2004 (Figure 6.8). Thus, the number of individuals who will need assistance may increase during the next 20 years.

The factor that bears the greatest share of the blame in the health decline is the proportion of the populace that is overweight or obese. The proportion that is fit, in that they are not overweight or obese, has declined dra-

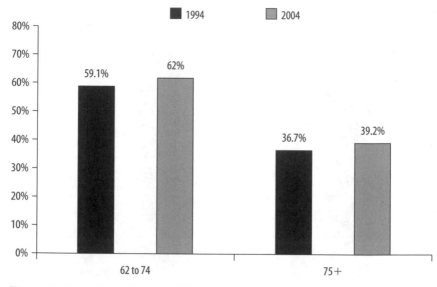

Figure 6.7. Proportion of the population age 62+ who receive more than 50 percent of their income from sources other than Social Security

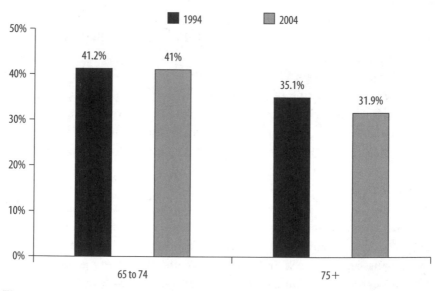

Figure 6.8. Proportion reporting their health as "excellent" or "very good"

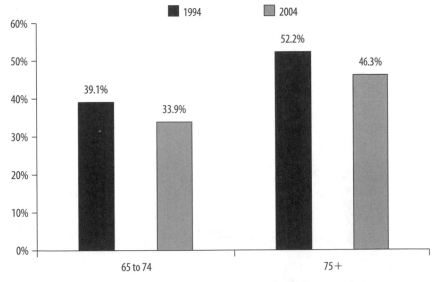

Figure 6.9. Proportion reporting they are not overweight and are not obese

matically in the past decade (AARP, 2006). The proportion who are not overweight or obese dropped from 39 to 34 percent of the 65–74 age group between 1994 and 2004, and from 52 to 46 percent of the 75-plus age group (Figure 6.9). It is projected that the obesity epidemic will reduce recent gains in longevity.

Use of Technology

Technologies are likely to help enhance the quality of the living environment and improve service delivery in the coming years. Use of computers has increased dramatically (Figure 6.10). As another indicator, the American Association of Retired Persons showed that among those 65 years of age or more, cell phone adoption increased from 27 to 37 percent between January and December of 2003 (AARP, 2005). The primary reason these consumers acquired cell phones was for security in case of emergency (59 percent) and convenience (37 percent). Few intended to use cell phones on a daily basis but, rather, saw the device as a way of summoning help, even when they were at home. Despite these long-term prospects, the segment moving into assisted living during at least the first part of the next decade will be more likely not to have adopted these newer technolo-

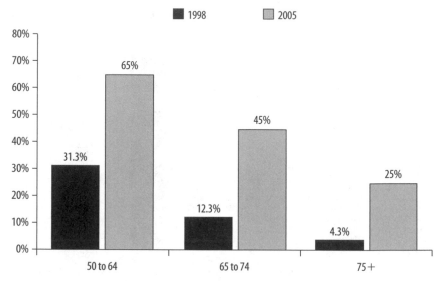

Figure 6.10. Proportion of the population age 50+ who access the Internet

gies. They may be less enamored with a "high-tech, low-touch" environment than future generations.

Further in the future, however, new and better technologies will emerge that will enable people to communicate better, more easily, and more affordably with each other, even at long distances. Assisted living residences that learn to take advantage of technologies to help provide opportunities for residents to have more rewarding interactions and intelligent discourse with family, friends, and professionals will help improve their prospects with future assisted living customers (see chapter 8).

Awareness and Acceptance of Assisted Living by Today's Customers

Awareness of assisted living among potential customers (residents) has increased rapidly in recent years. Since 1998, several studies have asked individuals 60 years of age or more whether they knew of an assisted living residence (National Investment Center for the Seniors Housing and Care Industry [NIC], 1998, 2001; ProMatura Group, 2006). Among respondents in the "middle-income and better" socioeconomic category, the primary target market for assisted living, awareness of an assisted living community rose from 58 percent in 1998 to nearly 87 percent in 2006 (NIC, 1998; ProMatura, 2006) (Figure 6.11).

Despite this significant increase in awareness during the past 8 years, there does not seem to be increased acceptance of assisted living as a residential alternative for individuals who need assistance. A 2006 nationwide study of 3,524 households age 60 or more revealed that, although 87 percent are aware of assisted living residences and about 25 percent of individuals in this age group have visited an assisted living residence to look at it as a place they might live, only about 12 percent said they were "likely" or "very likely" to consider a move into this option should circumstances warrant it (Figure 6.12) (ProMatura Group, 2006).

Awareness has also increased among younger adults, probably because of media attention and the increase in the proportion of individuals who knows someone who lives in an assisted living residence. In a 2000 telephone survey, some 17 percent of 1,500 adults 45–64 years of age said a parent, other relative, or other person for whom they felt responsible lived in an age-qualified community for adults 55 years or more or 62 years or more (NIC, 2000). In a 2006 survey, approximately 3 percent of adult children in this same age bracket who have a living parent, stepparent, or parent-in-law reported that at least one of these family members is currently in an assisted living residence; and slightly more than 19 percent

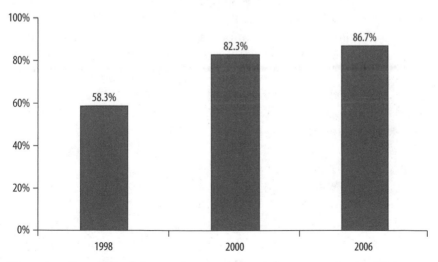

Figure 6.11. Proportion of the population age 60+ who are aware of assisted living residence

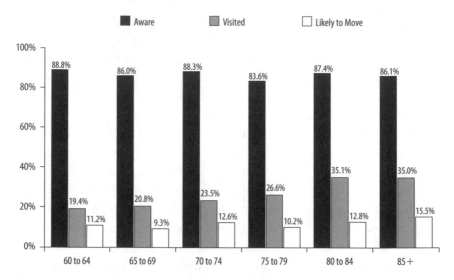

Figure 6.12. Proportion of the population age 65+ who are aware of, have visited, or are likely to move to an assisted living residence if circumstances warrant a move

had a parent, stepparent, or parent-in-law who lives in age-qualified housing (ProMatura Group, 2006).

The proportion of adult children who have learned about an assisted living residence because their parent or another relative, a friend or colleague told them about it, or know someone who lives in an assisted living residence has increased significantly in the past six years (Figure 6.13). In 2000, 6.3 percent of the adult children said their parents or another relative told them about the assisted living residence (NIC, 2000); in 2006, that figure was 30 percent (ProMatura Group, 2006). Similarly in 2000, 14 percent of adult children surveyed said they knew someone who lived in an assisted living residence (NIC, 2000) compared to 21 percent in 2006 (ProMatura Group, 2006).

Customers' Acceptance of an Assisted Living Residence, 2006–2026

Many factors will influence customers' acceptance of assisted living in the years to come. Whether the future will bear out the fundamental prediction that a greater proportion of physically and cognitively frail elders will be served by assisted living remains to be seen. This section speculates about the future customer's acceptance of future assisted living residences based on conclusions drawn from primary and secondary data analysis; observation of and discussions with hundreds of assisted living residents and their families; work with front-line employees, management, and owners of assisted living residences; and my own experience as both a provider and a customer.

The evidence suggests that prospective customers will continue to want to remain in their current home and avoid moving to a property that is perceived as a "care" facility. That said, at least five forces are likely to influence the size of the market for assisted living: the availability of a labor force willing to provide care for others, the rise of active adult housing, the change of the assisted living model from rental to ownership, the increase in accessible residences, and customers' attitudes toward aging. Although some of these factors examined next might individually suggest that more consumers will seek out assisted living, taken together they are likely to contribute to *less,* rather than more, overall demand for assisted living in the next two decades.

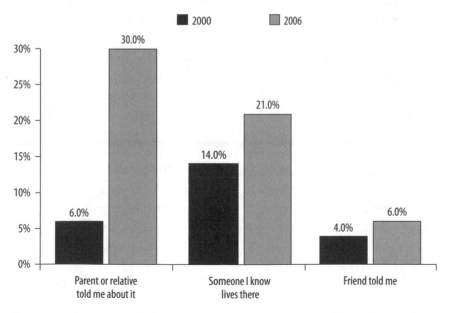

Figure 6.13. Proportion of adult children with a parent in assisted living, by how they first learned about assisted living

The Changing Labor Force

In the next 20 years

- Baby boomers will leave the work force in increasing numbers;
- The oldest old will continue to be the fastest growing segment of all age groups;
- Immigration will peak around the year 2010 as a result of the 1986 Immigration Reform and Control Act;
- Youth participation in the labor force will decline; and
- The disparity in the dependency ratio (the proportion of working individuals to support those who are not working) will grow (Toossi, 2005).

Two of these trends are especially relevant to assisted living. First, the number of available workers is shrinking relative to the number of people who need services. The annual growth rate of the 55-plus age group is projected to be nearly four times greater than the growth of the overall labor force. A smaller work force means that it will be harder to find employees willing to perform distasteful jobs. Second, the work force is becoming more culturally diverse. A work force that has greater cultural diversity means that the consumer looking for help at home must be prepared to interact with a multi-cultural work force or to be prepared to accept services from the agency that is adept at managing this work force.

In the end, however, it is projected that, because of the shortage of personnel, the cost of private domestic help and personal care may be too great for the majority of individual households to afford in their own homes. Consequently, they will be driven to purchase these services from an assisted living residence. The dynamics of the labor force, then, would seem to favor predictions about increasing reliance on assisted living.

Active Adult Housing

The Silent Generation is the predominant market for active adult housing today. The boom in the active adult housing market, which has begun in this decade and will likely continue for the next 20 years, will affect the demand for assisted living. An active adult housing community provides many of the basic ingredients that people need when moving to an assisted living residence: social contact, a sense of safety and security, access to resources, and an accessible residence that promotes easy living in a maintenance free environment.

Active adult communities used to be considered a sunbelt-targeted resort product dependent on attracting thousands of homebuyers to large developments. Today active adult communities are being built in every state, varying in size from two dozen to several thousand homes and located in towns of just a few thousand inhabitants to the large populated center cities of metropolitan areas. These attributes of active adult communities, the concentration of many 55-plus adult households in proximity to each other, and the desire of homeowners to remain in their homes will create environments likely to compete directly with assisted living residences.

Most consumers of active adult housing move to these communities between the ages of 62 and 79 for three primary reasons: the single-level floor plan, freedom from responsibility for household maintenance and upkeep, and the opportunity to enjoy a lifestyle in which getting together with others is simple. When active adult communities are built, the homes are sold to people of about the same age. In time, the community gets older together, whereupon greater numbers of its members require services and help with daily living. As this occurs, they tell their neighbors about the resources they are using. Before long, the service agencies establish a presence in or near the community and provide the resources many need to remain in their homes longer, perhaps even indefinitely. The service agencies find the enclaves with higher proportions of adults who require assistance or care to be a cost-effective environment because they can deliver services to multiple customers within a limited geographic area.

Depending on the size and location of the active adult community, the homeowner may be able to obtain most of the goods and services he or she needs without using a vehicle. Some active adult communities attract retail and service establishments that cater to this market sector and other communities have built near these resources. Clever homeowners recognize the advantages of being able to walk or travel to a grocery store in a golf cart or on a three-wheeled bicycle.

Change of the Assisted Living Model to Home Ownership

We noted at the outset that consumers age 70 or more prefer to own their homes. This trend is not likely to change, first because consumers remain enamored with home ownership and the sense of control it gives them, and second because many developers of age-qualified housing are catering to the homeowners' market. New models of assisted living residences offer condominium or fee-simple ownership, with the promise that if the homeowner needs assistance, the residence's professional managers will arrange and oversee provision of services to the customer in his or her home.

Customers understand the advantages of home ownership, and despite the inevitabilities of an aging body, they are reluctant to give up this level of control. Thus, the ownership model is likely to have significant appeal and could change the future assisted living customer at initial buy-in from someone who is older and frailer to someone who is slightly younger and who has fewer limitations.

Increase in "Easy Living" (Accessible) Homes

The demand for and acceptance of design- and architecturally accessible housing is increasing and consumers will expect to have better choices of environments that will enable them to overcome their frailties. The accessible housing movement has been slow to establish because most builders and homebuyers have equated accessible housing with wheelchair use by people with specific disabilities, not with functional design for persons with a range of different limitations.

The building industry is beginning to recognize, however, that, by 2011, more than 50 percent of the homeowners in the United States will be more than 55 years of age (Emrath, 2006). The industry is also learning that an easy living design—such as fewer stairs, low or no thresholds, stacked closets, adaptable to the introduction of home elevators, spacious showers with seats—is desired by home buyers. As the number of homes designed for easy living increases, however, more purchasers will be able to remain in their homes longer, thereby reducing the demand for assisted living.

Consumers Will Continue to Open the Front Door and Say, "I'm not ready yet"

More than ever, we want to stay young, so well evinced by the increased demand for cosmetic surgery. The American Society of Aesthetic Plastic Surgeons reported that between 2003 and 2004 there was a 44 percent increase in the number of cosmetic procedures overall; and the number of procedures for women increased by 49 percent (American Society of Aesthetic Plastic Surgeons, 2004).

Becoming older does not increase one's desire to live among those who are frail. Prospective customers of assisted living will size up future neighbors and determine whether these are the people they want to see everyday. The reality is that they will open the doors of assisted living residences and see people who are frailer and less able than themselves, whereupon they will close the door and go home and hang on for as long as they can in their homes where they are not constantly reminded of human limitations.

Assisted Living Regulation Will Increase

Competition is healthy. Many consumers welcome having different options, and they are helped in their efforts by providers who are willing to push the envelope and satisfy eclectic life-styles rather than complying strictly with regulations. Indeed, many in the industry would argue that it needs to be driven more by consumers' preferences and less by minimal standards set by the government.

Consumers are not enamored with government regulations. According to a 2004 AARP survey, only 31 percent of those born between 1900 and 1924, 34 percent of those born between 1925 and 1942 (the Silent Generation), and 34 percent of baby boomers (born between 1946 and 1964) believe there should be more government regulation (Love, 2004). One 2005 poll revealed that 62 percent of 1,004 randomly selected likely voters held negative views of the government's handling of health care issues (Zogby, 2005).

The imposition of government regulations creates "Catch 22" environments. The consumer wants something different, but the property does not provide it because the response would not be compliant with regulations or because they do not want to expend the effort and they blame it on the regulations. The consumer wants to complain but does not want to get the residence into trouble, and thus regulation designed to protect may succeed in holding back better service, warmer environments, change for the better, and spontaneity—all of which could make life more fun, interesting, and worth living.

If assisted living becomes more heavily regulated, the most successful providers will be those who know how to make the regulations transparent to the consumer and can offer creative responses that camouflage regulations. Although the Silent Generation is supposed to be compliant and accepting, when it comes to living with something that is believed not to be working, this group has demonstrated the verve to escape from a bad situation. Options and competition yield power to the consumer.

Big versus Small and the Meaning of Home

Except those catering to high-end niche consumers, smaller, freestanding, independent "mom-and-pop" assisted living residences will slowly give way to larger, professionally managed assisted living buildings. But during the next 20 years customer acceptance of larger residences will be mixed as a result of the interplay of three factors: the fact that people want to feel "at home" regardless of where they live; that homeownership among households age 70 or more is at an all-time high and is growing; and that a greater proportion of the growing number of future customers are buying condominiums in multifamily, multistory buildings.

In and of itself, the larger, "more professional" assisted living community managed by a corporation may not play well with consumer's expectations. The extent to which these corporations can manage the customer experience will determine whether these properties will continue to be successful. Satisfaction surveys to date have shown that a higher proportion of residents who live in small rather than large assisted living residences are very satisfied. Moreover, managing the customer experience must go beyond creating luxurious apartments, having the appropriate levels of care, and providing delicious and nutritious meals. The most successful providers will be those who can create and sustain "home."

Consumers will not flock to larger, more professionally managed properties unless they are perceived as homelike. When the relationship of the

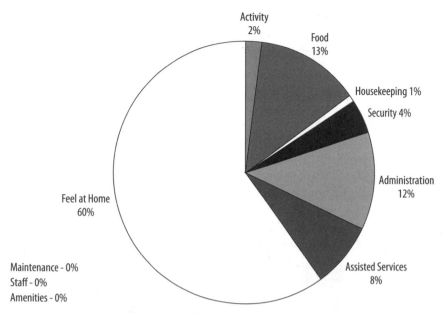

Figure 6.14. Results of satisfaction surveys of assisted living customers (residents) and the extent to which feeling at home and each service area correlated with "overall sense of satisfaction"

assisted living customers' ratings of the extent to which they feel "at home" in the assisted living residence is analyzed with other service components (Figure 6.14) to see the relationship of each attribute to their sense of satisfaction, we observe that "feeling at home" has the strongest impact on the experience of assisted living. It is the single strongest determinant of their willingness to recommend the assisted living residence to a friend, their sense of value for the money spent, their overall satisfaction with the services they receive and their overall sense of satisfaction with their quality of life in the community. Even as customers want a sense of "home," however, we still have much to understand about what creates this sense of contentment before providers of a multiple-property corporation can systematically create the appropriate conditions.

Most satisfaction surveys have concentrated on the traditional service areas: staff performance, the activities available to residents, food services, housekeeping services, maintenance, safety and security, administration (administrator and front office staff), amenities, and personal care services. Few address the relationship between customers' overall sense of satisfac-

TABLE 6.1

Attributes of Assisted Living Residence and Their Relationships to the Assisted Living Customers' Sense of Feeling at Home

Variation (%)	Attribute
11.0	The opportunity to pursue my own interests (variety and number of educational programs and the quality of social activities)
10.5	Friendliness and courteousness of staff
9.9	The quality, variety, and frequency of fitness programs
8.7	The quality and variety of food and the overall dining experience
8.1	The quality and timeliness of maintenance services
6.5	The sense of safety and security
6.0	The quality, variety, and frequency of day trips
5.0	The quality and timeliness of housekeeping services
4.8	The extent to which friendships have been formed with other residents and staff
4.5	The friendliness and courteousness of the executive director
4.3	The friendliness and courteousness of the dining room servers
4.0	The opportunity to volunteer outside of the assisted living residence
2.6	The quality and timeliness of personal care services
86.0	Total variance explained among those who strongly agreed they "feel at home"

tion and the extent to which they "feel at home" and in turn the extent to which they "feel alive."

What best explains assisted living customers' sense of "feeling at home"? To address this question, a factor analysis (a type of multivariate statistical analysis) was used to identify the key clusters of correlates of why respondents strongly agreed with the statement that, "They feel at home in the assisted living residence." We identified thirteen factors that explained 86 percent of the response variation (Table 6.1). The attributes of the assisted living residences and the percent of variation each explained are shown in Table 6.1.

These results suggest that it is the quality of daily living, and not necessarily the quality of care, that creates happy customers. The results are extremely limited, however, because they were derived from surveys that have only begun to address quality-of-life issues. More work is required to define what it takes to improve the sense of feeling at home in an assisted living community.

A New Paradigm for Assisted Living

The importance for customers of feeling "at home" suggests the need for a new paradigm for assisted living. It embodies a culture of customer service that not only sustains the technical quality of care but also ensures that residents' interactions with staff and their overall experience offer that vital sense of "home." By thinking in terms of residents' "living of daily life" and focusing on the components of high-quality customer service, assisted living residences can better meet the many challenges the future holds.

A Culture of Quality Customer Service Focused on Living of Daily Life
Living of Daily Life

Table 6.1 showed that the attributes of an assisted living community that influenced the "sense of home" were pursuing one's own interests, opportunities to do something interesting during the day, and the friendliness and courteousness of the residence's employees. The industry needs to see these components of "Living of Daily Life" (LDLs) as something they can and should address, just as they do with responding to their residents' activities of daily living (ADLs). If they understand these customers' wants, they will be more successful at creating the assisted living "home."

Individuals' LDLs should not be projected solely from their physical capabilities, but rather should be based on their wants. This approach is unlikely to require a cadre of new employees. It will, however, require better understanding of the individual, better education and empowerment of employees, and greater facilitation of individualization and freedom among customers. It means learning more about our customers, and creating a culture for employees that recognizes it means more to the customer to have the employee spend a few minutes chatting with them than carefully making up his or her bed. Improving the LDLs for customers will require culture change among most of today's assisted living residences.

Customer Service

The assisted living industry has made great strides in providing high-quality care but has not yet centered on customer service. As is true for other services, it is necessary to focus on the individual as a paying customer in control of his or her purchase of assisted living services. The person is buying our services and is not one of "our" residents. We do not own the customer; rather, he or she decides to purchase or not to purchase our services.

To date, the assisted living industry has more or less left customer service up to the individual employee, but has provided this staff person with little guidance. Employee education now includes learning about the changes in aging, the rules and methods for providing service, the dos and don'ts of the particular community, and emergency procedures. In contrast, customer service is left to chance or to a belief that if we treat our employees well, they will treat our customers well.

It is not that owners and most managers do not know what constitutes high-quality customer service. They themselves have experienced it in fine restaurants and hotels, on cruise ships, and in good department stores, but many, if not most, frontline employees may never have experienced top quality customer service. How will they know how to deliver a service they have never known? Your frontline employee most likely does not know how to say, "I don't know, but I'll find out and get right back to you" or "I'm really sorry, but I'm not allowed to help you with that. Please let me call someone to assist you."

Residents will not tell someone about how they were assisted with their bath, but they will communicate that the aide took a few extra moments to warm the bath towel in the dryer. A resident is not likely to pay too much attention to the way an employee brought the dining tray to her room when she was not feeling well, but she will be delighted when that employee says, "Is there anything that I may do for you before I leave?"

Instead of "customer service" being a once-per-quarter in-service program or maybe a few pages in a notebook, it must become a process incorporated into every aspect and level of the community. An effective culture of customer service will take the form of a fundamental outlook and set of standards and practices used by every employee to provide service of consistently high quality. Specifically, a culture of quality customer service is one in which:

1. All employees believe in its processes and benefits.
2. The procedures incorporated in the customer service program produce immediate results.
3. All employees recognize the benefits of the program and adopt the standards as their own.
4. The components of the customer service can be learned and assimilated readily into daily practice.
5. The performance of high-quality customer services can be observed, measured, and rewarded.

6. Is self-sustaining because it is right, it is good, it is teachable, and the results realized by the employee are sufficient reinforcement for them to repeat the level of quality service again.

A high-quality customer service program yields many benefits:

1. Increase in resident and family satisfaction.
2. Increase in occupancy.
3. Increase in personal job satisfaction and happiness of employees.
4. Reduction in employee turnover.
5. Improved services.
6. More and better communication among all parties: staff, management, residents, and families.

Components of a High-Quality Service Program

Management must introduce several components if an effective, culture-changing program of high-quality customer service is to be assimilated into an assisted living residence. These include promise keeping, employee education, ways to make the program self-sustaining, and performance measures.

Promises

The first necessary component is the core set of promises that will be kept. These core promises are the high-quality service initiatives that will be delivered every time the opportunity to practice them arises. These are promises that every employee can positively and absolutely deliver at each opportunity.

A promise may be something as simple as "Always greet someone who comes into your space." Your space is defined as a room, an area out of doors, or a corridor, anywhere you are within speaking range of an individual. The customer service that will be adhered to by every employee all of the time is that you will look up, make eye contact, smile, and greet or welcome any person who comes into your space.

Another simple promise is that, regardless of what you are doing, you will always acknowledge someone's presence, even if you are unable to speak to him or her at the moment. In conducting hundreds of mystery hunts of assisted living residences where a researcher posed as an adult child seeking an assisted living residence for her parent, it has been disheartening to observe the number of times the shopper has been kept standing in front of a receptionist's desk without the receptionist even so much as looking at the visitor, even though it is obvious the receptionist knows the visitor is there. The receptionist does not have to do anything but look at the visitor, smile, and hold up a finger to indicate it will be just a bit before she can get to the visitor. To ignore someone is an unforgivable offense to an individual. Yet I have observed this behavior countless times in community after community.

Method to Educate Employees and Help Them Communicate with Customers

The effective customer service program must use a variety of education methods, particularly self-paced methods, to train employees and continually provide them feedback on their progress. There should be easy and multiple reminders throughout their day of when, where, what, and how to deliver quality customer service.

Employees must be taught the words that will help them improve their service, they must be given an opportunity to practice the right words, and they should be rewarded for working to improve their skills.

Method to Keep the Program Self-Sustaining

A high-quality service program will become part of the culture of an assisted living residence only if it is self-sustaining. If it depends on management to line up in-service "training" sessions, it is likely to falter. The educational program must be incorporated into the daily routines of the community and assimilated by employees to the extent that they teach new employees by example and have a sense of pride in saying, "This is the way we do it here."

Method to Measure Progress and Reward Performance

Frontline employees are assisted living's key to success, yet they are the lowest-paid and least-recognized employees. When employees are surveyed to learn what they want most as "rewards" for adopting high-quality customer service procedures, they were most excited by an opportunity to advance. They did not need trinkets or cash incentives to be motivated; they just wanted an opportunity to succeed and for their success to be recognized.

Steps to Develop a Lasting High-Quality Customer Service Program

1. Get everybody on board. Absolutely everyone in the organization, from the bottom to the top, must believe in, practice, and support the program.
2. Determine what your promise(s) will be. Pick key promises that everyone will deliver. They should be visible; have an immediate, positive effect on customers; and be easy to keep consistently, correctly, and repeatedly.
3. Determine how you can always deliver on those promises. These fundamental, faithfully kept promises form the foundation for your program. If you cannot figure out how these fundamental promises can be always honored, you need to identify other promises that you absolutely and positively will keep.
4. Develop educational programs to teach skills and attributes that will ensure your promises are kept. You will need to invest in these educational programs. This does not mean that they must be expensive or require elaborate audiovisual materials. You need to invest in them to ensure they provide palatable education that is rewarding and empowering for your employees.
5. Make the education easy, progressive, self-paced, individualized, and accessible.
6. Post reminders (subtle and specific) everywhere, including in employees' pockets or as part of their name badge. Give your employees easy tools they can use so that they are reminded of what to do, when to do it, and the right words to use. It is usually the right words that your employees have difficulty finding. So give them the right words to say something negative in a positive manner. Give them the words so that they can be comfortable in an uncomfortable situation. Give them the gift of the right words so they feel strong in a situation where they may have felt tenuous.
7. Develop the process for one employee to teach or share with other employees. If the quality customer service program can be learned, practiced, and assimilated by every employee, each employee should be capable of mentoring a new employee. Give them the opportunity to be the experts.

8. Create opportunities for people to be rewarded. There are many rewards that fit well in a customer service program. Ensure that your rewards are meaningful and distributed fairly among all levels of employees.
9. Include a method for your employees to advance (position, pay, benefits, stature, educational opportunities, etc.).

Conclusions and Implications for the Future

Future customers will have many choices. There will be consolidation in the assisted living industry and its products and services will continue to evolve. Successful providers will be those who know their customers and how they can enhance customers' lives.

Customers will increasingly measure their satisfaction with their assisted living experience based on how well their residential environment and services improve their living of daily life. If they live their daily life in a manner that is consistent with their sense of self, are provided with quality service that affirms their existence, and are known as persons, for who they were, are, and still can be, they are likely to be customers who say, "I'm home."

REFERENCES

American Association of Retired Persons. 2005a. *Beyond 50.05: A report to the nation on livable communities creating environments for successful aging.* Washington, DC: American Association of Retired Persons.
American Association of Retired Persons. 2005b. *Older persons and wireless telephone use.* Washington, DC: American Association of Retired Persons.
American Association of Retired Persons. 2006. *The state of 50+ America 2006.* Washington, DC: American Association of Retired Persons.
American Society of Aesthetic Plastic Surgeons. *Highlights of the ASAPS 2004 statistics on cosmetic surgery.* www.cosmeticplasticsurgerystatistics.com/statistics.
Emrath, P. 2006. *Profile of the 50+ housing market, 50+ demographics, 50+ housing council.* www.nahb.org.
Love, J. 2004. *Political behaviors and values across the generations: A summary of selected findings.* Washington, DC: American Association of Retired Persons.
National Investment Center for the Seniors Housing and Care Industry. 2000. *NIC national survey of adult children: How they Influence their parents' housing*

and care decisions. Annapolis, MD: National Investment Center for the Seniors Housing and Care Industry. www.nic.org.

National Investment Center for the Seniors Housing and Care Industry. 2001. *NIC national housing survey of adults 60+.* Annapolis, MD: National Investment Center for the Seniors Housing and Care Industry. www.nic.org.

National Investment Center for the Seniors Housing and Care Industry. 2006. *NIC MAP 30 MetroMarket Benchmarker: Data from the thirty largest metropolitan statistical areas, quarter Ending March 31, 2006.* Annapolis, MD: National Investment Center for the Seniors Housing and Care Industry.

ProMatura Group, LLC. 2006. *Proprietary study of 5,000+ households headed by someone 45+ years of age: Their current home, their plans to move, and their parents' current home and their plans for parents.* Oxford, MS: ProMatura Group.

Toossi, M. 2005. Labor force projections to 2014: Retiring boomer. *Monthly Labor Review,* November, pp. 25–44.

U.S. Department of Commerce. 2002. *Census of the United States.* Washington, DC: Government Printing Office.

Zogby International. 2005. *Zogby American poll, October.* www.zogby.com.

CHAPTER 7

Family Care and Assisted Living

An Uncertain Future?

DOUGLAS A. WOLF, PH.D.
CAROL JENKINS, PH.D.

Throughout the years, there have been numerous assertions that emerging social trends threaten the functioning—and even the existence—of "the family" and, in particular, its capacity or willingness to serve as a source of care for elderly individuals. In the 1970s a great deal of geronto-logical research aimed at refuting the myth that family members had abandoned their older members (Shanas, 1979). During the 1980s and 1990s, research turned to documenting the burdens borne by family members involved in providing informal elder care (Anthony-Bergstone, Zarit, & Gatz, 1988). The most current evidence confirms that the family remains the bedrock of long-term care despite studies showing the adverse social, health, and economic consequences associated with caregiving.

Nonetheless, concerns continue to be expressed regarding the sustainability of the family-care system. For example, Angel and Angel expressed fears that "the greater occupational and geographical mobility, higher female labor force participation, lower fertility, and rising family disruption that characterize our modern world must inevitably affect the family's ability and willingness to provide support to the elderly" (1997, pp. 88–

89). Depending on one's perspective, the growth of assisted living appears to pose yet another threat to the family's place in the world of elder care or a new source of relief from the burden of family caregiving.

Promotional materials for assisted living emphasize "independence"— the Assisted Living Federation of America's online "Guide to Choosing an Assisted Living Residence" (ALFA, n.d.) uses the word (or variations on it) six times on just its first page (see chapter 9). Moreover, assisted living typically offers housekeeping and transportation services as well as congregate meals and help with such daily activities as eating and dressing, many of which are activities in which family caregivers ordinarily play a major role (Wolf, 2004). "Independence," however, need not preclude family care; the same ALFA document notes that assisted living "encourages the involvement of a resident's family and friends."

Although assisted living's sales pitch appears to encourage substitution of formal for family care, there are some countervailing factors. For example, assisted living residences are likely to not retain residents with moderate to severe cognitive impairments or with behavioral symptoms associated with dementia, such as wandering (Hawes et al., 2003). In contrast, family members—especially spouses and children—are deeply involved in the supervision and care of community-dwelling older people suffering from such conditions.

This chapter explores the relationship between assisted living and family care and the direction in which that relationship is likely to evolve as assisted living continues to grow. We draw on both recent literature and the results of our analysis of data from the Health and Retirement Survey to form an image of what the world of family care will look like in 15–20 years. That world will be shaped by the context in which decisions to move to an assisted living residence are made, including major trends in several factors that influence those decisions. It will also be influenced by the unique characteristics of assisted living residents compared to elders living in the community and in nursing homes. We must also understand what research tells us about how family members are currently involved in providing care for residents in assisted living. We conclude with some reflections about how further growth in the assisted living sector might be accompanied by changes in family care during the coming years.

The recent literature reveals that family care does not end with an older person's entry into assisted living. The families of assisted living residents continue to provide care and also monitor the care and services provided as part of the assisted living package. Depending on the type of residence, family members help with a variety of activities ranging from housework, laundry, and transportation to personal care. They sometimes participate in the health-related care received by the resident, particularly end-of-life care. They want to participate in care and treatment decisions and are more satisfied when they can do so. Family members often focus on the quality of care provided to older relatives and are especially concerned about safety issues. They want to see their older relatives living in a home-like situation and ensure that they have a clean personal space. Such involvement suggests that families have the potential to affect the future of assisted living significantly, including how it is regulated, how quality of care is defined and assured, and what services are offered.

The Nature of Family Care

Family care—a type of "informal," unpaid care—is generally contrasted with formal, or paid, services. Both categories of care can take place in community settings, in assisted living residences, and in nursing homes or other specialized settings. For family care, however, it is much more difficult to distinguish between caregiving—that is, giving "aid or assistance to other family members beyond that required as part of normal everyday life"—and the "aid given as a part of the normal exchange in family relationships" (Walker, Pratt, & Eddy, 1995, pp. 402–403). The specific tasks typically mentioned in accounts of caregiving include activities of daily living (ADLs), such as eating, dressing, bathing, using the toilet, and transferring (in and out of bed or chair), and instrumental activities of daily living (IADLs), which include shopping, housework, laundry, and meal preparation. Particularly with respect to the latter tasks, family members often help out even in the absence of need for help or of disability; thus, the measurement of family care involves some arbitrariness and ambiguity.

It should also be noted that, whereas "living arrangements" and "care arrangements" are conceptually distinct, they are nonetheless closely related dimensions of the organization and quality of life for older people. Much of the literature on the living arrangements of older people focuses exclusively on the presence or absence of others—especially family members—in the household. Co-residence with adult children clearly facilitates the provision of informal care and, indeed, often occurs for exactly that reason. Institutional residence, in contrast, necessarily implies a heavy reliance on formal care, although it does not rule out informal care by family members. Finally, many older people live alone while receiving help from formal caregivers, informal caregivers, or both. Because an older person's living arrangement may include both family members and other helpers, decisions regarding living and care arrangements are often complex.

We use the term *community dwelling* to refer to older people living in nonspecialized housing, whether alone or with others and whether or not that housing may have been modified or adapted (e.g., with ramps, grab bars or other equipment) to meet the needs of individuals with functional difficulties. The community setting, which is commonly associated with the capacity for self-care or independent living, lies at one end of a continuum, whereas the nursing home represents the other, most dependent, end of this continuum. Assisted living residences fall somewhere between these extremes, depending on the services they offer and the needs of their residents.

The Changing Context of Elder Care Decisions

The decision to move into assisted living, as well as whether to continue family involvement in care, depends on several factors, including the older person's needs and preferences for care, the family's ability and willingness to provide care, and available alternatives to family care. The factors that give rise to older people's needs for care and the living and care arrangements that arise in response to those needs create a highly dynamic situation—and thus one whose future is quite uncertain.

The Need for Care

How much and what kind of care elders will need in coming decades is difficult to predict. Different trends in health status among the older population tend to pull against each other. Disability appears to be decreasing at the same time that the incidence of chronic illness is rising.

The prevalence of disability among the older population fell during the 1980s and 1990s (Manton & Gu, 2001; Freedman et al., 2004; Spillman, 2004). The prevalence of cognitive impairment (including various types of dementia), which is closely linked to disability and the need for care and supervision, has also declined (Freedman, Aykan, & Martin, 2002;

Liao, McGee, Cao, & Cooper, 2000; Manton, Stallard, & Corder, 1998). By themselves, these trends suggest shrinking needs for family care, at least in a relative sense (see chapter 2).

Other, concurrent, trends, however, argue for caution in extrapolating these recent declines in disability. For example, during the same period that disability rates fell, the prevalence of several chronic diseases and conditions associated with disability—for example, osteoporosis, hip fractures, cancer, stroke, and diabetes—actually *rose* (Crimmins, 2004; Freedman & Martin, 2000). Still other conditions associated with care needs, such as vision and hearing problems, showed no apparent trends upward or downward during these years (Desai, Pratt, Lentzner, & Robinson, 2001; Lee, Gómez-Marín, Lam, & Zheng, 2004). Attempts to explain the recent improvements in disability at older ages often point to the role of education, noting the rising levels of educational attainment of older people over time (Freedman & Soldo, 1994; Zimmer & House, 2003), but others have cautioned that because there is a limit on the potential educational attainment distribution for any given cohort the trend toward improved educational levels will gradually taper off (Wolf, 2001). As the trend toward improved educational attainment tapers off, the trend toward reduced prevalence of disability may taper off as well. In view of the available evidence, then, we cannot say with certainty how needs for care are most likely to evolve among elders and thus what impact need for care will have on care and living arrangements.

The Family as a Source of Care

Although the family remains the principal source of care and assistance for older people, its place in the elder care system is shaped by numerous dynamic factors. Among the most important are demographic changes, reflected in the age structure of the population as well as in family structure and familial and social attitudes toward elder care.

Demographic Change

Possibly the best-known contemporary demographic fact is that the population is growing older. Both the average age of the population and the proportion of the population older than 65 are growing and are projected to continue growing. According to U.S. Census Bureau projections, in the two decades between 2010 and 2030, the population of individuals

65 or older will grow rapidly as a proportion of the total, from 13.0 percent to 19.6 percent (He, Sengupta, Velkoff, & DeBarros, 2005). In contrast, before 2010 and after 2030 the projected decade-to-decade change is more gradual.

All things being equal, growth in the percentage of the population older than 65 can be expected to increase the overall level of family caregiving. As the population gets older, the ratio of older people—those with the greatest care needs—to younger people—those likely to provide care—grows. The increased longevity that contributes to population aging also implies that a greater proportion of older people will have a living spouse. Because spouses, along with children, provide a majority of family care, the aging of the population is likely to encourage growth in family care.

The rapid demographic change projected to occur between 2010 and 2030 is, of course, a consequence of the passage into "old age" of the baby boom generation, a phenomenon nearly universally expected to place unprecedented strains on public budgets. Population aging is widely viewed as a threat to public programs that contribute to late-life well-being, especially Social Security and Medicare. Any cutbacks to these major programs would further increase the pressure on family members to provide care and services that might otherwise be collectively provided (see chapters 11 and 14).

At the same time, however, other demographic trends suggest possible erosion of family care. One such trend is the growing prevalence of childlessness. Figure 7.1 shows trends in childlessness among ever-married women age 40–44 from 1940 to 2002. Trends for 40–44 year old women of all marital statuses are also shown, although the latter series is available only from 1976 onward. Few women have their first child after age 44, so the percentage of women childless at age 40–44 provides a very accurate picture of childlessness in the population. As Figure 7.1 shows, the prevalence of childlessness reached its low point around 1980. For women in this cohort, their years of peak childbearing coincided with the baby boom. Since 1980 the percentage of women ending up without children has grown, although it appears to have leveled off after 2000. The implications of these fertility patterns for care in old age, however, arise only after a considerable delay. For example, those 40–44 in 1980—a group with relatively high fertility—will be 80–84 in 2020. Only after 2020 will the ranks of the "oldest old" exhibit a growing prevalence of childlessness.

Other demographic trends may also tend to decrease family caregiving.

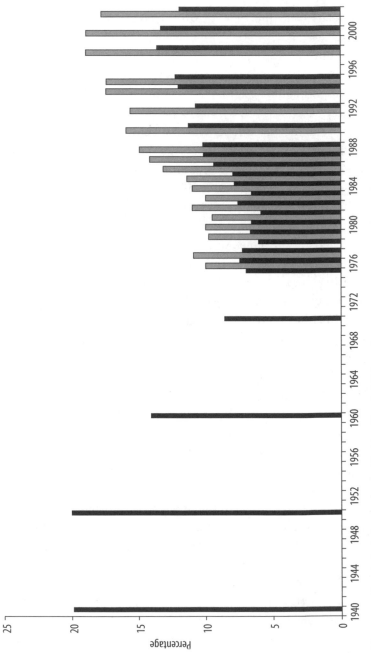

Figure 7.1. Proportion of women age 40–44 without children, by year

For example, the average age at which women have children has also risen for more than two decades (Mathews & Hamilton, 2002). Later childbearing, all things being equal, will create a larger pool of women "caught in the middle" between simultaneous claims on their time from their parents and their children. Also, divorce has become more common within the older population. Divorce not only removes a potential spousal caregiver but also tends to reduce the quality and quantity of parent-child contacts (Lye, Klepinger, Hyle, & Nelson, 1995), with implications for the availability of care from adult children. Similarly, the continued trend toward greater labor force participation by women may strain their capacity to serve as caregivers within the family.

Norms and Attitudes

Attitudes and beliefs regarding giving and accepting care influence care decisions. Within the family, care decisions are made in the context of norms of responsibility, reciprocity, and affection. The availability of supportive formal care, which is influenced by societal attitudes about who is responsible for caring for frail elders, affects these decisions as well, and because living and care arrangements are so closely related, attitudes about household structure will also influence care decisions.

Differences in living arrangements and household composition among racial or ethnic groups in the United States and elsewhere have been attributed to cultural factors and differing norms of behavior (Burr & Mutchler 1993; Wilmoth, 2001; Tomassini et al., 2004). The fact that many white elders in the United States live independently—that is, in a private home or apartment, with or without additional help from others—may have much to do with preferences to live separately from adult children. There is little agreement about changing trends in norms or preferences. Some researchers suggest that long-term trends toward smaller households and independent living arrangements are associated with changing norms or preferences (Burch & Matthews, 1982); others argue that preferences have remained fairly stable, whereas the capacities and resources that support independent living have grown over time (Beresford & Rivlin, 1966; Schoeni & McGarry, 2000). For our purposes, what is relevant is the fact that preferences in favor of independent living remain very strong (Mack et al., 1997). Furthermore, people not presently living in nursing homes have a strong aversion to entering a nursing home (Kane & Kane, 2001).

Together, we expect that these attitudes will encourage, and be reinforced by, continued growth in the availability of assisted living options.

Public policy can also be influenced by attitudes about caregiving. For example, Silverstein and colleagues found that people's stated willingness to expand public benefits for older people decreased throughout the 1980s and 1990s (Silverstein, Angelelli, & Parrott, 2001). There is, however, also a high level of public support for government programs that support family caregivers (Silverstein & Parrott, 2001). Thus, declining support for government assistance, in general, appears to be coupled with growing support for "family-friendly" policies. Such support, generally, may reflect both a general belief that providing care for elders is primarily a family, as opposed to a societal, responsibility and a willingness to make public resources available to aid families in that endeavor. We are not aware of any research on trends in older people's attitudes about accepting, or younger people's attitudes about providing, informal care. Whatever those attitudes might be, informal care remains a highly prevalent behavior.

Alternatives to Family Care

The availability of other ways of providing care also has implications for how direct a role families play in elder care. In particular, the evolution of assistive technologies and the design of living environments to accommodate various levels of disability, along with incentives for and against family care created by public policies, shape the context in which decisions are made.

Assistive Technology and Environmental Features

Assistive devices and technology constitute a broad category of items ranging from the long-standing and "low-tech," such as canes and walkers, to more recent "high-tech" innovations such as robotic assistants (see chapter 8). Environmental features designed to mitigate the effects of disability include home modifications, such as grab bars, showers with integral seating, or mechanical lifting devices. Many older people with health or physiological conditions that limit their functional capacity are able to fully meet their care needs using these assistive strategies, while others make use of a combination of human and mechanical assistance.

Of particular relevance to the question of trends in family care is recent research indicating that people who use assistive technology use fewer hours of informal care (Agree et al., 2005). Trends in the use of specific devices are mixed: from 1980 to 1994, the use of crutches and artificial limbs declined, while the use of other relatively low-tech devices such as leg or foot braces, canes, walkers, and wheelchairs increased (Russell et al., 1997). New types of devices—for example, sensors that detect falls, or computers that monitor adherence to medication regimens—are continually being introduced, however, which suggests that overall the extent and range of technology-based elder care is growing, a trend that will, no doubt, continue. As assistive technology becomes more widely available and a more likely coping response to frailty, community-based living is likely to become more feasible even for individuals with higher levels of need; this, in turn, could serve to suppress the demand for assisted living residences.

The Role of Public Policy

Policies at all levels of government—federal, state, and local—have the potential to influence the level and nature of family care. Policies that change the relative attractiveness of, or access to, different residence types, such as nursing homes or private housing, indirectly affect family care given the significant differences across these residence types in the involvement of family members in care. Policies that subsidize or improve access to home-care services—or that reward, encourage, or even require, family care activities as a condition of programmatic eligibility or benefits—have more direct effects. Policies that regulate, subsidize, or otherwise influence the assisted living industry are relevant as well, of course (see chapter 13).

Changes over time in some federal programs have been linked to changes in living or care arrangements. For example, increases in the real value of Social Security benefits have been linked to the substantial increase in independent living by older people during the second half of the twentieth century (Michel, Fuchs, & Scott, 1980; Schoeni & McGarry, 2000). The contemporary politics of the Social Security program suggest, however, that the trend toward more generous benefits not only has ended but is also not likely to resume in future decades (see chapter 11).

At the state level, officials have considerable latitude to adopt policies that alter the relative attractiveness of different living and care arrangements for older people, with the result that state programs vary considerably in their components and their consequences. The main such program is Medicaid, through which much of the nation's nursing home and home-based long-term care costs are reimbursed. Changes in Medicaid with respect to reimbursement levels, coverage of medically needy individuals, adoption of the personal care option, and participation in waivered home health programs have all carried implications for individuals' and families' decisions about long-term care (see chapters 11 and 13).

Research has shown that other policy tools, such as certificates of need and prospective payment requirements, also affect the supply of long-term care, including both the variety of settings in which care is available and people's access to them. For example, Harrington and colleagues (Harrington, Swan, Nyman, & Carillo, 1997) found that states that used a "certificate of need" process to approve new nursing homes reduced the growth of nursing home beds between 1981 and 1993. Other research has shown that the lower the ratio of Medicaid nursing home reimbursement rates to private-pay levels, the lower the chances that a Medicaid-eligible person will be admitted to such a facility (Cutler & Sheiner, 1994; Harrington Meyer, 2001). On the other hand, states' adoption of the "medically needy" option, by which people can be eligible if their medical expenses brings their "net income" below the threshold for Medicaid, enhances access to nursing homes (Cutler & Sheiner, 1994) and promotes use of home health services (Harrington et al., 2000). Very little research has addressed whether state-level policy choices such as these have any effects on informal care activities. However, Wallace and colleagues (Wallace, Levy-Storms, Kington, & Anderson, 1998) found that states' imposition of a moratorium on expanding the number of Medicaid nursing home beds increased the chances that an older person would rely exclusively on informal home care services.

Public policy also has very direct effects on assisted living: several states have begun to provide some Medicaid coverage of assisted living services. As of 2001, 38 states covered such services, mainly through home and community-based service waivers, and six states covered assisted living services under their basic program (Mollica, 2001). This coverage, however, does not extend to the basic assisted-living fees for room and board; thus, nearly all assisted living residents are on a private-pay basis.

State policies in other areas also affect the choices people make about living and care arrangements. One example of such a policy is the supplementation of Supplemental Security Income (SSI) benefits (Social Security Administration, 2005). Those states that have chosen to supplement SSI have adopted a wide range of supplementation levels. To date, however, research has not demonstrated a direct effect on whether older people choose to live independently (Favreault & Wolf, 2004). Staffing requirements for nursing homes are another area in which state policy affects care choices. Because these requirements directly affect the cost of providing nursing care, they can have a major impact on the supply of nursing home beds or on access to them. In addition, the provision of social services, such as home-delivered meals, transportation services, housekeeping and chore services, and congregate meals, all of which are largely a matter of state-level initiative, can promote independent living in the community (Krivo & Chaatsmith, 1990).

Finally, many states have developed new programs aimed at supporting family caregivers following implementation of the 2000 National Family Caregiver Support Program, which provides federal funding for caregiver support programs. Before that policy was implemented, only a few states had undertaken such programs on their own. Among the services provided under these programs are respite care, information and referral services, support groups, case management, transportation, housekeeping and chore services, counseling, cash grants, and other services, although, as of 2004, states varied considerably in the levels and types of services offered (Feinberg, Newman, Gray & Kolb, 2004). Interventions have been shown to reduce caregiver distress or depression (Burns et al., 2003; Mittelman, Roth, Coon, & Haley, 2004; Zarit, Stephens, Townsend, & Greene, 1998) and prolong the period of informal care and delay nursing home placement (Mittelman, Schulman, Steinberg, & Levin, 1996). The latter finding is of particular interest, as it indicates the potential for public programs to encourage informal caregiving by providing more, rather than fewer, services.

Differences in the Characteristics of Older People by Type of Residence

In view of the selective nature of the factors influencing the move to assisted living—a reflection, in part, of the distinctive services and amenities that such residences offer—it is not surprising that the assisted living population differs from both the community-dwelling and institutionalized (nursing home) populations. The distinctive characteristics of assisted living residents are an indication of future demand—and of possible changes in the demand—for assisted living residences. Such comparisons also help to illuminate the place of assisted living on the continuum of housing choices available to older people. Among the salient distinguishing characteristics of the occupants are their family structure, notably marital status and number of children (if any), and health status, especially level of disability.

Family Structure

Family structure has significant impacts on where an older person resides. Individuals who are unmarried, whether they have children or not, are more likely to move from a community residence (e.g., private home or apartment) to assisted living than are individuals who are married and have children. Persons who are both unmarried and do not have children are most likely to make that transition (Waidmann & Thomas, 2003). A study of residential care facilities in Oregon showed that compared to nursing home residents, older people in assisted living residences were more likely to have one or more living children (Reinardy & Kane, 2003).

The Oregon study also found that assisted living residents were much more likely to have moved from a community setting, such as a private home or retirement apartment, whereas nursing home residents were more likely to have transferred from another nursing home or an acute care setting, indicating their need for skilled care (Reinardy & Kane, 2003). Many residents reported that their decision to move was influenced by family members, while the primary decision makers for nursing home residents were professionals, including doctors, hospital discharge workers, and case managers.

Data from the Medicare Current Beneficiary Survey (MCBS) yield a similar profile of assisted living residents (Spillman, Liu, & McGilliard, 2002). They tended to be older, white, and widowed. In addition, they had higher incomes than nursing home residents. The MCBS data also reveal changes in the family characteristics of assisted living residents during the six-year period from 1992 to 1998. The proportion of assisted living residents who were ever married increased, while the proportion of those who had never been married decreased. This suggests a growing potential availability of family care for assisted living residents.

Health Status

In terms of disability, the Oregon study found that compared to nursing home residents, assisted living residents had significantly fewer ADL needs and better cognitive function (Reinardy and Kane, 2003). The MBCS data similarly indicated that assisted living residents had lower levels of disability and more were in "excellent" or "very good" health compared to nursing home residents (Spillman, Liu, & McGilliard, 2002). Trends in disability showed increasing frailty over time, with the proportion of assisted living residents who reported difficulties with only one or two ADLs decreasing from 38.5 percent in 1992 to 32.5 percent in 1998, whereas the proportion of residents who had difficulties with three or more ADLs rose dramatically, from 34.6 percent to 52.1 percent. Health status changed in a similar manner, with fewer residents reporting "excellent or very good" health and more reporting "fair or poor" health in 1998.

Findings from the Health and Retirement Survey

As a contribution to the literature on differences in individual characteristics by type of residence, we present results from our own descriptive analysis of data from the 2002 interviews conducted as part of the Retirement History Survey (for details on this data source see http://hrsonline .isr.umich.edu/). Our findings confirm the established general picture of how populations differ across living and care arrangements. Our data similarly locate the assisted living population between the community-dwelling and nursing home populations. As Table 7.1 shows, with respect to average age, percentage of residents who had a spouse or partner, and number of children, our sample of assisted living residents was more similar to the nursing home population than to community-dwelling older people, although differences in the average numbers of children were quite small.

With respect to difficulties with ADL tasks, the differences between assisted living residents and community-dwelling elders were dramatic: The assisted living population had greater care needs for each of the six ADLs included in our data set than did the community-dwelling population and was about twice as likely to have *any* ADL needs (36 percent

TABLE 7.1

Need and Family-Care Attributes of HRS Respondents Age 65 or Older, 2002,
by Type of Residence

	Type of Residence		
	Community	Assisted Living	Nursing Home
Unweighted count (%)	10,237 (94.2)	127 (1.2)	504 (4.6)
Weighted count	33,547,675	457,788	NA
Mean values of			
Age	74.4	81.1	84.1
Has spouse/partner (%)	59.7	33.1	21.2
Number of nearby children[a]	0.84	0.75	0.70
Number of additional children[a]	4.67	4.54	3.44
Has difficulty with			
Bathing (%)	8.6	19.7	72.5
Dressing (%)	10.8	19.7	61.5
Eating (%)	3.8	7.1	40.8
Transfer (%)	6.4	10.3	50.4
Toileting (%)	6.4	11.0	50.0
Walking (%)	8.4	17.3	60.0
Any ADLs (%)	20.4	36.5	79.8
Has any ADL difficulty and			
Gets help from spouse (%)	18.4	8.7	2.6
Gets help from child(ren) (%)	17.4	13.0	15.4

[a]Includes stepchildren and children-in-law.

versus 20 percent). Differences between the assisted living population and the nursing home population also followed the pattern seen elsewhere, with greater care needs among nursing home residents. The prevalence of difficulty with individual ADL tasks was much higher in the nursing home population—as much as six times higher for eating—and was more than twice as high overall (80 percent) in the nursing home as in the assisted living population.

Family Care for Assisted Living Residents

Family involvement in the care of assisted living residents begins before the individual moves to assisted living, as family members play an integral role in the decision-making process. Studies show that a large proportion of residents, perhaps as high as 90 percent, receive help in making their relocation decision and that most of that help comes from family members, particularly adult daughters and daughters-in-law (Hawes, Phillips, & Rose, 2000; Reinardy & Kane, 2003). Many owners and operators have thus begun marketing their homes directly to adult children (see chapter 6). One CEO of a large company that operates homes across the United States estimates that his company directed as much as 30 percent of its advertising dollars toward marketing to adult children (Smith, 2002).

Family members continue their involvement with older relatives after the transition to assisted living. Much of the assistance older people receive is specific to their individual needs, especially their disability level. Older and frailer residents receive both more help overall and a wider range of help from family members (Gaugler & Kane, 2001). Older residents tend to get more help with IADLs, with spouses providing most of this type of assistance (Gaugler, Anderson, & Leach, 2005). Older age and increased frailty are also associated with more frequent monitoring of care by families (Gaugler, Anderson, & Leach, 2005). Families with fewer living children are more likely to direct staff in care than are larger families, who are more likely to participate in providing care; moreover, family participation in providing assistance is enhanced in homes that encourage positive relationships between family and staff and that offer family-friendly activities (Gaugler, Anderson, & Leach, 2005).

Our analysis of HRS data shows that in all three types of residences only a minority of individuals who have difficulties with ADLs got help from a spouse or one or more children. As expected, because each type of residence is associated with progressively higher levels of formal care, the percentage of residents getting family care falls as we move from community to assisted living and from assisted living to nursing home. One surprising finding is that fewer assisted living residents who have difficulties with ADLs received help from any children (13 percent) than did nursing home residents (more than 15 percent) even though assisted living residents had both more children in total and more children living nearby, than did nursing home residents. In light of the small size of our assisted living sample (127 individuals), however, it is not clear whether this finding is generalizable.

The characteristics of assisted living homes may also influence informal care behavior. Given the wide array of available services, family members may not feel the need to provide large amounts of hands-on assistance, the most personal form of personal care. The environment in some homes may actually present disincentives for family participation. Homes that provide high-quality care by professional staff are likely to inspire a positive attitude about the home and its staff on the part of family members, which has been shown to lead to reductions in both instrumental and personal help (Gaugler & Kane, 2001).

Approximately one-third of residents remain in the assisted living residence until they die (Sloan et al., 2003). Thus, some residents will receive end-of-life care in assisted living and many providers encourage families to participate in making decisions and providing care at the end of life. Family members involved in such decision making are likely to be more satisfied with the care offered by their assisted living community (Sloane et al., 2003).

Nonetheless, there can be tension among family members and staff over the degree of family involvement, with administrators for assisted living residences tending to want more help from families than some either can or will give (Cartwright & Kayser-Jones, 2003). For their part, family members may express concern about the capability of staff to provide necessary care, especially appropriate pain management (Cartwright & Kayser-Jones, 2003). Although family satisfaction with end-of-life care is significantly higher for assisted living residences than for nursing homes (Sloane et al., 2003), a majority of families expect their older relative to move to a nursing home when care needs become greater than the assisted living provider can meet (Cartwright & Kayser-Jones, 2003).

Conclusions and Implications for the Future

The central question motivating this chapter was what the world of family care for frail elders would look like after 15 more years of growth in the assisted living industry. Taken in isolation, many trends appear clear. The reduced demand for personal assistance brought about by lower disability rates, the spread of assistive technology, and even the growth of the assisted living industry itself suggest that family care will likely decrease. Other factors, more associated with the supply of than with the demand for care, might reinforce this decrease in informal care—for example, the growing prevalence of childlessness, increasingly common divorce, and women's increasing participation in the labor force.

Yet there are also powerful forces working in the opposite direction: the sheer aging of the population implies that in the future there will be more person-years of need for elder care per potential caregiver than at present, with some portion of that need met by family members. Public policy also has the potential to affect family caregiving significantly, whether acting to encourage or discourage it. For example, states may continue to extend their coverage of assisted living services through the Medicaid program on the rationale that this promotes a lower-cost alternative to nursing homes. Demographic pressure on the social safety net, principally such high-cost items as Social Security and Medicare, however, would seem to render unlikely any major new expansions of long-term care programs, with their potential to encourage substitution of formal for informal care. Indeed, one of the newest growth areas in federal support of long-term care is the National Family Caregiver Support Program, which supports interventions intended to promote and extend family caregiving, but actual funding for the program remains relatively low, leaving states facing a demand for services that far outstrips the current supply.

In light of such offsetting trends, it is tempting to avoid attempting to predict the likely future of family care. It seems reasonable to argue that that future will not differ markedly from the present. In fact, that is our prediction. Our rationale, however, goes deeper than a simple counting up of offsetting trends. First, and most superficially, we must remember that trends do not operate individually but jointly, producing in some cases mutually reinforcing synergies and in others negative feedback loops. Second, a closer look at the several trends reveals difficult and unresolved questions concerning just what is cause and what is effect, and, therefore, which trends can be expected to continue. For example, some have argued that the downward trends in disability at older ages observed during the 1980s and 1990s are partly a consequence of the growth of new assistive technologies (Spillman, 2004), including, under a broad conceptualization of "technology," assisted living itself (Wolf, Hunt, & Knickman, 2005). It has also been suggested that demographic trends such as growing divorce rates and women's labor force participation have already begun to shrink the supply of informal caregivers, prompting greater reliance on other care modes, including assistive devices and self-care (Wolf, Hunt, & Knickman, 2005).

As we narrow our focus to the future of assisted living itself, the picture becomes still more complex. We can envision two relatively contradictory scenarios. In one, the assisted living industry caters to a population that has higher disability levels and needs. In the other, the industry draws in a population with higher activity levels and a preference for a more active lifestyle.

The first scenario derives from the fact that with respect to disability and need for care, there is considerable overlap between the populations of assisted living homes and nursing homes (Morgan, Gruber-Baldine, &

Magaziner, 2001; Zimmerman, Sloane, & Eckert, 2001). At the same time, nursing homes serve a population that has higher levels of ADL impairment and cognitive dysfunction. It is possible that, for some older people, an assisted living home serves as the place where they "spend down" their assets at the same time that their disability is increasing. Those with sufficient income to purchase extra services, such as skilled nursing care, will be able to remain in their assisted living home even as their need for care increases. Those who are unable to continue paying for assisted living care at the level they need may find themselves eligible—both physically and financially—for nursing home care. This suggestion is supported by research showing that of the 72 percent of live residents who leave assisted living, nearly half transfer to a skilled nursing facility (National Center for Assisted Living, 2001).

Medicaid's recent arrival as a source of financing for assisted living care is likely to further increase disability levels and needs for care among residents in assisted living. Many states have begun using their Medicaid waiver programs to finance personal care in assisted living homes for residents with nursing home-level needs, thereby providing necessary care less expensively than if the same residents were in nursing homes. This practice is likely to become more widespread as states continue to grapple with budget shortfalls. As a result, assisted living homes may begin to look more like nursing homes, at least in terms of their resident characteristics. This would have an adverse effect on assisted living's image as a place of "independence."

The growing prevalence of disability among residents in assisted living is not an indication of changes in disability in the general older population; indeed, as we have seen, the prevalence of disability is falling in the older population as a whole. Rather, it most likely reflects responses on the part of assisted living owners and operators who must survive in an increasingly competitive environment. Early in the history of assisted living, many chose—and were able—to provide services only to individuals who showed little evidence of dementia and had relatively light care needs. As the supply of assisted living residences grew, some of these suppliers experienced turnover rates of 50 percent or more as their residents' needs for care increased and were forced to move to facilities that accepted residents with higher levels of disability (Moore, 2000). Many owners and operators were compelled to loosen their restrictive admission and retention criteria to remain competitive. Increases in the supply of special care

Alzheimer's units within assisted living residences are another response on the part of owners and operators to enhance their competitive stance.

The increasing availability of assisted living to persons with higher levels of physical and cognitive disability may influence family decisions about providing care in the community. Nursing homes as settings in which to place older relatives have held negative connotations for families and are often considered the choice of last resort for long-term care. This does not appear to be the case for assisted living residences. Family members are an integral part of the decision process, and indications are that they support the move into an assisted living residence. Some of the characteristics most widely used in marketing assisted living are its homelike environment and its support of residents' independence—aspects that have great appeal for family members. Thus, there are strong arguments supporting the position that assisted living residences of the future may resemble more closely today's nursing homes.

As the popular media continually remind us, however, the baby boom cohort is poised on the transition into retirement and is unlike earlier cohorts in numerous respects. This suggests a different scenario for the future of assisted living. Among the distinctive features of boomers are their considerable assets, their high level of activity and "lifestyle" characteristics, and their independence and self-sufficiency. Were it to remake itself in response to the opportunities seemingly presented by the passage of the baby boom cohort into and through old age, the assisted living industry could undergo dramatic changes. If assisted living residences were to cater to an "active retirement lifestyle," associate themselves with desirable retirement destinations—located in the amenity-rich types of areas already identified with retirement migration (Duncombe, Robbins, & Wolf, 2003)—they might achieve higher levels of growth than in recent years. As a by-product of occupying this new niche, the assisted living world would house a healthier, fitter, and more independent population with relatively low care needs. This would make it seem like the growth of assisted living is associated with a reduction in the role of family care. That association, however, would be spurious, because it would be a result of the lifestyle demands of the baby boomers, not the lifestyle offerings of the assisted living industry.

Even if assisted living continues to house an increasingly disabled population, it will presumably continue to emphasize its appeal to those seeking independence, including the independence associated with receiving services from staff rather than from family members. Yet this need not imply any diminution of family care, especially in light of the still comparatively small size of the assisted living sector. Those residents in assisted living whose needs are met by their complex's optional services rather than by family members might not have been cared for by family members even had they remained in their own home; there may, in other words, be a "selection effect" underlying these residential and care decisions.

In the presence of selection effects, evolving practices regarding the placement and retention of people with greater needs for care, continued technological evolution, and a changing policy environment, assisted living can be seen as simply one more element in a complicated—even increasingly complicated—environment in which care needs arise and care-provision decisions are made. For many years the range of choices and opportunities facing those with care needs has grown, and there has been a general tendency for new developments to promote independence and self-care. In spite of these changes, family members have remained the most important source of care and support for older people unable to fully address their care needs. The specific components of "care" have, and will continue to, evolve—consider, for example, the previously unknown task of providing assistance with configuring Web browsers—while the prominence of family members in the overall constellation of caring remains. We see no reason to suppose that further growth of assisted living in the coming several years will change this basic fact.

REFERENCES

Agree, E. M., Freedman, V.A., Cornman, J. C., Wolf, D. A., & Marcotte, J. E. 2005. Reconsidering substitution in long-term care: When does assistive technology take the place of personal care? *Journal of Gerontology: Social Sciences 60B,* S272–280.

Angel, R. J., & Angel, J. I. 1997. *Who will care for us? Aging and long-term care in multicultural America.* New York: New York University Press.

Anthony-Bergstone, C. R., Zarit, S. H., & Gatz, M. 1988. Symptoms of psychological distress among caregivers of dementia patients. *Psychology and Aging 3,* 245–248.

Assisted Living Federation of America. No date. Guide to choosing an assisted living residence. www.alfa.org/public/articles/ALFAchecklist.pdf.

Beresford, J. C., & Rivlin, A. M. 1966. Privacy, poverty, and old age. *Demography 3,* 247–258.

Burch, T. K., & Matthews, B. J. 1987. Household formation in developed societies. *Population and Development Review 13*, 495–511.

Burns, R., Nichols, L. O., Martindale-Adams, J., Graney, M. J., & Lummus, A. 2003. Primary care interventions for dementia caregivers: 2-year outcomes from the REACH study. *Gerontologist 43*, 547–555.

Burr, J. A., & Mutchler, J. E. 1993. Ethnic living arrangements: Cultural convergence or cultural manifestation? *Social Forces 72*, 169–179.

Cartwright, J., & Kayser-Jones, J. 2003. End-of-life care in assisted living facilities. *Journal of Hospice and Palliative Nursing 5*, 143–151.

Crimmins, E. M. 2004. Trends in the health of the elderly. *Annual Review of Public Health 25*, 79–98.

Cutler, D., & Sheiner, L. 1994. Policy options for long-term care. In D. Wise (Ed.), *Studies in the economics of aging* (pp. 395–434). Chicago: University of Chicago Press.

Desai, M., Pratt, L. A., Lentzner, H., & Robinson, K. N. 2001. Trends in vision and hearing among older Americans. *Aging Trends, no. 2.*

Duncombe, W., Robbins, M., & Wolf, D. A. 2003. Place characteristics and residential location decisions among the retirement-age population. *Journal of Gerontology: Social Sciences 58B*, S244–252.

Favreault, M., & Wolf, D. A. 2004. *Living arrangements and Supplemental Security Income receipt among the aged.* Boston College Center for Retirement Research Paper No. 2004-03.

Feinberg, L. F., Newman, S. L.,Gray, L., & Kolb, K. N. 2004. *The state of the states in family caregiver support: A 50-state study.* San Francisco: Family Caregiver Alliance.

Freedman, V. A., & Soldo, B. J. 1994. *Trends in disability at older ages: Summary of a workshop.* Washington, DC: National Academy Press.

Freedman, V. A., & Martin, L. G. 2000. Contribution of chronic conditions to aggregate changes in old-age functioning. *American Journal of Public Health 90*, 1755–1760.

Freedman, V. A., Aykan, H., & Martin, L. G. 2002. Another look at aggregate changes in severe cognitive impairment: Further investigation into the cumulative effects of three survey design issues. *Journal of Gerontology: Social Sciences 57B*, S126–131.

Freedman, V. A., Crimmins, E., Schoeni, R. F., Spillman, B., Aykan, H., Kramarow, E., Land, K., Lubitz, J., Manton, K., Martin, L. G., Shinberg, D., & Waidmann, T. 2004. Resolving inconsistencies in old-age disability trends: Report from a technical working group. *Demography 41*, 417–441.

Gaugler, J. E., Anderson, K. A., & Leach, C. R. 2005. Family involvement and quality of life in residential long-term care. www.mc.uky.edu/Permeability/Reports/Final%20Report.pdf.

Gaugler, J. E., & Kane, R. A. 2001. Informal help in the assisted living setting: A 1-year analysis. *Family Relations 50*, 335–347.

Harrington, C., Swan, J. H., Nyman, J. A., & Carrillo, H. 1997. The effect of certificate of need and moratoria policy on change in nursing home beds in the United States. *Medical Care 35*, 574–588.

Harrington, C., Carillo, H., Wellin, V., Miller, N., & LeBlanc, A. 2000. Predicting state Medicaid home and community based waiver participants and expenditures, 1992–1997. *Gerontologist 40*, 673–685.

Harrington Meyer, M. 2001. Medicaid reimbursement rates and access to nursing homes: Implications for gender, race, and marital status. *Research on Aging 23*, 532–551.

Hawes, C., Phillips, C. D., & Rose, M. 2000. *A national study of assisted living for the frail elderly: Final summary report.* Washington, DC: U.S. Department of Health & Human Services. http://aspe.hhs.gov/daltcp/reports/finales.htm#chap 3B.

Hawes, C., Phillips, C. D., Rose, M., Holan, S., & Sherman, M. 2003. A national survey of assisted living facilities. *Gerontologist 43*, 875–882.

He, W., Sengupta, M., Velkoff, V. A., & DeBarros, K. A. 2005. *U.S. Census Bureau, Current Population Reports, P23-209, 65+ in the United States, 2005.* Washington, DC: U.S. Government Printing Office.

Kane, R. L., & Kane, R. A. 2001. What older people want from long-term care, and how they can get it. *Health Affairs 20*, 114–127.

Krivo, L. J., & Chaatsmith, M. I. 1990. Social services impact on elderly independent living. *Social Science Quarterly 71*, 474–491.

Lee, D. J., Gómez-Marín, O., Lam, B. L., & Zheng, D. D. 2004. Trends in hearing impairment in United States adults: The National Health Interview Survey, 1986–1995. *Journal of Gerontology: Medical Sciences 59A*, 1186–1190.

Liao, Y., McGee, D. L., Cao, G., & Cooper, R. S. 2000. Quality of the last year of life of older adults: 1986 vs. 1993. *Journal of the American Medical Association 283*, 512–518.

Lye, D. N., Klepinger, D. H., Hyle, P. D., & Nelson, A. 1995. Childhood living arrangements and adult children's relations with their parents. *Demography 32*, 261–280.

Mack, R., Salmoni, A., Viverais-Dressler, G., Porter, E., & Garg, R. 1997. Perceived risks to independent living: The views of older, community-dwelling adults. *Gerontologist 37*, 729–736.

Manton, K. G., Stallard, E., & Corder, L. S. 1998. The dynamics of dimensions of age-related disability 1982 to 1994 in the U.S. elderly population. *Journal of Gerontology: Biological Sciences 53A*, B59–70.

Manton, K. G., & Gu, X. 2001. Changes in the prevalence of chronic disability in the United States black and nonblack population above age 65 from 1982 to 1999. *Proceedings of the National Academy of Sciences 98*, 6354–6359.

Mathews, T. J., Hamilton, B. E. 2002. *Mean age of mother, 1970–2000.* National vital statistics reports vol. 51, no. 1. Hyattsville, MD: National Center for Health Statistics.

Michael, R. T., Fuchs, V. R., & Scott, S. R. 1980. Changes in the propensity to live alone, 1950–1976. *Demography 17*, 39–53.

Mittelman, M. S., Ferris, S. H., Schulman, E., Steinberg, G., & Levin, B. 1996. A family intervention to delay nursing home placement of patients with Alzheimer disease: A randomized controlled trial. *Journal of the American Medical Association 276,* 1725–1731.

Mittelman, M. S., Roth, D. L., Coon, D. W., & Haley, W. E. 2004. Sustained benefit of supportive interventions for depressive symptoms in caregivers of patients with Alzheimer's disease. *American Journal of Psychiatry 161,* 850–856.

Mollica, R. L. 2001. State policy and regulations. In S. Zimmerman, P. D. Sloane, & J. K. Eckert (Eds.), *Assisted living: Needs, practices, and policies in residential care for the elderly* (pp. 9–13). Baltimore: Johns Hopkins University Press.

Morgan, L. A., Gruber-Baldini, A. L., & Magaziner, J. 2001. Resident characteristics. In S. Zimmerman, P. D. Sloane, & J. K. Eckert (Eds.), *Assisted living: Needs, practices, and policies in residential care for the elderly* (pp. 14–72). Baltimore: Johns Hopkins Press.

Moore, J. 2000. Assisted living views market niche options. *Provider,* September. www.ncal.org/news/provider/pdf/mgmt-9-2000.pdf#search='provider%20 assisted%20living%20niche%20market'.

National Center for Assisted Living. 2001. *Facts and trends: The assisted living sourcebook. Report by Health Services Research and Evaluation Group.* Washington, DC: National Center for Assisted Living.www.ahca.org/research/alsource book2001.pdf#search='demographics%20assisted%20living%20residents'.

Reinardy, J. R., & Kane, R. A. 2003. Anatomy of a choice: Deciding on assisted living or nursing home care in Oregon. *Journal of Applied Gerontology 22,* 152–174.

Russell, J. N., Hendershot, G. E., LeClere, F., Howie, L. J., & Adler, M. 1997. *Trends and differential use of assistive technology devices: United States, 1994.* National Center for Health Statistics, Advance Data No. 292. Atlanta: National Center for Health Statistics.

Schoeni, R. F., & McGarry, K. 2000. Social Security, economic growth and the rise of the elderly widows' independence in the twentieth century. *Demography 37,* 221–236.

Shanas, E. 1979. Social myth as hypothesis: The case of the family relations of old people. *Gerontologist 19,* 3–9.

Silverstein, M., & Parrott, T. M. 2001. Attitudes toward government policies that assist informal caregivers: The link between personal troubles and public issues. *Research on Aging 23,* 349–374.

Silverstein, M., Angelelli, J. J., & Parrott, T. M. 2001. Changing attitudes toward aging policy in the United States during the 1980s and 1990s: A cohort analysis. *Journal of Gerontology: Social Sciences 56B,* S36–43.

Sloane, P. D., Zimmerman, S. Hanson, L., Mitchell, C. M., Riedel-Leo, C., & Custis-Buie, V. 2003. End-of-life care in assisted living and related residential care settings: Comparison with nursing homes. *Journal of the American Geriatrics Society 51,* 1587–1594.

Smith, R.A. 2002. Assisted-living centers court the family: pitches include adult kids, who are helping seniors make housing choices. *Wall Street Journal,* July 3, B6.

Social Security Administration. 2005. State Assistance Programs for SSI Recipients, January 2004. Washington, DC: Social Security Administration Office of Policy.

Spillman B. C. 2004. Changes in elderly disability rates and the implications for health care utilization and cost. *Milbank Quarterly 82,* 157–194.

Spillman, B. C., Liu, K., & McGilliard, C. 2002. Trends in residential long-term care: Use of nursing homes and assisted living and characteristics of facilities and residents. Washington, DC: Urban Institute. http://aspe.hhs.gov/daltcp/reports/rltct.htm.

Tomassini, C., Glaser, K., Wolf, D. A., Broese van Groenou, M. I., & Grundy, E. 2004. Living arrangements among older people: an overview of trends in Europe and the USA. *Population Trends 115,* 24–34.

Waidmann, T. A., & Thomas, S. 2003. Estimates of the risk of long-term care: Assisted living facilities and nursing home facilities. Washington, DC: Urban Institute. http://aspe.hhs.gov/daltcp/reports/riskest.htm.

Walker, A. J., Pratt, C. C., & Eddy, L. 1995. Informal caregiving to aging family members. *Family Relations 44,* 402–411.

Wallace, S. P., Levy-Storms, L., Kington, R. S., & Andersen, R. M. 1998. The persistence of race and ethnicity in the use of long-term care. *Journal of Gerontology: Social Sciences 53B,* S104–112.

Wilmoth, J. M. 2001. Living arrangements among older immigrants in the United States. *Gerontologist 41,* 228–238.

Wolf, D. A. 2001. Population change: Friend or foe of the chronic-care system? *Health Affairs 20,* 28–42.

Wolf, D. A. 2004. Valuing informal elder care. In Folbre, N., & Bittman, M. (Eds.), *Family time: The social organization of care* (pp. 110–129). London: Routledge.

Wolf, D. A., Hunt, K., & Knickman, J. 2005. Perspectives on the recent decline in disability at older ages. *Milbank Quarterly 83,* 365–395.

Zarit, S. H., Stephens, M. A. P., Townsend, A., & Greene, R. 1998. Stress reduction for family caregivers: Effects of adult day care use. *Journal of Gerontology: Social Sciences 53B,* S267–277.

Zimmer, Z., & House, J. S. 2003. Education, income, and functional limitation transitions among American adults: Contrasting onset and progression. *International Journal of Epidemiology 32,* 1089–1097.

Zimmerman, S., Sloane, P. D., & Eckert, J. K. 2001. Emerging issues in residential care/assisted living. In S. Zimmerman, P. D. Sloane, & J. K. Eckert (Eds.), *Assisted living: Needs, practices, and policies in residential care for the elderly* (pp. 317–332). Baltimore: Johns Hopkins University Press.

CHAPTER 8

Technological Tools of the Future

Contributing to Appropriate Care in Assisted Living

DAVID M. KUTZIK, PH.D.
ANTHONY P. GLASCOCK, PH.D.
LYDIA LUNDBERG
JACK YORK, B.S.

Any time technology is used as a focus for an article, whether in academic or popular press, the expectation is that there will be an emphasis on gadgets, newer gadgets, and future gadgets. It is as if the technology, the gadgets, will somehow leap up and begin to provide care, without humans being involved or involved only at a distance. This approach can be termed robocare: some high-tech device doing the work quicker and cheaper than humans can. Robocare is neither the focus of this chapter nor the wave of the future. Care is our topic and, in particular, how technology can be used as a tool to enrich the lives of older people and those with disabilities as well as provide better and more cost-effective care. Therefore, the people involved—those receiving and giving care—take center stage in our discussion. On the surface, this approach appears obvious, but older people, their friends, family, and paid caregivers are often left out of discussions of the use of technology. It is as if the humans and the technology occupy different spaces in the caregiving environment. Consequently, it is not surprising that seniors and caregivers are often reluctant to adopt and use new technologies and often fear that the goal of the new technology is to replace human relationships with some new gadget, a well-grounded fear if one believes the pie-in-the-sky scenarios about the future of high-tech care.

In contrast to the futurists' approach, technology should be viewed as simply a tool that enables a person to accomplish a particular task. Thus, a pencil is a tool, a thermometer is a tool, and a microprocessor is a tool. In each of these examples, the particular tool helps a person bring about a specific result. Technology applied to care provision must be viewed in the same way: it is a tool that helps a person with disabilities to accomplish activities or get the support they need and want. From this perspective, all "new technologies" must be evaluated by how they are to be used to enrich the lives of those receiving supportive services and whether they allow for more satisfying, efficient, or cost-effective care than the currently used tools. The purpose of this chapter, then, is to explore how technology is likely to affect the way services are provided in assisted living settings, and the impacts these changes may have on the industry as a whole.

Technologies That Will Affect Assisted Living's Future

With this focus, the first objective is to review a variety of existing technologies that are being used to aid in the provision of care in assisted living environments: (1) computer-based rehabilitation, cognitive stimulation, entertainment, and interpersonal communication systems; (2) resident assessment, data, and medical record software; (3) traditional emergency call systems; (4) passively activated call systems; (5) wandering prevention and tracking systems; (6) vital signs monitoring; (7) fall detectors; and (8) more comprehensive activity monitoring systems. After this review, the critical steps that providers need to keep in mind when they begin to integrate new technologies in their buildings will be considered, as well as a glimpse into a future in which these technologies serve as caregiving tools as opposed to stand-alone high-tech panaceas.

Computer-Based Rehabilitation, Cognitive Stimulation, Entertainment, and Interpersonal Communication Systems

The personal computing revolution has produced a range of technologies for frail elderly and disabled population as end users. In recent years, personal computer–based systems have been deployed in assisted living environments. These systems provide opportunities for enhanced social interaction, cognitive stimulation, and in some cases, mental and/or physical rehabilitation. This section discusses key design challenges for making computer technology accessible for frail older persons and then briefly reviews some examples of the personal computer-based communication and rehabilitative technologies recently developed and deployed in assisted living residences.

The world of e-mail and the Internet opens doors of participation for frail elders that provide remarkable opportunities for socialization and exploration: correspondence with family and friends; participation in online communities; shopping; and video teleconferencing are all finding their way into the everyday lives of assisted living residents.

The challenge, though, is to overcome the aversion that many older people feel when faced with computers, because frequently they find the keyboard-mouse configuration is very difficult to use. It is necessary to keep in mind that persons lacking very specific skill sets, such as touch typing, find themselves in an uphill climb just to try out a computer. For this reason, computers in assisted living settings should not be viewed as an entertainment unit that residents will automatically use but rather the focus of highly structured activities, the core of which is one-on-one training. The point of this training is to both motivate and enable older persons to be users of the computer-based technology, whether e-mail, web surfing, or specialized rehabilitation programs.

This is especially true for the many residents of assisted living facilities who experience difficulties with sight, coordination, and cognition. Hardware and software developers have created a variety of interface alternatives that serve a range of disabilities. These include replacement of the standard keyboard with an alphabetized large character keyboard, the replacement of text prompts with large image icons, and the use of touch-screen clicking, rather than using a standard point-and-click mouse. A wide variety of nonstandard equivalents of the mouse exist, such as larger stationary units with a track ball, which some individuals find easier to control. For visually impaired persons, there are enlarged and color-shifted monitor displays and even speaking interfaces that allow the user to listen and speak to the computer directly (Assistive Technologies, n.d.).

Although these alternative interfaces are useful in compensating for physical and perceptual disabilities, the key to creating a user out of a nonuser remains individualized training, beginning with specialized assessment to determine the exact fit between the user and the interface tools as well as individual training on how to use them. The point is that, when it comes to assisted living residents as computer users, the most important factors are neither the hardware nor even the software, but rather the training and structured activity. In terms of products currently available, notable is the In-Touch system (Mattern, 2005). Created and distributed by Never2Late, Inc., the core of the system is individual assessment and training, tailoring a variety of programs and devices to the needs of individual users. Users are assessed for special needs and then trained both individually and in group activity sessions on a variety of computer skills such as e-mail, web surfing, and relatively standard games and programs. Typically, icon-based touch-screen navigation is used with assisted living residents to enable them to easily use the computer. In addition, a variety of cognitive and physical training/rehabilitation programs are provided. In one of the group activity programs, participants use a bicycle pedal interface and take part in a virtual bicycle race projected on a large viewing screen. Thus, they get a workout while being involved in a group activity. Trainers provided by the distributor work on-site with residents and staff to implement the programs and activities (It's Never 2 Late, n.d.).

Several other systems targeting cognitive disabilities and computer-based rehabilitation are moving from the lab to the market. One example of a cognitive training and rehabilitation system developed specifically for dementia residents is the [m]Power system (Dakim, n.d.) This system uses a computer with a touch-screen interface plus specialized software to generate a wide variety of interactive games designed to assess and enhance cognitive performance in a variety of domains. Designed by neuropsychologists, the intention is to custom fit each user with a series of interesting, entertaining, and progressively challenging interactive games that closely match the individual user's strengths and weaknesses while constantly adjusting the games to maximize this fit. Using video and music clips, as well as a wide ranging library of topical areas of interest, the user is able to tailor the content of the exercises to suit their own preferences to maximize continued engagement. Following the "use it or lose it" dictum, the intention of the developers of this and similar systems is to maximize the cognitive ability of persons in the early stages of dementia by offering daily challenges.

Finally, though not requiring the user to control a computer per se, an entertainment device designed for dementia clients which uses a series of large jukebox-like buttons and icons is worth mentioning. The Memory Lane Media system (Olsen, Hutchings, & Ehrenkranz, 2000) provides an easily learned interface for patients to cue music and audio programming from the time periods corresponding to their youth, providing a basis for a variety of group activities focused on shared reminiscence.

Resident Assessment, Data, and Medical Record Software

While many assisted living providers still use paper records for most resident data, a number of software products are now available. Nearly all of these function as an integrated data base, which allows providers to generate both resident-specific and summary data. In some cases these products have embedded assessment capabilities, and most support the recording and updating of service plans. One feature that makes such software particularly useful within the assisted living context is its ability to capture aggregated resident service hours, thereby allowing providers to plan for adequate numbers of appropriate staff. These software products also allow providers, in some cases via data entry at point-of-service devices, to capture the specific amounts of services a particular resident is using, thereby ensuring that the resident's service plan and billing rates are accurate reflections of their needs. Web-enabled versions of these products also allow for real-time aggregation of data for quality-assurance purposes, as well as the potential for assisted living providers to communicate health information to residents' health care providers if so instructed by the resident.

There are currently several such software packages available. One example is AlphaPLAN Resident Centered Assisted Living Software (AlphaPLAN, n.d.), which includes a marketing/tracking capability; a service planning and assessment system that is designed to meet the various approaches of different assisted living providers; a broad range of customizable services; rent roll and invoicing capability; and staffing and quality improvement modules. These types of software packages could, at some future date, be tied to real-time monitoring, family communications, and electronic medical records, all of which have the potential to improve the services available to assisted living residents.

Call Systems

Call systems traditionally consisted of a pull cord connected to a hard-wired call box that signals a central monitoring station. These call boxes are usually placed in the bathroom and within reach of the resident's bed. Originally developed for hospital patients, such systems have been in use since the early twentieth century. In its most basic form, the pull chord triggers an auditory alarm and an indicator displays the room number of the signaling individual in a central location staffed by responders. When an alarm is signaled, the appropriate staff person is dispatched to the resident's room. The alarm remains active until reset by the staff at the same location from which the alarm was initiated.

A variant of the hospital call system has been the community based social alarm, widely deployed in the United Kingdom and Scandinavia. Originally developed for elderly public housing complexes, the alarm signals community nurses or "wardens" to call the distressed individual by phone, sometimes using a specially designed speaker phone installed in the resident's home for this purpose (Stenberg, 1992).

In the past dozen years, existing call systems have undergone an evolution spurred by cost-effective telecommunication and computer technologies. Wireless systems are widely available, vastly reducing installation costs while increasing reliability in the event of fire and other potential disruptions. Some call systems are bundled with two-way voice communication through which the resident and care provider can hear and talk to each other by means of a sensitive speaker phone (Lifeline, n.d.). In this way, immediate communication can be established between the resident and staff. Furthermore, the simple buzzer and blinking light has been replaced by a computer, with its ability to display the location and nature of the alarm as well as to log all alarm information accurately.

The advent of networked wireless communication systems allows for the integration of the stationary call box with other devices. Several systems provide personal emergency response system (PERS) pendants and wristbands enabling the resident to activate the alarm when out of reach of the pull chords, while others integrate wireless smoke and motion detectors to alert staff of a variety of possible problems in addition to resident initiated alarms, thereby bundling the call alarm with fire and security functions (Visiplex, n.d.). Other systems use open platforms to send text messages directly to caregiver cell phones, thus eliminating the central monitoring system in a traditional sense (Spectralink, n.d.). The result is a wireless telephone and pager system adapted to the assisted living environment but essentially similar to mobile communication systems found in other commercial settings with the added feature that alarms are cancelled at the site of origin thereby assuring staff response.

It is likely that in the next decade wireless systems will come to dominate the institutional call alarm market. The shift from wired to wireless call systems, though underway, is governed by state and local regulations resulting in some localities requiring fully wired systems, others allowing the communication channel to be wireless while requiring the device to be hardwired to an AC power source, whereas other localities now allow for the substitution of PERS-type units in place of the traditional call boxes.

The most important aspect of call systems is not their technological basis but rather their use as a tool for care giving. In other words, what is the impact of call systems on the caregivers and the residents? How does one implement a call system so that it is seamlessly integrated into the care giving practice and the business plan of the particular institution? Although there is published research on call system usage in acute hospital environments, as well as a copious literature on social alarms (Dibner, 1992; Thie, 1998), there is no comparable body of third-party research yet available for such call systems in the assisted living environment. Rather, what is available is largely in white paper form: short, small sample, single site studies conducted by the provider or the technology vendor (Ostland, 2002).

In sum, the technologically modern version of the traditional call system combines centralized monitoring and decentralized wireless paging, the ability to establish two-way voice communication with the resident very quickly, as well as the ability to integrate PERS and other devices into the network.

Passively Actuated Call Systems

Call systems are considered passively actuated in that they require no change in behavior or special interaction with the system on the part of the resident such as pushing a button or wearing an electronic device. These systems represent a refinement of the call systems because they use a variety of detectors (e.g., motion sensors, pressure sensors, ammonia sensors) and computer software to actuate an alarm based on the automated collection of information about the behavior of the residents. Thus, ammonia sensors in the sheets can signal the presence of urine; pressure sensors on the mattress and on either side of the bed can determine whether the resident is in or out of bed; and the motion sensors, strategically placed, enable the system to establish whether the resident is moving around. These systems are dependent on specific software that employs pattern recognition rules to translate the raw data signaled by the sensors into information about the sleep status of the resident. Hence, the presence of urine or the pattern of a person out of bed and exhibiting much movement back and forth in her or his room triggers an alarm condition and sends the information to the pagers carried by the staff. This type of sophisticated call system can not only be actively actuated by the resident pushing a call button but also can be passively actuated by resident behaviors.

A commercial version of the above described system is produced by Vigil Healthcare Solutions, of Victoria, British Columbia, and has been deployed in dementia units in both North America and Australia. Vigil reports that their system allows care facilities to decrease the number of night staff while increasing efficiency of response (Myers Research Institute, n.d.). By closely monitoring select behaviors of residents through the night in their own bedrooms, it is possible for the provider to maximize both independence and security simultaneously. By automatically generating alarms based on resident behavior rather than depending on the resident to push a call button, it is far more effective for persons suffering confusional states associated with dementia. Furthermore, the automated record keeping of the system allows for the production of a clinical record of the calls and responses, logging the interaction of staff and residents as it takes place in real time.

Wandering Alarms

The problems of wandering and elopement are well known. Several kinds of wandering alarms and resident tracking systems are currently deployed in the assisted living environment. These systems typically use various kinds of electronic radio frequency identification (RFID) tags attached to the resident to enable sensors in the environment track their movements. Most RFID devices are transponders, miniature transmitters that send a unique identification code via a low-power radio signal when triggered by a proximity detector in close range. Usually these tags are worn as bracelets, wristwatches, and other accessories, although they can be attached to clothing, wheelchairs, and other physical objects tied to the monitored individual.

The most basic kind of system consists of an RFID tag in the form of an electronic bracelet worn by the resident and proximity detector built into an alarm box (Stanley-Blick, n.d.). The bracelet is put on the person to be monitored. It contains a battery-operated low-power radio frequency (RF) transmitter that broadcasts an identity code to a receiver in an alarm box that is placed at every door opening to restricted areas. The box contains both an RF receiver to detect the presence of a bracelet wearer at close range as well as a sensor to determine whether the door is opened. Alarms are typically triggered when both a bracelet and an open door are detected at the same time. In this way, staff, visitors and unrestricted residents can pass through the doors without triggering an alarm.

This basic system consists of individual alarm boxes strategically placed on doors in the residence. A more sophisticated system exists that networks these units so that each communicates with a centralized computer that simultaneously monitors groups of doors and groups of residents. Such a networked system (Secure Care, n.d.) is capable of being linked to a call system, like those described in the previous sections, thereby signaling through a staff pager system instead of, or in addition to, generating audible and visual alarms.

It is most useful for a networked wandering monitor system to divide the building into permitted and restricted zones and use RFID tags to track individuals through controlled doorways. Thus, different individuals can be permitted different degrees of free access throughout and in and out of a building by programming their individual codes into the tracking software controlling the alarm. These permission levels can be altered as needed, depending on the changing behaviors of residents.

In addition to sounding an alarm or sending a routed pager/telephone alert to the appropriate caregiver, several systems automatically lock designated doors when a restricted resident comes within range and several such commercial products have been marketed to assisted living providers. It should be noted that these systems have built-in override functions to ensure that the doors are able to be quickly opened as needed by attending staff persons or in case of fire and that the usage of automatic door control is strictly regulated by local safety and fire ordinances.

Key to the proper use of any wandering tracking system is the valid assessment of the wandering risk for individual residents. In general, it does not make sense to tag every individual resident to prevent wandering, but only those who have a history of such behavior. New residents with an ambiguous history can be assessed with wander tracking for a period of time to determine whether they, in fact, have the need for this type of support. It is also possible to use these systems to provide different types and levels of care dependent upon the discerned behavioral patterns of the residents wearing RFID tags. Those residents who exhibit moderate levels of safety awareness and wayfinding ability can be given greater freedom and access to more areas within and around the building, whereas those individuals displaying less ability can be supervised more closely and their access more limited.

Although a number of ethical concerns have been raised about the potential restrictiveness and stigmatization of requiring certain residents to wear RFID bracelets (O'Neill, 2003), the emerging consensus is that such technologies permit greater freedom for cognitively impaired residents and have resulted in the reduction of the proportion of persons in dementia units (Hughes & Louw, 2002). The key question is how to use these tools to maximize the resident's autonomy and dignity while enabling the caregiver to both reduce the risk of the person wandering off as well as continuously assess their wandering behavior.

Vital Signs/Health Status Monitoring

The monitoring of physiological parameters such as heart rate, blood pressure, glucose, and oxygen saturation in a person's residence rather than the doctor's office has become increasingly commonplace. The data obtained from the proper use of these devices, together with body weight and sometimes temperature, are a potentially powerful tool in the hands of a skilled caregiver. This is especially true in relation to managing chronic disease states relatively common among frail elderly people, such as congestive heart failure or adult-onset diabetes. The problem with these consumer versions of devices formerly found in doctors' offices is that they are often difficult to use effectively. Even the best consumer blood pressure cuffs and glucometers are anything but foolproof. A misaligned cuff or an uncalibrated glucometer will repeatedly result in invalid data. Even more problematic is the interpretation of these data: translating them into information about a person's health status and knowing when and how to take appropriate action when necessary. Accurate measurements are of no use unless they lead to correct caregiving action.

With these issues in mind, there are several design approaches aimed at making physiological monitoring practical and effective for the frail elderly. They begin from the premise that individuals should not have to collect, interpret, and take action on their own but should be assisted in the different steps of this process by human and technological supports.

Perhaps the best-known approach of comprehensive monitoring of vital signs targeted at the elderly population is the remote nurse visit. Using a combination of vital sign monitoring tools and video conferencing equipment, a face-to-face remote visit takes place between a nurse in her office and the older person in her home. Proceeding in real time, the nurse and patient converse and view each other over a two-way video system. While watching the action of the screen, a nurse can instruct patients, step by step, how to take their blood pressure. During this process, a nurse-patient dialogue can take place that affords a potentially high level of caregiving similar in quality to an in-person home visit by the nurse (Philips Medical Systems, 2003). Although various remote nurse visit products have been available for a decade, it has only been in the last several years that a dramatic decline in cost and improvement in video conferencing quality have made the systems practical. One system (Philips, n.d.) attaches a device similar to a cable box to the patient's existing television and provides two-way calling so that the older impaired person can call the nurse, as well as the other way around, while seamlessly integrating the unit into the home entertainment system's infrastructure.

Although a remote nurse visit in the resident's room is not a likely fit with an assisted living environment, a variant of this approach would place a telehealth kiosk in a common area where residents can, on a periodic basis, check their vital signs. Such a system shared among the residents has two definite advantages: first, it reduces equipment costs by eliminating the need for every monitored individual to have a dedicated system; and second, it creates the setting for human support and supervision during a session. An example of a commercially available unit suitable for an assisted living environment is the Viterion 500 Lifecenter Telehealth Kiosk (Viterion, n.d.). This unit connects to a web-based patient information management system that schedules, tracks, and summarizes the vital sign information for each resident providing staff and potentially health care professionals with a variety of useful reports and records. Because, with the exception of blood sugar, most physiological monitoring need not be done on a daily basis, but rather one or two times a week, it is possible for a large number of residents to use the same kiosk efficiently.

In addition to vital sign monitoring requiring the user to interact with special devices, there is considerable research on unobtrusive techniques that can monitor weight or heartbeat by embedding special detectors in the environment. For example, researchers at the University of Virginia are working on a sensor-laden mattress pad that can measure pulse, respiration and sleeping positions (NAPS, n.d.). Several groups are perfecting means for detecting weight using mattress pads or load sensors connected to the bed (Elite Care Technologies, n.d.). Still others, extending advanced technologies developed for the military and NASA, plan to embed clothing with an array of sensors capable of real-time, simultaneous tracking of heart rate, blood pressure, and respiration as well as other functions relating to hazardous environmental exposure or severe trauma (Mundt, 2004).

It is likely that some of the methods of these emerging technologies may prove to be of practical use with assisted living residents in the near future; however, simultaneous tracking of multiple vital signs in real time is unnecessary, except for research subjects, critically ill individuals, and those in unusual environmental situations, such as astronauts. Thus, the nonintrusive embedding of sensors in clothing, mattress pads, and other objects in the environment, if valid and reliable, could provide helpful intermittent health status and disease state information.

Fall Detection

A variant of the monitoring systems described above are those designed to detect falls and potential falls. Perhaps no other event has greater catastrophic impact on frail older persons than the effects of a fall, and nothing is of greater importance than early detection to maximize the chances of recovery for the resident. In the past decade, there have been a variety of tools developed to automatically detect whether or not a resident has fallen. These systems involve a range of sensors, some of which are worn by the resident and others embedded unobtrusively in the surrounding environment.

Wearable Devices

The most common approach is derived from man-down alarms used in industrial sites where a worker is at risk of being overcome by toxic substances. These typically are small devices, about the size of a pager or cell phone, which are worn by the resident in a special holster. The device contains instruments that sense the pattern of velocity changes consistent with a fall as well as determine whether a person remaining in a prone position and not moving follows this pattern. When this happens, it sends a wireless signal to a receiver that then actuates an alarm indicating that a fall has occurred for the individual wearing the particular detector unit sending the alert. Commercially available versions of this device typically integrate a PERS call button into the unit (Tunstall, n.d.). Although these devices were developed with the community-based independent living market in mind, they fit well in independent, congregate, or assisted living buildings where the alarm is routed directly to the staff paging system.

It is likely that the next generation of wearable fall detection will include a locator function using either global positioning or embedded RFID tag technology to pin point the location of the fall victim automatically. The global positioning approach would enable the individual to be located within 20 feet virtually anywhere in the world, whereas an embedded RFID approach could indicate the room or approximate present or past location of the individual within a residence or campus. In either case, an automatic locating function would extend the usability of such systems beyond the resident's apartment.

Nonwearable Fall Detectors

The alternative approach to fall detection involves the use of sensors embedded in the resident's environment so that the resident need not wear anything special. A variety of very high-tech systems have been developed in the lab, each seeking a reliable way of determining whether a person has fallen, without having any contact with her or his body. Several systems use computerized video image processing, where small TV cameras are placed throughout the environment and very sophisticated software attempts to spot the telltale signs of a person having fallen. Another system uses ultra-high-frequency sound waves to see changes in gait and body position indicating falls. Still others use configuration lasers to remotely sense body position (Biswas, 2006).

The most reliable systems for real-world application, however, are those that use common motion, pressure, and vibration sensors. For example, data generated from motion sensors can indicate that a resident entered the bathroom but did not exit. A monitoring system can be programmed to generate a possible bathroom fall alert if the individual does not come out of the bathroom before a predetermined time limit. A commercially available system, QuietCare, has been designed to detect both bathroom falls, as well as other significant problems connected with very long bathroom stays in the assisted living environment (see section on activity monitoring for more detail on QuietCare).

Another approach to nonwearable fall detectors listens to the subsonic vibration fingerprint of a fall. By use of specialized vibration-sound detectors connected to the floor in strategic locations, it is possible for a computer using software to correctly identify falls under test conditions (Alwan et al., 2006). By use of an approach analogous to speech recognition, not only is the thud of the fall determinable but possibly also subtle changes in gait indicative of the onset of problems that place a person at risk for a fall may be noted. Deployment of such a fall-detection system in the apartments of persons in an assisted living environment may, in the near future, be a useful alternative to wearable detectors.

Dependability

No fall-detection approach can be expected to be 100 percent accurate all of the time. Perhaps the most critical issue in the design and implementation of such systems concerns the management of error, both false positives and false negatives. False positives occur when there has been no fall but an alarm is generated, whereas a false negative error is produced when there is in fact a fall but the system fails to generate an alarm.

From a design point of view, these two types of errors are related in opposite ways to sensitivity: the more sensitive the instrument is for detecting falls, the higher the likelihood of generating an alarm when there has been no fall, a false-positive error, whereas the less sensitive the instrument is, the higher the chance of the device not triggering when there has indeed been a fall, a false-negative error. Achieving a proper balance between the two types of errors entails the impact of each on a caregiving system. In an assisted living environment, false positives would be generally preferable to false negatives: it is better to send a staff person scrambling to someone's apartment to find out that there is no problem than to not detect a person lying on the floor for several hours.

How dependable are fall detectors? This is a difficult question to answer, because published material reporting on the reliability of such devices shows that they have been tested only in the laboratory environment. These laboratory tests appear to indicate that the differential reliability of a wristwatch-like device in detecting falls of different kinds—forward, backward, and sideways—is relatively high (Degan et al., 2003), as is the reliability of nonwearable devices (Sixsmith & Johnson, 2004). At this time, however, there appear to be no tests of commercial products outside of the laboratory.

Activity Monitoring

Activity monitoring automatically gathers information about a person's routine behaviors and presents the information to caregivers in a way that helps them provide better care. Depending on the specific system, motion detectors, RFID transponders, infrared tags, vibration sensors, either worn or embedded in their environment, are used to collect data. These data are processed by analytical software that translates the sensor data into information about what residents are doing and not doing, even behind the closed doors of their apartments. Are they sleeping through the night? Is there a change in bathroom usage? Are they preparing or eating meals on a regular basis? Do they seem to have experienced an overall decline in activities?

From a narrow technical standpoint, activity monitoring may seem to be an extension of the passively actuated out of bed or frantic behavior alarm system. The essential difference, however, is that activity monitoring is focused on the production of reports for caregivers about the performance of a variety of daily activities indicative of the health and wellness of individuals. Although some of these systems do generate alarms calling for immediate attention (e.g., Elite Care and QuietCare), the emphasis is on providing the caregiver with a continuous baseline assessment of the resident with respect to selected functional activities. Caregivers can, therefore, combine information received from the monitoring system with information about the resident obtained from all other sources, direct observation or interaction, and discussion with other staff members to help them better understand the changing needs of the resident.

To date, several activity monitoring systems have been tested in settings across the continuum of care. Beginning in the late 1990s, home-based lifestyle monitors and wellness-assurance systems were tested in Europe as potential supplements to social alarms in independent living environments (Miskelly, 2001). These systems generally triggered an alarm if there was an extended period of unexpected lack of motion. By 2000, systems tracking such activities as eating, sleeping, and toilet use were undergoing tests in the United States, Europe, and Australia. In 2005, at least two different systems were implemented in assisted living residences with promising results in terms of potential for increased quality of care.

Two basic designs are used in activity monitoring and wellness systems: maximalist and minimalist. The maximalist approach to hardware uses many, sometimes literally hundreds of, sensor and detector components networked together into an impressive infrastructure. Likewise, the maximalist software designs employ extremely computationally intensive activity pattern recognition ontologies that attempt to guess not only what the person may be doing but also what he or she is intending to do next. The design philosophy underlying this maximalist approach is to provide various forms of cognitive assistance, reminders, and interventions automatically without the intervention of a human caregiver (Haigh & Yanko, 2002).

On the one hand, it appears that the driving force behind the maximalist approach is the development of products that may become practical a decade or so in the future. On the other hand, the minimalist approach to software and hardware design is to tightly focus on specific types of activities. Thus, the hardware employed is most often limited to only a half dozen components, whereas the software uses a small number of rules that can examine very specific patterns of sensor data to see if a carefully chosen narrow range of activities have occurred. This minimalist design philosophy has allowed for extremely practical systems to be developed that are already deployed in assisted living residences.

Two such systems are CARE, developed by Elite Care of Milwaukie, Oregon, and QuietCare, developed by Living Independently Group, of New York City. CARE, which relies on a person-tracking type system that uses wireless ID tags, has been installed at Oatfield Estates, in Milwaukie,

Oregon. Oatfield Estates employs a sophisticated hardware infrastructure derived from asset management and process tracking industrial applications (Elite Care, n.d.). It uses state-of-the-art combined infrared and radio frequency-based systems for tracking, whereby embedded devices in the ceilings and walls can identify the inventory number of each personal ID tag (Stanford, 2002). In this system, all members of the community wear infrared/radio frequency (IR/RF) tags, staff and residents alike, thereby reducing the stigma attached to wearing these devices. The resident badge also includes a push-button emergency call functionality providing an extra level of protection. Using a system of embedded IR receivers in every room, as well as in the common areas, it is possible to identify, pinpoint, and track every individual in real time.

The IR/RF data collected by the system are converted into caregiver-relevant real-time information to allow caregivers to determine where a given resident is at the present moment and, to a certain extent, know what he or she is doing. Location is determined by the position of the IR/RF badge within the building. In addition, resident weight and sleep patterns are gauged using special weight-sensitive load cells placed under each leg of the resident's bed and programmed activities and socialization are inferred by the timing, duration, and location of the resident in relation to specific activities. For example, if time is spent in a specific common room between the hours of 10:00 and 11:00 a.m., it can be inferred that the residents are involved in an exercise class. In addition, further activity information entered into the system's database by staff and the residents themselves via wireless personal digital assistants and touch-screen terminals creates a more comprehensive record of the activity experience. Finally, all alarms triggered by the call buttons carried by the residents are logged into the database along with information on who responded, the nature of the help requested, and the length of time between the alarm's being sent out and the response.

The Oatfield Estates' administrative portal is based on the system's internal network and provides management with a comprehensive picture of the position, likely activity, and the security status of each resident and staff person. Thus, it is possible to view the identities of staff and residents to discern with whom and where they are spending time. This provides the basis of a variety of staff-resident interaction reports. In addition, staff work task logs are automatically generated in the form by means of an electronic timecard allowing for validation of the staffs' own work

Current Status ❓ As of 12:28 pm on 01/09/2004

Resident	#	Wake Up	Bath Falls	Meds	Meals	Activity	Night Bath	Sleep	
Carol Finster	1	○	○	●	○	○	○	○	VIEW
Irma Queen	2	○	○	●	●	○	○	○	VIEW
Charles Brown	3	●	○	●	○	○	○	○	VIEW
Leslie Munson	4	○	○	●	○	○	○	○	VIEW
Barbara Rouche	5	○	○	●	○	○	○	○	VIEW

Figure 8.1. QuietCare daily event summary page

log reports. By contrast, the family portal uses a pin-secured website to allow the family to view the status and activity history of their loved ones. The intent is to give family members a greater sense of peace of mind, while at the same time, more closely involving them in the care of their elders by providing an open window into the daily activities, call alerts, and interactions of their elder.

A second activity-monitoring system, QuietCare, developed by Living Independently Group, of New York City, is more minimalist in its hardware and software design than is CARE. QuietCare consists of two components: a residential data-collection unit consisting of motion detectors and a base station and a web-based server that periodically uploads these sensor data to a website that analyzes current conditions and especially over-time behavioral trends and translates them into information about the monitored individual's status and behaviors (QuietCare, n.d.).

Personal identification number–secured portals are provided, giving easily interpretable and timely advice to the caregiver. Thus, the website's pages display the information on each activity as simple icons and clear narrative statements that relay the most important trends as simply as possible (see Figure 8.1).

Present-day information is automatically compared to previously collected activity data to determine changes in activity. Green indicators are displayed when the data show no significant deviation in the frequency and/or timing of data for a given activity; yellow status indicators are displayed when the frequency and timing of a given activity is higher or lower than expected; and red status indicators are displayed when a still higher threshold of deviation is recorded. Yellow and red indicators represent alerts and are sent to staff and designated family by means of e-mails, pager, or text messaging that direct the caregiver to take action and to check the website for additional information about the monitored individual.

Designated caregivers have the ability to access more detail on the status and behavioral history of the resident (e.g., length of stay in the bathroom, exact time that medication box was opened) by pointing and clicking on the icons. Moreover, the caregiver can examine month-to-month comparisons of selected activities to discern subtle trends that would not be observable by reviewing the information on a daily basis. Thus, a resident who has undergone a slow decline in eating or experienced a slow but steady increase in overnight bathroom use too subtle to trigger alerts will reveal these patterns of change when their activity data is graphed out over a series of months (Glascock & Kutzik, 2006).

Within assisted living residences, QuietCare provides the staff with information about nonpublic activities, such as sleeping, eating, and bathroom usage, which would remain invisible under normal circumstances. Supervisors at Lakewood Commons, an assisted living residence in Maplewood, Minnesota, have used the system to document scheduled late-night bathroom assists and bed checks. In addition to an increase in staff accountability, information provided by this system was then used to assess care needs of new residents during their first month of stay as well as document evidence of higher care needs requiring additional services for both the provider and the family members of the resident. Also, the staff were alerted to the onset of a range of problems with individual residents as they unfolded. The list of problems uncovered and investigated by the nursing staff during a trial period included the following: sleep disturbance, "sun downer syndrome," acute urinary tract infection, prostate problems, insufficient hydration, stomach flu, residents stuck in bed or chair because of mobility problems, behavioral changes related to medication issues, social isolation, and excessive heat or cold in the dwelling area. The staff concluded that each of these problems would have remained unknown for hours, days, or even weeks without behavioral monitoring technology (Ecumen, 2005).

Conclusions and Implications for the Future

Although many of the technologies discussed here are new, in that they have been developed and employed within the last decade, none of them falls into the category of robocare: a futuristic desire for some high-tech device that will provide care better, quicker, and cheaper than humans can. Instead, each, in its own way, is a tool that employs existing technology to help people provide better and more cost-effective care. Whether it is a wireless call system that precisely records the time of the call and of the response or an activity monitoring system that tracks changes in behavior over time, each of the systems has been integrated into an existing care environment rather than replacing a care model. Yes, this integration has required that caregivers do their job differently, because the technology provides more complete and timely information than has been available previously (e.g., blood pressure data from a kiosk on a daily basis, rather than only when the person visits the doctor).

This results in the caregivers having more information to assess, more decisions to make, and more actions to take. In addition, this information can now be time stamped, stored and retrieved, thus increasing accountability at every stage of care giving. Supervisors can now retrieve precise data on needs and responses. When caregivers do not respond appropriately, they and their organization are both potentially liable. Thus, with this increase in information, the users of the technology have had to reassess their business models and weigh the costs incurred against the benefits derived. However, no assisted living provider can afford to ignore these new tools and so it is not a question of whether to use these technologies but, rather, which ones to use and in what combination.

This brings us first to a consideration of the near future—not the technological breakthroughs that may come about two decades hence, but what most likely will occur in the next few years. There appear to be two major trends that will shape this short time horizon. The first is fairly obvious: the continued incorporation of technology into all care environments. This will be driven by both the decline in the cost of available technologies and the advent of new technological applications, as well as the public's expectation that residences will use such technology in providing care. It is perhaps this latter point, the public's expectations, that will drive the inclusion of technology in assisted living residences the most. The ubiquitous use of computer technology in everything from cell phones to automobiles will drive expectations on the part of both the assisted living residents and, perhaps more important, the families of the residents. People today just assume that there are technologies out there that will provide better and more timely care. "If I can get text messages about sporting events on my cell phone, why can't I get text messages about whether my mother has taken her medication?" Questions similar to this are being asked today and tomorrow even more demanding questions will be asked, and woe to the assisted living provider who cannot answer these questions in the affirmative.

The second trend is that these various technologies are increasingly being combined, and this integration will accelerate in the next few years. PERS are being combined with activity-monitoring systems as well as with fall-detection systems; vital signs and activity-monitoring systems are being merged for specific disease states (e.g., congestive heart failure); and call systems are being merged with passively activated alarm systems. This integration will continue and at some point in the next few years, assisted living residences will have the ability to select from a technology tool kit the best combination of functions for their particular business model. This is not a pie-in-the-sky prediction, but only the logical continuation of the trends that are currently taking place. The only questions for assisted living companies will be, what type of technology makes the most sense and how soon can I get it installed?

Pushing out the time horizon to a somewhat more distant future, say a dozen years from now, is to engage in a far more speculative and, hence, fictional exercise. Nevertheless, this is an intriguing thought experiment that fits well within the rubric of this volume. It is likely that the integration of technologies over the next few years will accelerate and that qualitatively new tool kits will emerge, with the essential point of integration being a comprehensive, self-updating, and automatically analyzing electronic care record. Where will these tools come from? As with the technologies described in this chapter, they will tend to come from outside of assisted living, mostly from home and the workplace settings. So the question becomes, what will be in the homes and workplaces of twelve years from now which will find customized application in assisted living settings?

Thoughtful speculation projects a vision of living and work environments characterized by a full unfolding of the pervasive computing revolution, a condition cleverly dubbed "Everyware" (Greenfield, 2006). In the world of Everyware, hardware, firmware, middleware, and sensor systems will be embedded in our appliances, entertainment systems, security systems, personal and business phones, organizers and computers and even walls, clothing and disposable food and medicine containers. In such an environment, both the activity of our devices and ourselves will be reported, recorded and analyzed in an ongoing dialogue of machines talking to machines.

This is not science fiction. Already the "meshed" networking protocols are in place for dishwashers and microwaves to report their maintenance status over the Internet just as printer toner is already automatically ordered in most offices. Indeed, it is likely that even the lowly light bulb will talk to the network and ask for replacement! So, a dozen years from now, it may well be common for the refrigerator to report the need to buy milk and apples and even, if so instructed, to automatically order these from the grocery store. Furthermore, in such a world, people will have years ago accustomed themselves to living in an environment where machines, monitor not only machine actions, but human actions as well. After all, appliance usage alone could be used to construct a remarkably detailed picture of an individual's daily routine (Glascock & Kutzik, 2000).

In this future will also have evolved a work culture transformed by automated employee monitoring. After all, it is already commonplace for employers to monitor every keystroke and mouse click of an employee's behavior, and many categories of workers are required to routinely electronically log and timestamp their work activities. Today, position locating systems that can track packages and people anywhere on earth within a ten-foot radius are widely used in many types of industrial work sites. Putting aside what to us seem glaring ethical issues of personal privacy, our point is that automated tracking and analyzing of human behavior will have become so commonplace at home and work in a dozen years time that most people will view this as normal or even desirable.

This brings us to the issue of cohort cultural shift. The attitudes toward technology and the skill sets for using technical tools of assisted living clients in the future will be considerably different than they are today. They will carry with them their experiences and expectations of the home and work technical environment into the assisted living environment. These future elders will be used to working with computers and expect to be reminded to do things by a little digital device. They will certainly expect that their assisted living residences will have a similar technological environment—smart appliances and personal managing assistance will be, after all, very much a part of their sense of being at home.

So it is without a great leap of imagination to envision an assisted living resident going about her daily routine and having her vital signs, physical activities, and social interactions tracked, analyzed, and presented to both family and professional caregivers. It is easy to imagine daily or even hourly status updates on residents accessible by staff and family in the form of reports, using data collected both inside and outside the residence. We would not be surprised by what might seem to us today to be a disappearance of interface hardware, in that ubiquitous sensor and voice and activity recognition systems need only to receive spoken words or gestures or gait from the users in order to operate. We would certainly expect a fusion of personal computing, wellness monitoring, personal management, telecommunications, and entertainment to greatly reduce the number of disparate gadgets into a single carry-along device and a single stationary home unit system.

Finally, in this world, despite the cultural shifts entailed by adaptation to an Everyware environment, we would expect caregiving to remain caregiving. Caregiving will continue to be provided by people. It will remain intimately human. The technological tools of the future will help caregivers provide the appropriate amount of care at the appropriate time by the appropriate person. Technology will neither replace the caregiver nor do too much for the care recipient. In other words, it will not become robocare, and assisted living will remain a homelike environment where people manage their lives, albeit with new tools and capabilities.

REFERENCES

AlphaPLAN Resident Centered Assisted Living Software. No date. www.ivyhall seniorliving.com/AlphaPLAN.

Alwan, M., Rajendran, P. J., Kell, S, Mack, D., Dalal, S., Wolfe, M., & Felder, R. 2006. A Smart and Passive Floor-Vibration Based Fall Detector for the Elderly. Paper presented at the Second IEEE International Conference on Information & Communication Technologies: from Theory to Applications. Damascus, Syria. http://marc.med.virginia.edu/pdfs/library/ICTTA_fall.pdf.

Assistive Technologies. No date. Information on computer products and user interfaces for persons with physical and cognitive disabilities. www.assistive technologies.com/.

Biswas, J. 2006. Agitation monitoring of persons with dementia based on acoustic sensors, pressure sensors and ultrasound sensors: a feasibility study. Paper presented at the International Conference on Aging, Disability and Independence, Orlando, FL.

Dakim, Inc. No date. Information on the [m]Power system. www.dakim.com/solution.html.

Degen, T., Jaeckel, H., Rufer, M., & Wyss, S. 2003. SPEEDY: a fall detector in a wrist watch. *Proceedings of the Seventh IEEE International Symposium on Wearable Computers (ISWC'03)*, pp. 184–187.

Dibner, A. 1992. Introduction. In A. Dibner (Ed.), *Personal response systems*. Binghamton, NY: Haworth Press.

Elite Care. No date. Information on Elite Care installation at Oatfield Estates. www.elite-care.com/oatfield.html.

Elite Care Technologies. No date. Active Relationship-Based Care. Received via email on June 18, 2006, from Lydia Lundberg.

Glascock, A., & Kutzik, D. 2006. The impact of behavioral monitoring technology on the provision of health care in the home. *Journal of Universal Computer Science 12*, 1, 59–79.

Glascock, A. P., & Kutzik, D. M. 2000. Behavioral telemedicine: a new approach to the continuous non-obtrusive monitoring of activities of daily living. *Telemedicine Journal 6* (1), 33–44.

Greenfield, A. 2006. *Everyware: the dawning of the age of ubiquitous computing.* Berkeley, CA: New Riders.

Haigh, K., & Yanco, B. 2002. *The role of intelligent technology in elder care: a survey of issues and technologies.* AAAI technical report WS-02-02, 39-53. www.cs.cmu.edu/~khaigh/AAAI02.html.

Hughes, J. C., & Louw, S. J. 2002. Electronic tagging of people with dementia who wander. *British Medical Journal 325,* 847–848.

It's Never 2 Late. No date. Description of products and program resources for computer-based rehabilitation. www.IN2L.com.

Lifeline. No date. Lifeline e-call product descriptions. www.lifelineseniorliving.com.

Mattern, J. 2005. In-Touch: An evaluation of an adaptive computer system for LTC residents in nursing homes and assisted living for dementia. Myers Research Institute of Menorah Park Center for Senior Living. Received as email attachment from It's Never 2 Late, Inc. August 11, 2006.

Miskelly, F. G. 2001. Assistive technology in elderly care. *Age and Ageing 30,* 455–458.

Mundt, C. 2004. Lifeguard: a wearable vital signs monitoring system. http://lifeguard.stanford.edu/lifeguard_writeup_medium.pdf.

Myers Research Institute. No date. Executive Summary. *Menorah Park Center for Senior Living.* www.vigil.com/products/case-studies/myers-research-executive-summary.pdf.

NAPS: Non-intrusive Analysis of Physiological Signals. http://marc.med.virginia.edu/projects_naps.html.

Olsen, R., Hutchings, B. L., & Ehrenkranz, E. 2000. Media Memory Lane: Interventions in an Alzheimer's day care center. *American Journal of Alzheimer's Disease 15,* 3, 163–176. http://aja.sagepub.com/cgi/reprint/15/3/163.pdf.

O'Neill, D. J. 2003. Tagging should be reserved for babies, convicted criminals and animals. *British Medical Journal 326,* 281. www.bjm.com.

Ostland, B. 2002. Social science research on technology and the elderly: does it exist? *Science Studies 17,* 2, 44–62. www.sciencestudies.fi/filestore2/download/266/Östlund.pdf.

Philips. No date. Telemedicine product information on Motiva system. www.medical.philips.com/main/products/telemonitoring/products/motiva.

Philips Medical Systems. 2003. TEN-HMS study demonstrates clinical and financial efficacy of home telemonitoring. www.medical.philips.com/main/products/telemonitoring/assets/docs/TEN-HMS_White_Paper_FINAL.pdf.

QuietCare. No date. QuietCare product information. www.quietcaresystems.com.

Secure Care. No date. Secure care model 135DE product information. www.securecare.com/135de.htm.

Sixmith, A., & Johnson, N. 2004. A smart sensor to detect falls of the elderly. *IEEE Pervasive Computing 3,* 42–47.

SpectraLink. No date. Linknet product line descriptions. www.spectralink.com.

Stanford, V. 2002. Using pervasive computing to deliver elder care. *IEEE Pervasive Computing 1,* 10–13. www.elitecare.com/pdf_files/elder-care.pdf.

Stanley-Blick. No date. WanderGuard product information. www.blickcommunications.com.

Stenberg, B. 1992. The Swedish model of social alarm systems for care of the elderly. In A. Dibner (Ed.), *Personal response systems* (pp. 135–147). Binghamton, NY: Haworth Press.

Thie, J. 1998. A pan-European social alarm system. *Journal of Telemedicine and Telecare 4* Suppl. 1, 60–61.

Tunstall Group, Ltd. No date. www.tunstall.co.uk.

Visiplex. No date. VS 3200 integrated system description. www.visiplex.com.

Viterion. No date. The 500 Lifecenter Telehealth Kiosk description. www.viterion.com.

CHAPTER 9

Enhancing Assisted Living

Are Collaborative Stakeholder Efforts Necessary?

DOUGLAS D. PACE, NHA
KAREN LOVE, B.S.

What role should advocacy groups play in the evolution of assisted living—and why should we care? Can providers, individual consumers, and state regulatory agencies be trusted to guide the ongoing development and operation of this important option in long-term care appropriately? Should we be concerned that the federal government might assume a new regulatory role? Are consumers adequately protected or represented?

The early successes and failures of advocates for seniors and persons with mental retardation / developmental disabilities (MR/DD) and the mental health community can help illuminate these contemporary questions. They have a cautionary tale to tell stakeholders seeking to influence the future status of assisted living, who might well learn from the work of others who faced comparable challenges and opportunities.

Historical Roots of Aging Advocacy

The Townsend Movement of the 1930s, largely responsible for providing the impetus for creating the public pension system, was one of our nation's first advocacy efforts on behalf of seniors. The passage of the Social Security Act in 1935 symbolized a historic change for Americans, heralding the federal government's entry into the social welfare arena for older adults. With this act, all Americans became entitled to public monies in "old age" (over the age of 64).

Not until the struggle to enact Medicare beginning in the late 1950s did organized efforts again coalesce around issues related to aging. Retired union workers concerned about health care became active advocates and eventually formed the National Council of Senior Citizens. The 1960s witnessed the first White House Conference on Aging (1961), after which major new federal programs supporting the interests of aging Americans were passed, including the Housing Act and Community Health Facilities Act (1961), Medicaid and Medicare (1965), and the Older Americans Act (1965), which established the Federal Administration on Aging.

The second White House Conference on Aging, convened in 1971, stimulated the creation of numerous special interest groups, including the National Caucus on Black Aged and the National Association for Hispanic Elderly. The National Association of State Units on Aging, the National Association of Area Agencies on Aging, and the Gray Panthers were also formed in the early 1970s. By the end of the decade, advocacy efforts around aging had become highly organized and a large, influential policy network was firmly in place. The increasing influence of such advocacy groups became highly evident by the 1981 White House Conference on Aging, when special interest groups began holding their own "miniconferences" to develop and put forth recommendations for the main conference. This trend grew to the point that in 2005 there were over 400 listening sessions, solution forums, and miniconferences leading up to the White House Conference itself.

The emergence of a large number of advocacy groups, each with its own specific agenda, not only spawned a new set of challenges, such as competition for access to decision makers and divisiveness over philosophical, political, and economic issues, but also a drive to carve out increasingly powerful fiefdoms. Arguably, the diversity and number of advocacy organizations diluted their ability to be effective. Compared to the first two White House Conferences on Aging, which ultimately resulted in landmark aging legislation, the past three have largely resulted in the compilation of increasingly voluminous recommendations from a multitude of special interest groups that have had little legislative impact. Special interest groups currently appear more intent on making their individual positions known than on working toward consensus solutions to common problems and agreeing on pressing issues facing America's senior citizens.

In addition, instead of being forums for catalyzing bipartisan agreement on public policy, the conferences have morphed into opportunities for both the reigning and minority political parties to publicly promote their agenda. Indeed, one of the 50 resolutions from the 2005 White House Conference serves as a glaring example of this partisanship: at the same time conference delegates voted overwhelmingly to increase the number of health professionals trained in geriatrics to meet the needs of increasing numbers of older adults, Congress was eliminating funding in the 2006 federal budget for the national network of geriatric education centers that provides this training.

It may be that lack of leadership more than multiplicity explains the loss of effectiveness among organizations for seniors. Without the commitment and willingness to put aside individual agendas and work toward consensus solutions, advocates cannot hope to improve the experience of aging in the United States. This is in considerable contrast to advocates for persons with MR/DD, who were faced with comparable challenges of divisiveness, but responded differently and thus have lessons to offer the assisted living community.

Lessons from the MR/DD and Mental Health Communities

Like the assisted living field, the MR/DD encompasses a widely diverse array of stakeholder groups, each with separate agendas, that has posed challenges to effective cohesive advocacy (see chapter 11). From birth to old age, the lifespan needs of individuals with MR/DD demand attention to schooling, transportation, job training, access to jobs, housing, discrimination, home health care, and personal care support, among others—and each has its own advocacy constituency. Elias Cohen, a noted, long-time legal advocate for persons with disability, explains that the MR/DD community strategically analyzed the various systems, barriers, and issues that needed to be addressed to improve the lives of the people they sought to help (Cohen 2004). That analysis, he contends, helped advocates understand the broad array of systems and laws that had to be changed and required action plans. Historic legislative changes resulted from these efforts, including the enactment of the Americans with Disabilities Act (1990), the Individuals with Disabilities Education Act (1975, 1997), the Rehabilitation Act (1973), and the Developmental Disabilities Assistance and Bill of Rights Act (2000).

In describing the importance of the collaborative process, Robert Silverstein, director of the Center for the Study and Advancement of Disability Policy, noted, "It is critical that various factions within the disability community work together and iron out differences in positions 'behind closed doors' while staying true to one's principle. Every major disability policy success in the last decade and a half is the direct result of the disability community sticking together" (Silverstein, 2000, p.1695).

The MR/DD community has not only successfully fostered effective collaboration among the array of stakeholder groups but has also done so while addressing a broad spectrum of issues. In contrast, the mental health community has not had similar success. Advocates have failed to develop the resources and programs needed to adequately house and care for the nation's population of individuals with mental illness. The mental health community seemed to have little understanding of the major changes in housing, expanded day care programs, and medical care systems needed to support those with mental illness. Stakeholder groups pursued individual special interests at the cost of focusing on the collective needs of the mental health community.

As a result, they missed a critical opportunity to catalyze their resources and put into place the infrastructure of programs and policies needed when policy makers sought to deinstitutionalize mentally ill men and women in the 1970s. Without adequate community-based resources to turn to, many people with mental illnesses have ended up homeless or in prison. One cannot help but wonder whether the outcome would have been different if the mental health community had worked together effectively to address and resolve the panoply of issues and needs facing those they purported to serve.

Why was the MR/DD community effective at addressing issues and needs while the mental health community was not? In our view, the critical difference is one of leadership and commitment. Able leadership and selfless determination ultimately brought great gains for MR/DD stakeholders. Lack of such leadership and commitment among stakeholders in the mental health community, along with unwillingness or inability to see the greater value of collaboration, left a weak and often ineffective infrastructure in place across our nation that failed to meet adequately the needs of individuals with mental health problems.

Assisted Living Stakeholders: Diversity of Purpose, Process, and Perspective
Divergent Stakeholders

To understand the diversity and divides of the various stakeholder groups in assisted living, it is important to understand how the field of assisted living evolved. During the mid-1980s, Paul and Terry Klaassen in Virginia and Keren Brown Wilson in Oregon separately began experimenting with a senior living option that would be an alternative to independent (congregate) living facilities, board and care, and nursing homes. Assisted living, as that experiment came to be known, experienced unprecedented growth over the next two decades, and by 2007 there were more than 38,000 licensed communities with close to one million residents nationwide. Both nonprofit and for-profit entities participated in this growth.

Assisted living properties ranged in size from small, homelike residences to large, multistory buildings. Settings also varied as to their health-related service offerings. Initially, assisted living emerged primarily as a housing (room and board) and a light social service model of care. It soon became apparent, however, that independent and active elders did not always view assisted living as an appropriate option, and instead it increasingly attracted elders with physical and cognitive disabilities, who required a full range of personal care and assistance. The question of whether assisted living properties can accommodate older persons with health care and nursing needs has been a long-standing issue. Whereas assisted living residents generally need assistance with activities of daily living such as bathing and grooming, which do not necessarily require nurse support, other residents need and are demanding that their properties administer medications to residents and address their unstable health care conditions. The lack of a clearly defined health care role and unified agreement about how to manage it has created a quasi–health care model of assisted living with state regulatory agencies given the ultimate decision-making authority. Thus, assisted living operates somewhat differently in each of the 50 states and the District of Columbia.

Some states have chosen to license and monitor assisted living within the same department that handles this responsibility for nursing homes while others have opted to associate assisted living with other service divisions, such as social services. Some regulate assisted living relying on a medical or nursing home model, whereas others regulate it more as a social or housing-with-services model. This variation has resulted in tremendous variations in the admission and discharge criteria used by different states. Furthermore, two national organizations represent state regulation activities related to assisted living, the Association of Health Facility Survey Agencies and the National Association of Regulatory Administration, also contributing to significant differences in regulation across the country (see chapter 13).

In the early years of assisted living, the primary stakeholders were providers (the owners and operators of assisted living residences) and consumers (the residents who lived there and their families, who often made the placement decision). As the field grew, so too did the types and diversity of stakeholders:

- Providers and provider organizations (Assisted Living Federation of America [ALFA], National Center for Assisted Living [NCAL], American Association of Homes and Services for the Aging [AAHSA], and the American Seniors Housing Association)
- Consumers and consumer advocates (AARP [formerly the American Association of Retired Persons], Alzheimer's Association, the Consumer Consortium on Assisted Living, the Paralyzed Veterans of America, National Senior Citizens Law Center, among others)
- Health and allied care professionals (including the American Assisted Living Nurses Association, the American Society of Consultant Pharmacists, and the American Medical Directors Association)
- Researchers in long-term care
- Regulators
- Accreditation entities (Commission on Accreditation of Rehabilitation Facilities [CARF]; as of January 2006 the Joint Commission on

the Accreditation of Healthcare Organizations (JCAHO) no longer
accredits assisted living.)
• Federal and state governments

Divergent Views

Although all stakeholders agree that the need for consistent, high-quality
care and services is paramount, each group has differing priorities, ob-
jectives, and perspectives about what this looks like and how to achieve
it. Sometimes there are even competing priorities within one group. For
example, the consumer group is comprised of residents, family members,
and other loved ones. Most prospective residents are initially (at least)
wary of moving away from their conventional homes. If a move into assisted living becomes necessary, they want good care, independence, and
savory, nutritious meals in a comfortable environment. Families, however,
are often initially focused on such elements as décor, ambience, medication assistance, and ability of the community to meet care needs. Both the
resident and the family's priorities may change substantially after move-
in, when such issues as aging in place or poorly trained or inadequate
staffing take priority—or when they are subjected to new charges for extra
care. Often these are issues that neither residents nor families considered
or perhaps even knew to consider before move-in. Indeed, such incomplete or inaccurate information has been the basis of consumer complaints
against particular assisted living property owners (see chapter 6).

Because assisted living emerged with a unique philosophy of supporting residents' independence, dignity, and choice, many providers felt that
their interests and concerns were not well represented by the traditional
national provider organizations in long-term care, the American Health
Care Association (AHCA) and AAHSA. ALFA was founded to represent
assisted living and its distinct philosophy. Providers who were already
members of AHCA or AAHSA that also developed assisted living generally
remained members of those organizations. In recognition of the distinction
between assisted living and nursing homes, AHCA created a separate division, the NCAL. Thus, providers are spread among three national organizations, leading to a situation in which the provider community has not
always been represented with a unified voice.

Consumer groups primarily representing the interests of nursing home
residents also look at assisted living through a different lens. Assisted liv-

ing's strongly held philosophy of autonomy and choice for residents has challenged the institutionalized decision making structure seen all too often in nursing homes. Advocates for nursing home residents and legal advocates for seniors (such as the National Senior Citizens Law Center, Legal Services, the National Citizen's Coalition for Nursing Home Reform, and long-term care ombudsmen) see the world differently. They often believe that the autonomy and choice offered by assisted living providers lead to unsafe resident care practices. Thus, there is often a strong conflict and a wide philosophical divide between the nursing home–oriented and legal advocates, on the one hand, and assisted living providers, on the other.

Providers and legal advocates, meanwhile, have vastly differing views on effective methods of quality control. Providers look to impose internal quality controls, whereby they continuously introduce improvements to fine tune their practices. Legal stakeholders, in contrast, promote external quality control methods, such as achieved by state monitoring and regulations. For the most part, legal and nursing home advocates have never worked in assisted living and so their understanding and perspectives are those of an outsider. This is comparable to someone who has never performed surgery weighing in on how an operation should be conducted, monitored, and evaluated. Of course, this same issue exists among the two stakeholder groups in the nursing home sector.

Researchers who study long-term care also generally do not have a good operational knowledge of assisted living. This often results in research on esoteric issues instead of areas that are operationally meaningful and could enhance providers' performance and outcomes. Collaborating with assisted living stakeholders would help researchers better define their projects, as some are beginning to appreciate. The Gerontological Society of America (GSA) now recognizes a special interest group for assisted living, which at the start of GSA's annual conference has held a one-day preconference session for the past several years. These preconferences have fostered discussions among researchers and other stakeholders, furthering dialogue and collaboration (see chapter 4).

Developing a strong and cohesive body of applied research in assisted living is also hampered by the lack of funding. Relatively few private foundations fund research in the elder care arena, and almost none commits monies to assisted living. Assisted living falls into the "red-headed stepchild" category of priority for federal research dollars as well. Large financially profitable providers of assisted living have also been reluctant to allocate a portion of their profits to research that would benefit the field as a whole rather than their special interests. This situation would be improved if stakeholder groups could work collaboratively to educate funding sources about the need and value of applied research.

State regulators are among the most influential stakeholders. They are responsible for the safety of residents and charged to ensure that residents are not abused, neglected, or exploited. Their oversight process is centered on site inspections to verify compliance with a given state's assisted living regulations—or lack thereof. Instead of taking a broad view of the plusses and minuses of a facility's operation, the process focuses on deficiencies or negative outcomes. It is the rare provider who does not feel defeated by the process, which contributes to antagonistic relationships between providers and regulators.

There is also a significant disconnect between national and local (state level) perspectives on the operation of assisted living. Individual states— for example, Pennsylvania—can choose not to require 24-hour staffing for assisted living communities, where from a national perspective stakeholders might assume that 24-hour staffing is the norm. This situation adds another element of confusion and challenge for the industry.

Assisted living providers themselves are responsible for some of the conflict among some stakeholder groups by taking an ostrich-like posture—namely, refusing to acknowledge publicly problems with quality of care, believing that what they do not own up to does not exist. Every industry has some bad apples that operate outside the boundaries of integrity and quality, and long-term care is no exception. This does not, however, excuse it from not putting up effective safeguards and peer-review systems to protect residents from harm and ensure that these outliers do not tarnish the reputation of the industry as a whole (Kane and West, 2005).

Although some difference of opinion is healthy for any field, the divide among stakeholders in assisted living has been counterproductive. A telling example of this is the stakeholders' inability to agree on a definition of assisted living. Every state defines assisted living differently. Indeed, not all states even use the term "assisted living," opting instead for terms such as "personal care homes," "shared housing establishments," and "residential care facilities," to name a few. The lack of cohesiveness in something as basic as defining what assisted living is has unwanted outcomes, including widespread consumer confusion over the potentials and limitations of this long-term care option (see chapter 15).

Studies in Collaboration

While the specific issues were different, the MD/DD community experienced many of the same kinds of disjunctions and conflicts assisted living stakeholders do today. The history of effective advocacy in the MR/DD community demonstrates not only that stakeholders must be willing to put aside their special interests at times and collaborate for the greater good of their community but also that there must be effective leadership to coalesce beneficial outcomes.

What would comparably effective collaboration actually look like in assisted living? In the following sections, we consider various case studies and examine them with this question in mind.

Accreditation for Assisted Living

Discussions to develop accreditation programs for assisted living began in July 1993. At that time AAHSA hosted a summit of provider and consumer organizations that recommended that a group of key organizations be convened to evaluate the potential of a national accreditation program. Numerous key organizations began meeting on a regular basis to explore viable avenues for accreditation. Ultimately, the group was unable to reach consensus on forming an accreditation program. In November 1995 AARP proposed launching a separate effort that focused on the wider realm of quality assurance, which led to the formation of the Assisted Living Quality Coalition (discussed further in Case Study 2).

While these collaborative accreditation discussions were under way, the Joint Commission on Accreditation of Health Care Organizations (JCAHO) was considering an accreditation program of its own. In April 2000 JCAHO introduced its first set of standards for assisted living accreditation developed in-house and without benefit of wide stakeholder collaboration. Separately and simultaneously, in late 1999 the CARF announced plans to develop its own program and in July 2000 CARF became the second national organization to offer accreditation for assisted living.

Despite these efforts, assisted living providers have been slow to adopt accreditation. As of mid-2005 CARF had accredited 48 communities and

JCAHO 118. Because of the lack of provider participation in its accreditation program, JCAHO decided to discontinue its program effective January 2006.

One wonders whether the results would have been different had the accreditation entities collaborated with key stakeholders during program planning and development. Through open-minded questioning and listening, they could have learned that there were significant issues and perceived barriers surrounding the acceptance of accreditation in this field. They might have better appreciated (and responded accordingly) that providers generally do not perceive the value of accreditation to outweigh the cost, time, and human resources involved in the process and that other stakeholders believe that the 3-year intervals between accreditation visits are too long to appropriately monitor a facility's performance.

Had the accreditation entities sought stakeholder input, they might have been able to allay these misgivings through a more inclusive decision-making process and more sensitive program design. A pilot project conducted in one test state with key stakeholder involvement (including the state regulatory agency, state provider associations, assisted living providers, consumer advocates, legal advocates, and researchers among others) could have rendered information and insights that led to a different course of action and outcomes.

The Assisted Living Quality Coalition

As noted above, the Assisted Living Quality Coalition developed as an outgrowth of one effort to consider accreditation for assisted living. In January 1996 six organizations joined forces to form the coalition: The Alzheimer's Association, AAHSA, AARP, the NCAL, the American Seniors Housing Association (ASHA), and ALFA.

Assisted Living Quality Coalition participants were united by two common purposes: (1) to promote the highest possible quality of life for older persons and consumers with disabilities by advocating for an assisted living philosophy of independence, privacy, dignity, and autonomy; and (2) to create a foundation for the continued growth and development of assisted living by fostering a quality improvement system that demands and rewards high-quality outcomes.

The Assisted Living Quality Coalition issued a report (Assisted Living Quality Coalition, 1998) that focused on two main areas: guidelines for state regulators and quality in assisted living. At the time many states were evaluating, updating, or creating an entirely new regulatory category for assisted living. The Assisted Living Quality Coalition's minimum standards were intended to serve as a roadmap for states.

The report recommended the creation of a national assisted living quality organization that would expand the work of the Assisted Living Quality Coalition and provide the framework and the forum to advance research, policy development, and consultation on quality improvement issues. A feasibility study commissioned by Assisted Living Quality Coalition was completed in the summer of 2001, by which time, however, discussions were already underway at the behest of the U.S. Senate Special Committee on Aging to bring together a larger, more diversified group of stakeholders to develop recommendations to assure quality in assisted living. The Assisted Living Quality Coalition disbanded once the Senate-mandated Assisted Living Workgroup effort got under way in the fall of 2001.

While the Assisted Living Quality Coalition efforts were beneficial in beginning discussions on issues affecting assisted living, limiting participation to only six organizations prevented participation by many of the other key stakeholders. Instead of their efforts serving to develop consensus on issues, the lack of wider stakeholder representation and collaboration was a significant shortfall.

The Assisted Living Workgroup

Spurred by problems with the quality of care as highlighted in the media, the Special Committee on Aging of the U.S. Senate held several hearings beginning in 1999. After the second hearing in 2001, the committee identified a number of key assisted living stakeholder organizations and charged them to develop recommendations for quality assurance in assisted living. The leadership of the committee recognized that collaborative efforts held the strongest promise for beneficial and acceptable outcomes. The committee mandated that the initiative be as inclusive as possible.

Fifteen organizations initially came together and formed the Assisted Living Workgroup and subsequently expanded participation to include more than 50 national organizations. The National Governors Association and the National Conference of State Legislators were invited to participate but declined, citing too great an investment of their staff's time.

The workgroup devised a system that promoted broad feedback from participating organizations and their constituents. Numerous opportunities were provided for all stakeholders to discuss each proposed quality recommendation in detail, including a democratic process requiring a two-thirds majority to decide whether a recommendation should go forward. Although this was a lengthy process, it ensured maximum stakeholder involvement and the opportunity to discuss each item from all stakeholder perspectives. In an April 2003 hearing before the Special Committee on Aging, the workgroup presented its final report, *Assuring Quality in Assisted Living,* which included consensus on 110 recommendations (U.S. Senate Special Committee on Aging, 2003).

In addition to creating an inclusive and balanced means for stakeholders to participate in the process, the Assisted Living Workgroup was also mindful of the need for inclusive and balanced leadership. A representative from both the consumer advocacy and provider sectors who was dedicated to collaboration facilitated the initiative. A steering committee representative of key stakeholders was also formed through a consensus process to oversee the effort and address problem areas.

The 18-month effort evidenced many of the features of successful collaboration; however, one element surfaced as a significant hindrance. A group consisting largely of legal advocates whose primary expertise was in nursing homes joined together and often voted as a block, violating the spirit of collaboration. At times, this tactic defeated the two-thirds majority needed for consensus agreement on a recommendation. A critical element needed for successful collaboration is the commitment and willingness of all participants to adhere to a jointly accepted collaborative process. This group, which represented only a small fraction of the participating organizations, lacked trust that the collaborative process could yield acceptable outcomes to them. The remaining organizations—the majority—however, felt the workgroup effort was very successful (see chapter 15).

In the five years since the release of the Assisted Living Workgroup report few states have actually used it to inform assisted living regulation. Nonetheless, it is an excellent resource as a benchmark against which states can consider their existing regulations or assisted living residences can strengthen their policies and procedures.

Center for Excellence in Assisted Living

The Assisted Living Workgroup represented a major advance in stakeholder collaboration for assisted living. Much like the earlier Assisted Living Quality Coalition collaborators, however, the promulgation of recommendations for the field was only a beginning. There remained an ongoing need for formal, sustained collaboration on quality assurance in assisted living, one that included stakeholders who had not participated in the workgroup, such as representatives from the assisted living research, finance, and governance sectors. In late spring 2003, 11 organizations began discussing the formation of a national "center for excellence in assisted living" (CEAL), which ultimately led to the creation of CEAL as a nonprofit organization in the fall of 2004.

CEAL was founded on the principle of collaborative participation by diverse stakeholders with knowledge of and expertise in assisted living. This was reflected in the composition of its 11-member board of directors:

- Four consumer/advocacy organizations—AARP, Consumer Consortium on Assisted Living, Alzheimer's Association, Paralyzed Veterans of America;
- Four provider associations—AAHSA, ASHA, ALFA, NCAL; and
- Three other stakeholder groups—National Cooperative Bank Development Corporation, Pioneer Network, American Assisted Living Nurses Association

An active Advisory Council comprised of representatives from more than 30 organizations around the country helps guide and shape the collaborative work of CEAL. Since its inception, CEAL has set a priority agenda to address key issues of assisted living, including quality and affordability of assisted living for low-income elders. CEAL's initial accomplishments speak to the power of dedicated professionals working in a climate of mutual respect and open-mindedness.

State-level decision makers are still not involved in this collaboration, however. This has created an enormous gap between what other stakeholders have identified as effective foci for state regulation and what actually happens in the states. While a few states in the past two years have considered the workgroup recommendations as they formulated their regulations, the vast majority has not taken advantage of their expansive and exhaustive collaborative work. Therefore, the participation of all key stakeholders is still lacking.

Accountability

Successful outcomes are also dependent on accountability among all stakeholders. As defined by *Webster's Collegiate Dictionary,* accountability is acceptance of responsibility for one's actions. Other than through state survey processes and voluntary accreditation, accountability has been lacking in assisted living. For example, consumers and consumer advocates typically become vocal only when a problem arises rather than working to prevent and resolve concerns before they escalate into crises. They generally do not perceive that they have a responsibility to work proactively to help ensure that problems do not arise in the first place. Rather, they delegate to state survey agencies or long-term care ombudsmen the responsibility to fix problems.

A system similar to parent-teacher associations (PTAs) could be very effective for consumers of assisted living. PTAs are formed for individual schools so that parents of students and teachers at that school can identify local needs and issues together and address them directly. Assisted living consumers could benefit from the same approach by forming individual "consumer-caregiver councils" for assisted living residences with participation only from consumers and staff at that particular residence. Beneficial outcomes would include more active participation and investment in the residence by consumers and mutual commitment to collaboratively address needs and issues as they arise.

As we have noted, providers have also generally not taken responsibility for proactively addressing systemic problems within their industry but instead behave like ostriches. They have left it to other stakeholders, including even the U.S. Government Accountability Office, to weigh in about significant, widespread, long-standing problems in the industry, such as medication management, insufficient staffing to meet residents' needs, inadequate staff training, inconsistent quality of care seven days a week, and questionable marketing and disclosure practices.

Similar examples could be provided for each stakeholder group, but the point is that none of the groups is stepping up to accept its full share of responsibility for the success of assisted living. Each tends to remain narrowly focused on its specific interests and/or immediate needs.

Collective accountability—the need for participants across all domains to account for their actions to one another and to the field as a whole—fares no better. In assisted living, stakeholders in the domains of practice, public policy, research, governance, and financing need to bridge the boundaries between their domains and integrate their efforts to benefit the industry as a whole. Although stakeholders in a single domain, such as public policy, may be highly accountable, without cooperation from other domains, whatever is achieved within the public policy domain is usually limited and often short lived.

The Assisted Living Workgroup offers an example of how a lack of collective accountability limited the outcomes of the initiative. The workgroup successfully involved most of the diverse stakeholders at the national level in the domains of *public policy* and *practice.* Outreach efforts were made at the start of the initiative to involve national counterparts from long-term care *research* (the American Geriatrics Society and GSA), *finance* (the Centers for Medicare and Medicaid Services, Department of Housing and Urban Development, and long-term care insurers), and *governance* (the National Conference for State Legislators [NCSL] and the National Governors Association [NGA]).

None of these groups, however, became invested in the workgroup's outcomes. For instance, the NCSL and the NGA involvement in promoting the final consensus recommendations among their constituencies would have been invaluable in influencing states to assess their regulations and systems of monitoring and oversight in light of these new recommendations. In its absence, only a few states reviewed the workgroup recommendations and fewer still have acted on them. Similarly, the research community has not initiated the needed studies identified by the workgroup in April 2003.

If leaders of assisted living are wise, they will find ways to enhance accountability among all stakeholders, at all levels, before a major crisis provokes massive public outcries and predictable, but potentially unwelcome, response from a dormant stakeholder—the federal government.

Conclusions and Implications for the Future

Given this uncertain future, two disturbing trends are emerging:

- In the face of massive budget shortfalls, states are increasingly stepping back from their responsibilities. They are carrying out less frequent (if any) inspections of assisted living residences, yet state inspection visits are currently the only means of monitoring operational performance for assisted living. As a result, frail, vulnerable residents are being compromised, and the prospects of federal regulatory presence are increased.

- Although 41 states currently use Medicaid to fund services in assisted living, in proportion to nursing home funding the amount allocated to assisted living is sorely inadequate. Without additional funding of Medicaid programs for assisted living, low-income seniors will not be able to access assisted living services.

Will stakeholders in assisted living step up to the plate as the MR/DD community did and set aside their agendas to respond to these threats? Or will they follow the ineffective path of the mental health community? Will they work collectively on issues to strengthen the whole field or will special interests take precedence?

The MR/DD community succeeded without a nationally recognized or famous leader. This offers an important lesson for assisted living, which lost its champion when Louisiana Democratic Senator John Breaux, former chair of the Special Committee on Aging and architect of the Assisted Living Workgroup, retired in January 2005. Like the MR/DD community, assisted living needs courageous individual leaders from within the community who can unite their stakeholder colleagues to pursue a common agenda that will strengthen the whole field, not simply promote the interests of a few.

Through CEAL, the assisted living profession has established the infrastructure to bring together the wide network of diverse stakeholders across domains to address pressing issues collaboratively. Although it can be devilishly hard to integrate effective and able leadership, collective accountability, and a commitment by all stakeholders to work jointly toward common purposes, there is no better time than now to do so. The assisted living industry is not currently under fire, and this is an ideal time for it to focus on strengthening and improving itself. Waiting until a crisis strikes to make needed changes is shortsighted and disingenuous.

If for no other reason, stakeholders may find common cause in keeping the federal government out of the business of overseeing assisted living. There is always a risk that Washington will step in with heavy-handed and potentially ineffective regulation. As the stakeholder most removed from the field and farthest away from delivery of care and services, the federal government is not well positioned to provide responsive, effective oversight. Perhaps one of CEAL's most valuable contributions could be to identify collaboratively other key areas of common cause to work continually and effectively toward strengthening the assisted living field.

Robert Frost may have put it best: "Two roads diverged in a wood, and I took the one less traveled by, and that has made all the difference." Assisted living could take the road less traveled and commit its collective and ample resources to holding itself accountable for the quality of services it provides. Otherwise, it will go the way of other industries, like nursing homes or mental health, that could not or would not rise above individual interests to champion the good of the whole.

REFERENCES

Assisted Living Quality Initiative. August 1998. Building a structure that promotes quality. Unpublished white paper. Washington, D.C.: Assisted Living Quality Initiative

Cohen, E. 2004. Advocacy and advocates: Definitions and ethical dimensions. *Generations 28* (1), 9–16.

Kane, R., & West J. 2005. *It shouldn't be this way: The failure of long-term care.* Nashville: Vanderbilt University Press.

Silverstein, R. 2000. Emerging disability policy framework: A guidepost for analyzing public policy. *Iowa Law Review 85* (5), 1695–1754.

U.S. Senate, Special Committee on Aging. 2003. *Assisted Living: Examining the assisted living workgroup final report, Hearing.* Washington, DC: Government Printing Office.

CHAPTER 10

Financing of Assisted Living Properties

Past, Present, and Future

ANTHONY J. MULLEN, M.S.
HARVEY N. SINGER, M.B.A.

The future of assisted living will largely be determined by the extent to which the financial community provides capital to the assisted living sector as opposed to alternate investment opportunities. Each lender and investor of mortgage debt and equity funding to the sector must make further decisions about the types of projects for their capital:

- Larger projects or smaller projects;
- Projects offering only modest assistance with activities of daily living (ADLs) or a service-rich environment for high acuity residents;
- Projects built to residential codes (for example, wood-frame construction) or to institutional codes (I-2, concrete and steel) to allow for alternate uses;
- Projects intended to be "affordable," or midmarket, or upscale;
- Projects in more densely populated markets with prospective residents, or in less densely populated (or less penetrated) markets without competitors.

When making these decisions, the financial community will react to both extrinsic factors, such as the state of financial markets supplying that capital, and factors more particular to assisted living—shifts in demographics and household markets, the regulatory environments, and public (government) and private sources of payment to pay for assisted living services.

Our objective in this chapter is to provide a sufficiently comprehensive review of the ways in which these crucial groups—the capital sources—view and respond to the assisted living sector. Our premise is that assisted living projects will continue to attract financing as long as their prospects for the return *of* and the return *on* investors' capital exceeds the perceived risk of employing the capital in the sector, especially when compared with other capital investment opportunities.

To make educated projections and statements about how the investment community views the future of assisted living, and how it influences its financing decisions, we must first look both to the past and current environment. In this exploration, we are fortunate to be able to draw on a dedicated source of information about the needs, sources, and flows of capital to the assisted living sector: data from the National Investment Center for the Seniors Housing and Care Industry (NIC, formerly the National Investment Conference for the Senior Living and Long Term Care Industry). The NIC was founded in 1991 to serve as an information resource for lenders of debt, for equity investors, and for others interested in the provision of capital to meet the housing and long-term care needs of America's aging population. Proceeds from NIC's annual conference (attended by more than 1,500 financial and operating executives) fund research and educational efforts supporting capital formation in the senior housing and long-term care industries.

Consistent with its mission, since 1994 NIC has undertaken lender and investor surveys of the industry's major financiers, to review lender/investor requirements and trends and discover how capital sources evaluate the sector's various product types. These surveys, conducted annually or biennially, also compile the prevailing lending terms for projects. Much of the information in this chapter that documents those capital flows is drawn from NIC's surveys.

NIC also maintains a unique database, updated each calendar quarter, which currently tracks more than 7,200 market-rate properties in the largest U.S. markets. This consists of more than a million units/beds across the complete spectrum of independent living, assisted living, dementia, nursing, and continuing care retirement communities. From this database, NIC compiles Market Area Profiles (MAPs), consisting of information about supply, demand, absorption rates, new construction, leasing pace, occupancy rates, rents, and concessions in these markets.

History of the Sector and Its Financing

Before 1950, seniors who could not stay at home were often either placed in small-scale boarding homes offering supervision, board, and care provided directly by the proprietors (rather than by professional staff), or were placed in mental institutions. More alternatives became available in the 1950s when government policies encouraged the building of more nursing homes.

From the mid-1960s, Medicare and Medicaid have had a significant influence on residential care opportunities for seniors, propelling dramatic growth in—and the need to capitalize—the nursing home sector. From 1965 to 1985, both the number of nursing homes and their population increased steadily. From the mid-1980s, the growth continued but at a much slower rate. This slow-down resulted from expanded options for seniors needing housing available to older consumers, from decreases in age-specific disability rates, and from states restricting the building of new nursing home beds. From 1991 to 1999, the number of properties offering skilled nursing services grew only by 22 percent, and the number of beds increased by only about 20 percent (NIC, 2000a).

In the mid-1990s increasing consumer affluence coupled with dissatisfaction with the heavily regulated, "medical model" of nursing home care propelled dramatic growth in—and the need to capitalize—assisted living properties, with their more "residential" orientation to care. In the 8 years between 1991 and 1999, the number of properties providing assisted living services increased by almost 50 percent, and the number of assisted living beds increased by 115 percent (NIC, 2000a).

However, overbuilding spurred by overabundant capital infusions (primarily but not exclusively from Wall Street and venture capital firms) and a lack of understanding among developers about the size and depth of the market for assisted living caused significant financial distress for many assisted living properties that opened between 1998 and 2002. During this period, a number of larger companies went bankrupt or were sold because of poor financial performance.

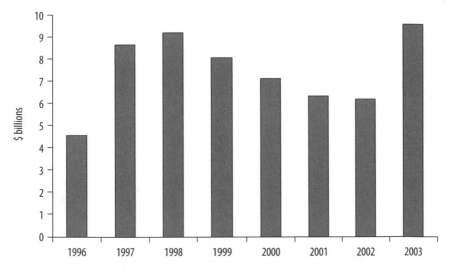

Figure 10.1. Total project financing provided to senior housing and care sector, 1996–2003

According to the most representative sample of national and regional developers available, new construction of assisted living dropped by almost 90 percent, from a high of 31,273 units under construction in 1999 to 3,627 units in 2002, before it began to rise again during the next 3 years, to approximately 6,000 units annually (American Seniors Housing Association [ASHA], 2005). Meanwhile, occupancy rates fell from a high of approximately 95 percent nationally in 1997, to 89.5 percent in 1999, to a low of 84.5 percent in 2001, rising back up to 88.5 percent in 2005 (NIC, 2006a).

NIC's lender/investor survey results over the past 10 years illustrate the changes in capital providers' perceptions of the senior housing and care sector, and the capital markets generally. Skepticism and caution played a role between 1994 and 1996, when many investors were first becoming aware of the available opportunities in this sector. In 1997 and 1998, there was marked enthusiasm for the industry, particularly for assisted living. In 1999 and 2000, and immediately thereafter, funding tightened as concerns about overbuilding and tightened reimbursements linked to Medicare's prospective payment system pervaded an industry already burdened by more widespread capital market restrictions (see Figure 10.1). Since then, although loan terms have remained relatively stringent, many lenders appear to be approaching the industry with renewed—although cautious—enthusiasm. Currently (as of 2006), the investment community has become relatively gratified with the performance of assisted living and the entire senior housing and care "continuum."

The demographics certainly appear favorable. Recent trend lines of key measures of income and wealth show an increase in the affluence of seniors. Census figures show, for example (U.S. Census Bureau, 2006, 2003, 2001),

- Households headed by individuals ages 65–74 have a higher net worth—largely home equity—than any other age group, and households headed by those older than 75 have the next highest net worth.
- Both median and mean net worth of households older than 75 increased by 20–30 percent from 1995 to 2000.
- Median and mean incomes of the population older than 75 have increased by approximately one-third in nominal dollars and almost 10 percent in real dollars—taking inflation into account—in the last decade. In 2004, the median income for these households was $20,467 and the mean income was $29,487.

While these incomes are generally *below* the typical annual costs of occupying assisted living residences in 2004, which are in the $35,500 median range (ASHA, 2005; NIC, 2006b), it is nevertheless the case that seniors are increasingly able to rely on financial sources other than their incomes to cover their housing and care costs. Several factors enable seniors to afford assisted living, including,

- Adult children who are increasingly willing and able to subsidize care—more than one in four of those whose relative was in assisted living said that they themselves (or other family members) had helped pay for those assisted living costs (NIC, 2000b);
- Seniors who are showing a greater willingness to liquidate owned assets (most notably, their existing homes) to fund service-oriented housing and care. The most recent data available show mean net equity in their owned home as $87,603 (median $81,075) for households over the age of 75, and their homeownership rate as 72.5 percent (U.S. Census Bureau, 2001).

The Current Environment
Supply of and Demand for Assisted Living Communities

Over the past 15 years, assisted living has received the most media and investor attention among the different segments of senior housing and care, but it is still a relatively small part of the overall continuum. According to such sources as ASHA (2004) and the NIC MAP reports (NIC, 2006b), assisted living units (including dementia care) represent just 20–25 percent of the continuum of properties that make up the senior housing and care industry. Nursing beds make up approximately 50 percent, whereas independent living units make up roughly another 20 percent of the total. If one were to add the growing segment of senior apartments (similar to independent living but without the bundled "communal/congregate" service package of meals, activities, transportation, and so forth), assisted living's share would shrink even more.

Industry studies (principally by NIC and the ASHA) have determined the existing stock of senior housing to be in the ranges shown in Table 10.1. Sufficient demand now exists to keep those units occupied at the 90 percent range and above (for stabilized properties, those beyond their initial fill-up).

The most recent studies by those same industry associations indicate the following current annual growth rates in the supply of senior housing options:

- Approximately 2 percent for senior apartments,
- 1–4 percent for independent living communities,
- 1–3 percent for assisted living properties,
- 1–2 percent for continuing care retirement communities (CCRCs), and
- One half percent for nursing homes.

The growth rate in new construction of assisted living has indeed diminished significantly from 1996 to 2003, when it averaged 8–10 percent per year or more, as compared with 2004–2005, when it averaged less than 2 percent per year (NIC, 2006b). That growth is in approximate balance with the 1–2 percent current annual growth rate of households over the age of 75 in the United States. Tables 10.2 and 10.3 provide examples of the best available supply and demand metrics from the NIC MAP quar-

TABLE 10.1
Senior Housing and Care Stock

	No. of Properties	No. of Units
Senior apartment	5,350	440,000
Independent living community	6,200	725,000
Assisted living residence	8,000	600,000
Continuing care retirement community	2,200	650,000
Nursing home	16,200	1,700,000

Note: These data report on units professionally owned and managed properties generally consisting of market rate properties that each have 25 or more units. If smaller properties, subsidized properties, and family-owned and -managed properties were to be included, the totals would be much higher (e.g., on the order of 1 million units of assisted living).

terly census of properties in the nation's 30 largest metropolitan areas (which account for approximately 40 percent of the nation's population).

Supply of and Demand for Capital to Finance Assisted Living Properties

The NIC's most recent survey (NIC, 2003) of nearly 100 of the sector's lenders and investors found that in 2003:

- There has been a decrease in the number of debt (loan) providers, but *not* a corresponding decrease in the *amount* of funding provided. This indicates that although the major financiers remain active, many of the marginal lenders have exited the industry; the experienced lenders are picking up the activity. (See Appendix 1.)
- Commercial banks and savings banks, along with mortgage bankers, represented approximately half of the active lenders responding. Pension funds (or their advisors) and mortgage brokers were frequent lenders; REITs (real estate investment trusts), insurance companies, credit finance companies, and investment bankers were less active providers of debt. In past years, investment bankers were much more active, to the point where (in 2000) they comprised about one-fifth of investment activity in the sector; however, since 1996, participation by other institutional financing sources and intermediaries has increased, supporting the position that capital for the senior housing and care industry has become more widely available and less restricted to local sources.
- Financing through less-traditional sources, such as Fannie Mae/Freddie Mac or loans insured by HUD, became more prevalent.

TABLE 10.2

Key Supply and Demand Metrics of the 30 Largest Metropolitan Statistical Areas in the United States, Fourth Quarter, 2005

Demand and Supply Metrics	Type of Housing or Care			
	Independent Living	Assisted Living	Dementia Care	Nursing Care
Demand:				
Median occupancy of stabilized properties	96.80%	95.80%	95.80%	94.00%
Mean occupancy of stabilized properties	92.70%	91.70%	91.20%	90.40%
Net monthly move-in rate of nonstabilized properties open <24 months	7.6	2.7	1.5	7.8
Increase or decrease in units occupied since last quarter	2.70%	1.80%	1.80%	0.80%
Supply:				
Total number of properties by type of service provided[a]	1,708	2,864	1,223	4,537
Total units/beds in inventory[b]	234,592	168,894	32,126	577,265
Penetration rate[c] of total units per 75+ households	5.10%	3.70%	0.70%	12.60%
Total number of new properties opened this quarter[a]	12	20	10	7
Completions (number of units in new properties opened)	1,371	1,145	208	596
Number of units under construction	8,097	4,580	919	3,430
Revenue:				
Median monthly revenue per occupied unit/bed[b]	$2,089	$3,000	$4,579	$5,173
Affordability index (ratio of price to income)	0.9	1.2	1.9	2.1
Property:				
Median age of property, in years	18	12	7	30
Properties reporting need to upgrade	25.90%	26.80%	24.00%	32.40%
Median number of units/beds per property	108	53	22	118
Properties for-profit	60.90%	70.90%	81.40%	71.30%
Properties that are part of chain	51.60%	51.00%	63.80%	49.00%

Source: 2006 National Investment Center for the Seniors Housing and Care Industry—Market Area Profiles

[a]A property is counted once for each type of service it provides. Therefore, the sum of properties across types is greater than the total of properties reported.

[b]Data are reported by unit for independent living, assisted living, and dementia care. Nursing care data are reported by beds.

[c]The supply of a type of unit (bed or apartment) relative to the number of 75+ households.

TABLE 10.3

Key Economic and Demographic Influences in the 30 Largest Metropolitan Statistical Areas (MSAs) in the United States, Fourth Quarter, 2005

Statistic	30 MSAs
Summary of Economic and Demographic Influences	
Projected annual growth rate of 75+ households	1.2%
Projected annual growth rate of 45–64-year-old households	2.6%
75+ households as percent of total households	9.4%
45–64-year-old households as percent of total households	37.1%
Median household income of 75+ age group	$29,244
Median household income of 45–64 age group	$68,753
Summary of Residential Real Estate	
Median home value	$338,453
Annual increase in price of existing homes sold from third quarter of 2004 to third quarter of 2005	13.6%

Source: 2006 National Investment Center for the Seniors Housing and Care Industry—Market Area Profiles

- More of the lenders had invested in freestanding assisted living or in nursing facilities than in other property types.
- The majority of lenders reported their intention to increase funding in the future (or at least to maintain previous levels of funding) to segments of the senior housing and care industry in which they have invested in so far.
- Funding was estimated at $9.75 billion or more during 2003, compared to $6–$6.5 billion in each of 2001 and 2002, and the total debt and equity funding outstanding was reported at $28 billion.
- With respect to *equity* investment, just as for debt lending, assisted living properties and nursing homes accounted for almost half of the investment activity, and most (63 percent) of the equity providers who responded expected to increase their future level of investment in the industry. Of these, 64 percent expected to acquire existing properties and 43 percent expected to fund the construction of *new* properties (though just about half of the transactions involved refinancing of existing property investments). (See Appendix 1.)
- Although nursing homes were listed as a favorite within the sector for future lending activity, lower-acuity projects (senior apartments, independent living or "congregate care" projects, and, especially, CCRCs) have gained popularity, and it was those lower acuity projects that were rated more highly from a risk/reward perspective. From the late 1990s into 2000, projects that offer higher levels of service, such as assisted living and nursing homes, had generally

been the favored investments. Nursing homes produced the strongest range of feelings among lenders—from very favorable to very unfavorable. Equity investors planned to fund more independent living and CCRC properties than either assisted living or nursing homes.

- Maximum loan-to-value ratios (LTVs) for permanent loans were in the 75–80 percent range (with very little change over the recent past), with higher acuity projects at the *lower* end of the LTV range. Construction loans required almost similar LTVs, but more leverage was accepted: almost half of the respondents indicated they would fund deals with higher than 80 percent LTV (that is, would provide sufficient loan capital to projects if developers were able to put up equity capital consisting of just 20 percent, or less, of the project's value). Minimum debt service coverage ratios (that is, the amount of cash flows after expenses, compared to the principal and interest payments required on the loans) ranged from just under 1.3-to-1 for lower acuity projects to almost 1.4-to-1 for nursing homes.
- For nursing homes, equity investors expected/required 16 percent rates of return for the "typical" nursing home investment made at 75–85 percent leverage. Sample sizes were insufficient to determine, with confidence, required rates of return for other project types.
- Most lenders required personal recourse (signature) on loans. Likewise, the majority of lenders required cross-collateralization (taking a lien on a borrower's other properties in addition to the one for which the funds were used). And 9 of 10 lenders would not lend to a prospective borrower who had not yet completed any projects.
- For "underperforming assets" (that is, those with nonexistent or negative earnings for which a capitalization rate based on earnings cannot be used as the basis for valuing the investment), value was most frequently determined as a function of selling price per bed (typically, $22,500 per bed for nursing home beds and $37,500 for assisted living beds).

There are a number of positive indicators and trends for capital formation in assisted living in 2006:

- Loan delinquencies are at the lowest levels since these records have been kept (NIC, 2006a).
- More debt capital was placed in the industry in the year 2005 than in any other year tracked (NIC, 2006a).

- One major provider of assisted living had an extremely successful initial public offering in the fourth quarter of 2005, demonstrating that the public equity markets liked the future prospects of assisted living and independent living.
- The NIC, whose information and services target the majority of financiers within the sector, had record attendance at its annual conference in 2005.
- In the fourth quarter of 2005, the values of properties as measured by (the inverse of) capitalization rates (capitalization rates being the most widely used measures to value income-producing real-estate-related business properties) were at the highest level ever recorded (NIC, 2006a).

What may be surprising to those not familiar with the financial aspects of assisted living is that the investment market has become so competitive for both debt and equity capital that investors are clamoring to find ever-smaller developers and operators to back. While larger providers (those with 10 or more properties) are especially sought out by financiers, there are simply too few of *them* in relation to all of the active financing sources. In the current environment, any company with at least two successful properties can be a candidate for financiers' attentions, although these providers will still need to meet criteria of sufficient liquid net worth of their owners and often also of obtaining some outside equity (more on this in the next section). But, as competition for use of capital intensifies, both debt and equity investors are forced to become less risk averse, and this is precisely what has happened in 2005 and 2006, even as the industry fundamentals improved (see chapter 1).

In what may be the most important financing-related development in the senior housing and care sector for the present and the future, the financial community has devised—and continues to devise—new techniques, models, and data sources to inform investment decisions. These new tools are designed to better analyze:

- *Market* feasibility (supply, demand, and resulting rents, pace of fill-up, and level of occupancy once that pace has stabilized) for new properties, or those whose operations and strategies have been reoriented; and
- *Financial* feasibility (revenues in excess of costs of construction, of

marketing, and of operations *given* the fill rate and level of market response to price levels indicated by the market feasibility analysis).

Improved feasibility analyses will in turn enable investors to determine
more accurately the likely profit and cash-flow outcomes of investments
in the sector—and so determine the likelihood of return *of* those investments and returns *on* those investments, which provide the sector's capital needs. (See Appendixes 2 and 3.)

Future Financing

Because of recent performance on such underwriting criteria, assisted
living looks quite promising to the investment community. The key question for investors is whether financiers and developers will be disciplined
enough to avoid another round of overbuilding. We believe the answer is
yes, for three important reasons:

1. Developable land has become more scarce, more difficult to obtain
   regulatory and building approvals for, and much more costly than in
   the mid- to late 1990s.
2. Construction costs went up significantly between 2004 and 2006,
   and there is still uncertainty about where they are headed in 2006–
   2007 (and beyond).
3. Equity capital (which is needed in addition to debt capital) for new
   construction is much more scarce today than it was between 1993
   and 1999. (Debt capital, however, is not necessarily more scarce.)

While these three factors may prevent overbuilding, they may also put
constraints on the expansion of assisted living. Given steadily growing
demand, these supply constraints also imply the likelihood of higher
future prices for residents.

In looking at the future of financing assisted living, a couple of key
"structural" issues with respect to financing in general and financing for
the senior housing and care sector in particular must also be understood:
the provision of new capital versus recycled capital, and what is called
"mezzanine" financing. These issues are likely to endure during at least
the next few years.

New Capital versus Recycled Capital

In understanding the potential for financing, one must understand the distinction between investing new capital (providing "new money") and recycling of outstanding capital ("refinancing," "recapitalizing," or "refunding").

In the financing of any new real estate or real estate–based business, such as senior housing and care, a physical asset must be created. Except in a few unique circumstances, both debt and equity capital are required to create the asset (land, buildings, equipment, soft costs, and so forth). Financing the creation of a new physical asset is considered a very risky proposition, which has caused a unique financing structure to evolve that takes into account the extra risk of a new asset. This structure is called "construction financing" (also termed "acquisition, development, and construction financing"). In construction financing, the debt or first mortgage position is usually provided by commercial ("merchant") banks or by savings banks, or by investment banks that sell tax-exempt bonds to mutual funds and other institutional investors and also to the public ("at retail").

Because there have been sufficient payback problems with construction loans in all types of real estate in the past 30 years, loan requirements have been made more stringent in order to reduce the risk assumed by construction lenders. The main change is that developers of new projects must put up more equity. In the last decades of the twentieth century, it was common for developers to put up 10 percent of the cost of a new project in the form of equity. In the first decade of the twenty-first century, all but the most successful developers need 20 percent (or more) of a project's cost in the form of equity (NIC, 2003). Banks are now subject to much harsher scrutiny by regulators on this issue.

In addition, these sources for construction funding normally require that the principals who are borrowing the money provide a personal guarantee of the construction loan up through the period of opening and fill-up of the property. Moreover, unless these principals have, *in addition,* a liquid net worth (e.g, cash or marketable securities) equal to 20 percent or more of the amount of the construction loan, they will find it difficult to obtain the construction loan—even if they can supply 20 percent of the cost of the project in the form of (other, less liquid) equity.

This means there will likely be less new development in general within senior housing and care, because equity is scarcer and more expensive (relative to debt). For example, in the 1980s a developer could build a 60-unit assisted living residence for approximately $4,500,000 by putting up about $450,000–$600,000 of equity. In 2006, this same 60-unit project would cost about $8,000,000 and so require at least $1,600,000 of equity (at 20 percent of the project's cost)—three times the amount of equity. It is difficult for many developers (or potential developers) of senior housing and care properties to raise this amount of equity.

The *recycling* of capital—also termed *refinancing* or *recapitalization* of properties—is, however, another matter. It will continue at a brisk pace, because of the ongoing consolidation of companies within the industry, their improved ability (given their greater size and concentration) to *qualify* for financing, their more sophisticated and professional financial staffs (which constantly seek to refinance in order to reduce their costs of capital), and increased competition among *sources* of capital to supply these entities with financing.

Mezzanine Financing

Because of the scarcity of outside sources of equity, one key trend that will likely accelerate during the next 10 years is the use of "mezzanine" financing for new construction and for acquisitions. "Mezzanine" financing here refers to financing structured "between" equity and debt: as "preferred" equity or as subordinated debt (with a second or third mortgage, and so forth, claim), which allows a developer to meet the equity requirements of a lender who holds the *first* mortgage. Several sources have been formed to provide this type of financing, and while it makes the financing process more complex and time consuming, it does allow new construction and acquisition projects to proceed that otherwise would not.

Mezzanine financing is one important example of the movement toward "structured" financing. It allocates different portions of a borrower's capital structure to separate financial sources that are willing to take on the different risks inherent in supplying capital for those various pieces, in return for a yield (a return on their investment) commensurate with the corresponding levels of risk that each portion entails. By dividing the debt into "tranches" (slices or segments), the *overall* cost of capital may be lowered and the financing process may become more rationalized—meaning that it provides each portion of the capital with a return on investment that is commensurate with the risk that is incurred by that portion—but it does not necessarily make the financing process easier. Although this structured approach is well established for recycling (debt) capital in the "public" debt market (that is, for bonds and debt securities), it has been slower to catch on for funding new construction or acquisitions in the *private* debt and equity markets (that is, with individual lenders and equity suppliers).

Few organized sources of common equity (that is, stock, or public secondary markets) for new construction exist in the senior housing and care field, but this situation will change as competition continues to grow among REITs, private equity, and venture capital firms generally devoted to real estate.

Other Structural Issues in Senior Housing and Care that Affect Financing

There is growing consensus that, although the stand-alone assisted living model, in which *only* assisted living but no other level of housing or care is offered, is still quite viable, it is less attractive to investors and to customers than it was twenty years ago. For one thing, it has been documented that the revenues per occupied unit or occupied bed in assisted living within properties offering assisted living *in combination* with other levels of care are significantly higher than those for stand-alone assisted living (NIC, 2006b). The same is true for assisted living within CCRCs: per-unit revenues are higher than for stand-alone assisted living (see chapter 1).

Many analysts believe the stand-alone model of assisted living has reached a point of balance between supply and demand in most markets and can grow at a compound rate of no more than about 2 percent per year for the immediate future—that is, at a rate no more than the demographic growth rate in the age groups who actually move to assisted living currently (Claritas, 2006). Any company growth above that rate will likely be due to mergers and acquisitions, or to new competition taking existing market share from existing competitors.

Granted, 2 percent compound growth should not be underestimated, because it can provide approximately 12,000 new units per year of market-rate assisted living across the United States. That amounts to about

200 new properties per year if we assume there are 50–60 units per property, which is currently typical. Each year there is also an opportunity for perhaps 8,000 new units of smaller "board and care" properties oriented toward lower-income residents, many of whom receive federal Supplemental Security Income (SSI). It is much more difficult, however, for board-and-care properties than for market-rate properties to attract capital for development and become financially feasible at less-than-market revenue rates (Howard, 2002). Historically, the majority of these properties have involved conversions of existing buildings.

The primary issues that will affect the *need* for additional financing, however, as well as the types of future financing, arise from developments in the senior housing and care markets as well as the progress of assisted living demand growth. In particular, demand growth and capital needs will be affected by

- Medicaid and Medicare budget pressures;
- Age of existing nursing homes, and their image;
- Segmentation of the market due to competition and customer choice;
- The market's image of *independent* living communities;
- New sources for private payment of assisted living costs;
- Technology; and
- Public and private partnerships.

Medicaid and Medicare Budget Pressures

It has been evident for some time that Medicaid and Medicare budgets will continue to come under pressure. The resulting cost reimbursement rates, especially for Medicaid nursing home stays, will make it increasingly difficult for providers to make an economic profit or will cause even greater losses from serving Medicaid residents in nursing homes. In fact, the Centers for Medicare and Medicaid Services (CMS) conceded that profits from Medicare (and private pay) residents fund the losses from Medicaid stays for the "average" nursing home in the United States (Van der Walde, 2003). In 2005, Medicaid residents represented about 65 percent of all nursing homes stays (CMS, 2005).

According to CMS data, occupied nursing beds paid by Medicaid reimbursement have actually declined, decreasing from almost 980,000 occupied nursing beds for which the primary payer was Medicaid in December 2001 to approximately 940,000 by December 2005, a reduction of 38,000 Medicaid-paid nursing beds or 3.9 percent in a 4-year period.

A few states have sought to use Medicaid dollars to move nursing residents to (much less expensive) assisted living by converting existing nursing beds to assisted living beds, or by encouraging the use of waivers that allow more Medicaid dollars to go to assisted living. The hope is that by reducing nursing homes stays overall, the cost to Medicaid will go down by an equivalent amount.

In recent years, however, only about 1 in 11 long-term care beds paid for primarily by Medicaid is in an assisted living property, and most of these are in the older "board and care" model of assisted living (Mollica, 2002); the remaining 10 beds are in nursing homes. The key question then becomes: do all 10 of those remaining residents *require* a nursing home level of care? The question has not yet been answered definitively, but there *are* studies that conclude that, at a minimum, 15 percent of nursing home residents could realistically be served in assisted living communities (e.g., Buttar et al., 2005).

Thus, as states continue to use waivers—what is being "waived" is the provision that Medicaid funds are to be used to pay for care only in licensed nursing facilities—under the home- and community-based services provisions of Section 1915(c) of the Social Security Act, the likely result will be to drive demand in terms of increases in the growth of new or renovated assisted living buildings, and so new capital for the financing of those buildings. This growth will likely be modest, but steady throughout the next 10 years or so. Such is the expectation, especially where states seek to convert existing nursing home beds eligible for Medicaid payment to assisted living beds eligible for Medicaid payment (see chapter 11).

Age of Existing Nursing Homes and Their Image

Closely related to Medicaid pressures, the median *age* of nursing homes is now about 30 years (NIC, 2006b). Many nursing homes built before 1975 are simply outdated today and suffer from physical obsolescence, thus making these facilities difficult to market to *any* customers, except those (primarily Medicaid residents) who have no choice. (So little is reserved for capital improvements—on average, only about $362 per year per bed

[NIC, 2003]—that it would take anywhere from 100 to 300 years to accumulate sufficient reserves to replace the property completely.)

A fair proportion of these properties, perhaps at least 10 percent of all existing nursing homes, will have to seriously examine the possibility of demolition or major renovation/refurbishment over the next 5–10 years. In light of their institutional feel and physically obsolete buildings, coupled with the poor image that the majority of seniors and their adult children have of nursing homes, it is likely that as many as 10 percent of nursing homes will be significantly renovated, converted to a related use (such as assisted living), or demolished for a new nursing home (or a non-seniors use) within the next 10 years. This possibility will necessitate creative financing approaches requiring both debt and equity capital. Already a major movement is under way through a joint venture of the National Cooperative Bank Development Corp., the Robert Wood Johnson Foundation, and the Center for Growing and Becoming, to bring a new nursing home model with a residential feel to as many sites as possible. According to Robert Jenkens of National Cooperative Bank, the joint venture expects to facilitate the construction or reconstruction of at least 50 new nursing homes, called "Green Houses," of between 40 beds and 100 beds each over the period from 2006 through 2010 (see chapter 3).

More such partnerships, between existing provider organizations and equity sources, will be needed to fund the transformation of older nursing homes. Although the overall stock of nursing beds will likely stay at the same level or decrease slightly in the coming 10 years, the amount of capital needed to replace or renovate 10 percent of the nursing stock will require a capital commitment of more than $5 billion (10 percent of 1.6 million beds, at a cost of at least $35,000 per bed). Most of this will be new capital, since many of the oldest nursing homes are debt-free and with equity investments that have been repaid.

New sources of equity capital will be needed to help renovate the previous generation of nursing homes and to build the next generation, many of which will have a more residential design. This shift will begin to blur the main distinction between nursing and assisted living. Both the need for capital to renovate last generation's nursing homes, and the potential increase in residential "feel" of newer, renovated nursing homes, may well have the effect of diverting capital that might have otherwise flowed to the financing of assisted living itself.

Segmentation Due to Competition and Customer Choice

As the senior housing and care sector climbs the demand curve of industry maturity toward its peak in 2021–2041 (when the baby boom generation reaches 75-plus years of age, the prime segment for entering facility-based housing and care), competition has intensified to the point where properties of all types must be truly customer focused. Unless they can provide real "customer value," where the benefits of the property are perceived to be equal to or greater than the price, many properties, especially "average properties," will lose occupancy and market share.

In efficient and free markets, heavy competition leads to further segmentation of the market for customers, as suppliers find unique niches where there is less price competition. This is precisely what has occurred, and it will continue to occur in senior housing and care during the next 10 years and beyond.

Independent living communities are unbundling their service packages and new "senior apartments" targeted to the mid-price and upper-middle markets are now starting to become an important niche in the market. Providers' own research shows that those new senior apartments are attracting a younger cohort, with an average age at entrance of 72. Many of these residents would likely have moved to all-ages apartments in the past, or simply waited until they were older to move to independent living. Research by the ASHA (2005), focusing on providers who are representative of the larger operators and developers of senior housing and care, showed that senior apartments have become the second-most-preferred type of new development: more senior apartment properties were under construction in 2005 than independent living *or* assisted living properties! As competition continues, we can expect more such segmentation (see chapter 1).

Consumers' demand for more choices and options can also have profound effects on the market and need for capital. For example, several larger developers and operators are now exploring resident-ownership arrangements for independent living units in the continuing care retirement communities. This will likely expand the market because some potential customers have heretofore opted out of the independent living market because there were too few opportunities for unit ownership.

Other customer value and consumer choice issues are exemplified in the success of the very large Erickson Retirement Communities that are now expanding into many major cities. These are CCRCs that normally comprise more than 2,000 units, of which 1,500 are usually independent living units.

The Erickson communities have grown at an extraordinary pace and have proven that there is untapped demand for independent living in every market that they have entered. Is it due to the 100 percent refundable entrance fee (an "equity-like" feature) that these communities offer and the good value in terms of benefits received for the price paid that they are perceived to provide? The economies of scale in its typical communities enable Erickson to offer more features (e.g., indoor pools) and more benefits (e.g., on-site doctors) for the price than can most other independent living or CCRC communities.

Its size and equity capital requirements make Erickson's model difficult to replicate, but there are several imitators getting started on a somewhat smaller scale. The Erickson phenomenon simply begs more study. The company plans to open more than 2,000 units of independent living every year for the foreseeable future—and has never had an unsuccessful project.

Image of Independent Living and Other Senior Care Communities

Data from the NIC show that as of 2000, older people had a mixed view of independent living communities, CCRCs, and assisted living communities. Almost half of potential residents found these communities to be undesirable or very undesirable places to live; only about 13 percent found them to be very desirable. This, then, would likely be the upper limit of demand (that is, penetration) among the age 60 or older household group. The proportion goes up just slightly if one examines just the age 75 or older household group (NIC, 2001). Likewise, only 10 percent of the age 60 or older household group *prefers* an age-restricted community with a minimum age requirement as a place to live. This research implies that demand has a potential limit, *but,* because only about 7 percent of the age 60 or older household group *lives* in age-restricted communities, and only about 9.5 percent of the age 75 or older household group lives in independent, CCRC, and assisted living communities combined, there *is* room for growth.

The wild card that could increase demand dramatically is if the desirability or image of these communities becomes more positive. As the senior housing and care industry further matures and begins consumer education and image campaigns, we could see the desirability or image change factor "tip," causing a significant growth in demand (Mullen, 2003). This would cause the amount of capital needed to go up proportionately; however, because assisted living by its nature is much more needs driven—and at least half of residents in assisted living say it was not their own idea to move into assisted living (National Investment Conference, 1998)—it is likely that we will not see the *same* proportionate increase in desirability for assisted living as for independent living or for independent living apartments in CCRCs.

New Sources of Private Payment

For assisted living, dementia, and nursing homes, there is a small but growing set of private payment mechanisms that could increase demand marginally over the next 10 years, and thus increase the need for financing capital. These mechanisms can be grouped into three main categories:

- Asset accumulation plans,
- Disability plans, and
- Long-term care insurance.

Asset accumulation plans—essentially the monetizing of existing assets to provide cash flow *before* a person's death—are relatively new and seek to use annuities and life insurance plan riders to accumulate or tap funds that can then be used to pay for long-term care needs.

Disability plans would seem to hold great promise. More than 35 million individuals have a short-term or long-term disability insurance policy (Insurance Information Institute, 2003), most provided by employers through group plans. If these policies had a small, excess premium in the years while the individual was working, going toward future long-term care, the premium could be held to a manageable level *after* retirement and so encourage policy holders to keep such policies in place through age 90, or for life. Instead of providing income, these plans could provide a similar amount for monthly or yearly payment for long-term care needs: for home health, assisted living, or nursing home care, once a person retired from work.

To date, the senior housing and care sector has been shaped largely by the fact that public monies, through Medicare, Medicaid, HUD, and other agencies, have served as primary of sources of payment for residents' costs of care and housing. Investors and administrators have tailored their products to meet the market-driven requirements of these programs. As *new,* private sources of reimbursement evolve, including managed care, private pay, and long-term care insurance—and bring with them new investors in properties to serve those markets opened up—is the magnitude of demand, perhaps even the nature of the product, likely to change radically?

Probably not. In the next 10 years, there *will* likely be a small increase in the number of households who move to senior care properties because of such payment mechanisms, but the consensus among analysts is that these will not become a significant influence until time frames beyond the next 10 years. Much of the value of such mechanisms will depend on whether current tax-favored policies remain in place and whether the federal government allows the costs of individual policies (as opposed to group policy costs deducted from employers' taxes) to be deductible from federal income tax.

Technology

The ability of technology to grow demand for senior housing and care properties (and therefore increase the need for property financing) is the subject of industry debate (see chapter 8). So far, there is no consensus.

The industry as a whole has been relatively slow to adopt technology to help manage properties. In the short term, we do not anticipate the advent of any technology that could meaningfully reduce the number of employees needed to perform the personal care functions of the property and execute the service and care plans that residents require. Certainly, handheld devices with appropriate software will help reduce paperwork and allow for more hands-on care time, but these devices are unlikely to reduce the need for employees.

If there is concern in the investment community about technology, it is that technologies may well allow people to remain independent in their current homes longer, especially if technology can help sustain meaningful social interaction, for example, through Web cams. It is the human interaction, the social connection, that may be the greatest benefit of these communal senior housing and care properties, and what is most difficult to duplicate through technology.

Public-Private Partnerships

There is little debate within the industry about the need for "affordable" senior housing and care properties. At issue, however, is whether it is possible to provide affordable care *and* earn a sustainable profit that exceeds the cost of capital as a for-profit company. There *are* for-profit companies seeking to provide affordable assisted living; there just are not many large ones, and the smaller ones do not necessarily seek publicity (see chapter 12).

The greatest opportunities to meet the demand for new affordable senior housing and care properties of any type are *partnerships* between non-profit owners and for-profit developers. This is especially likely where mezzanine financing can be used to replace or supplement equity from the nonprofit owner. Normally, a nonprofit owner can obtain lower cost (because tax favored) debt financing. But even given high demand, providing affordable housing and care exclusively may not generate enough revenues in excess of costs to yield sufficient margins to sustain the nonprofit and its "societal" mission (Jenkens et al., 2004).

The major obstacle faced by for-profit entities seeking to create affordable projects is that with the exception of modest "waiver" programs, Medicaid does not cover room and board outside of nursing homes. Thus, usually *several* subsidized programs must be put in place to make a project feasible. Pursuing such subsidized care can be extremely time consuming, and by their nature public subsidies are less likely to yield sufficient profits in excess of costs to justify the effort to obtain them. As a result, it is not-for-profit entities that usually are more willing to create such affordable assisted living projects (see chapter 12).

Conclusions and Implications for the Future

Although the future implications of all the financing mechanisms we have discussed merit further investigation, we can still make some predictions about likely near-term future of financing for assisted living and other modes of senior housing and care.

That future depends most fundamentally on the demand for assisted living, the demand for capital to finance that assisted living, and the supply of available capital. The *demand for assisted living* continues to grow, but, as we have seen, that demand is unlikely to grow much faster than 2–3 percent annually in the foreseeable future. The *demand for capital* will then grow at least at that rate, both to supply new physical facilities and to recapitalize existing facilities and those that may be converted from other senior housing uses, such as nursing homes. And the *supply of capital* is poised to respond to that growth in demand. In fact, the supply of capital could well grow even faster, because of

- New capital structures evolving to reduce investment risk;
- The availability of new data being pioneered by NIC and others in the industry that enable greater "transparency" and better assessment of investment risk; and
- The performance, that is, the satisfactory return of and return on invested capital in assisted living and other senior housing.

In the view of investors, the sector has performed as well as or better than alternative real estate classes to which that capital would otherwise be allocated (NIC, 2003); in turn, capital invested in real estate generally has performed better than in other asset classes to which it would otherwise be allocated (Figure 10.2).

Finally, the nature of financial markets will themselves affect the availability and terms of financing for the assisted living sector. For one thing, improvements in quantity and quality of market and performance data and more careful and complete analyses should encourage the allocation of capital to this sector versus others, because better research makes investments in assisted living both more "transparent" and less risky.

The nature of financial markets will determine not only *how much* capital is available to the assisted living sector but also *where* that capital flows within the sector. Investors have a fiduciary duty (as well as personal preference) to minimize the risk involved for a given level of return. Thus, they are more likely to support assisted living developers who stick to "tried and true" models (types) of assisted living for which the risks can be known with greater confidence. The result could be to reduce the variety of types of assisted living that get built.

Even more likely, however, than investors' reluctance to pioneer by financing new *types* of assisted living is the effect of investors' reluctance

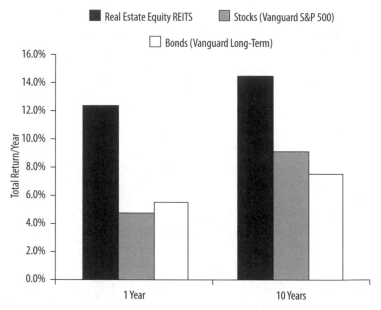

Figure 10.2. Real estate returns versus other investment options, year-end 2005.
Source: Nareit, Vanguard, Delta Associates, February 9, 2006

to pioneer by financing new *providers* of assisted living—providers that have not been tested in previous assisted living ventures. For this reason, the industry is likely to become more concentrated (more product produced by experienced providers). If there is to be innovation in product types of assisted living, it will therefore likely have to come from innovation by providers of existing products, rather than from innovation by new industry entrants.

APPENDIX 1. DEBT AND EQUITY FINANCING

Debt providers of investment capital provide loans to companies in the industry, where the loans typically carry a claim on the assets that are financed with that capital, and where the loan typically must be repaid, with interest.

Equity investment capital is in the form of "ownership"; that is, investment *in* a company. The investment is not required to be repaid with interest, as debt is, but the equity investment represents an ownership claim on the company; that is, it is a partial claim on the earnings of the company and on the sales proceeds when and if the company or its assets are sold.

Given the necessity for some equity (20 percent, plus or minus) to be provided even when debt financing is obtained, and given that debt financing (which uses "other people's money" without diluting company ownership) is usually less expensive than equity financing (and thus makes all-equity investments less desirable), financing providers and care providers alike must usually deal with both *debt and equity financing* issues—one is not any less important than the other.

APPENDIX 2. CURRENT STATE OF THE ART: HOW
CAPITAL PROVIDERS USE CURRENTLY AVAILABLE
INFORMATION TO ESTIMATE "SUSTAINABLE" RETURNS
ON INVESTMENT

(Material in this section is summarized from presentation to "Finance, Underwriting, and Investment Analysis for Seniors Housing and Care" course at University of Maryland, Baltimore County's Erickson School of Aging Studies by Christopher Simon, Senior Analyst at Health Care REIT, Inc.)

Capital providers determine their required return (depending on their cost of capital and their assessment of risk premium from the investment) and reduce the risk of not reaching the required return, by examining available information concerning demand, supply, rents, and vacancy from initial screens, using sources such as NIC MAP and then from more-detailed, "on-the-ground" market research.

The state of the art will take a quantum leap forward when reasonable information about profit margins and profitability become available to the industry, rather than having to estimate these crucial measures of the numerator—the "return"—in the quantity "return on investment" that is a crucial determinant of whether an investment is to be undertaken.

At present, the underwriting process that determines whether and how much capital will be provided, estimates the amount of return—sustainable earnings—based on evaluating the product type, the operator, the market's supply and demand, the particular property, the borrower's credit, and the regulatory environment.

The capital provider estimates the investment's "value" by dividing this estimated sustainable earnings by a so-called capitalization rate (which is nothing more than a ratio that compares sustained earnings to valuations). The provider's capitalization rate depends on its weighted average cost of capital (its own cost to obtain equity and debt, weighted by the proportions of that equity to debt in the capital structure).

The risk is assessed by analyzing macroeconomic factors (those that impact the entire economy) as well as

- Industry risk: for example, that risk stemming from the uncertainty of government reimbursement for costs of caring for residents; state and federal regulation, and liability, for the given property type;

- Property risk: the property's age, quality of design and construction, reputation, and location; and
- Operator risk: for example, the operator's liquidity and credit quality; whether it possesses sufficient organizational infrastructure and personnel to handle the investment in growth.

Sustainable earnings are figured as net income: revenues (rents times occupancy levels) less expenses—expenses of care labor, marketing and advertising, maintenance and repairs, food, necessary property taxes, insurance, and utilities, as well as management fees and reserves for capital expenses (the calculation to this point is the so-called EBITDAR—earnings before interest, taxes, depreciation, amortization, and rents), and then the expenses of interest on debt, income taxes, depreciation, and amortization.

To do this, the capital provider examines ("underwrites") the capital user's "operating model": reviews historical and forecast results; determines the probability of reaching that forecast EBITDAR, by analyzing key drivers of occupancy, rent revenue, and expenses; comparing those parameters with "benchmarks"; examining variances compared to historical performance and compared to similar operating models in local or regional or national markets.

Drilling down, underwriters examine "drivers" of occupancy, as influenced by supply and demand: rental rates, competitive position (as affected by the property's or operator's reputation and quality of care; its marketing team responsible for generating leads, and then converting leads to move-ins; its referral relationships (which can be either a gateway, or a barrier, to additional customers); services offered, physical plant, and microlocation.

Quality of care affects occupancy by increasing referrals (from residents, families, medical sources), reducing resident turnover, and reducing the risk of regulatory bans on admissions.

On the "rent" side of the equation of rents times occupancy levels driving revenue, underwriters examine the rental rates, payor mix (private-pay versus Medicaid versus Medicare versus private-insurance plans or health maintenance organizations), and other revenues (from community fees, respite care rents, rents charged to on-site service providers, and so forth).

For nursing facilities, in particular, payor mix and its concomitants have a significant impact on revenue, and so underwriters analyze Medicare proposed reimbursement rates; case mix refinements; they research state-by-state Medicaid payments, and estimate the rates for future periods by examining budgets and trends in states of interest (the outlook for surpluses or deficits; the proportion of total state budgets accounted for by Medicaid; the proportion of Medicaid budgets accounted for by nursing home reimbursements; and so on), as well as understanding the effects of acquiring (or of new financing for) a facility on its reimbursement rate basis, as well as determining whether delays in state payments require more working capital for sufficient cash flows to pay operating expenses and returns on capital.

For assisted living properties, the base rates as well as level-of-care fees (how they are determined and how often revised in response to care needs and cost changes) are significant determinants of revenue.

On the expense side, capital providers' underwriters examine, in particular, labor expenses; food expense; utilities; property taxes; insurance expenses; and, bad debt history. Labor expenses are impacted by staffing levels in comparison to other similar operations, and by labor rates per position staffed. Raw food expenses are typically compared to other properties in the same geographic region. Utilities are compared to other local properties and to the subject property's historical record; national benchmarks exist but provide little local guidance. Property tax changes can be triggered by reassessments upon the property's sale (or refinancing). Insurance expenses, driven by liability losses, had increased steadily throughout the last 15 years, and while they have now leveled off can be influenced dramatically by a property's risk management programs. Bad debt can be influenced by whether the operator obtains signatures accepting liability for fees from responsible parties beyond the resident.

Next, the capital provider underwrites (analyzes) the influence that the operator being financed has on the income (return) from an investment: the operator is seen as key to success or failure of operations, because the operator develops and implements strategy (for example, overall cost-and-price leadership, or product differentiation and positioning). The operator also determines an organization's culture (leadership, communications, and so forth), its infrastructure (accounting systems; marketing systems) and controls (expense monitoring, occupancy tracking and reactions, financial controls; tracking of resident care). Components of a well-thought-out business strategy include choices of product/service type, geographic focus, resident capacity and mix, and target markets (acuity level, price levels, etc.).

Underwriting market factors intelligently involves determining the demand for beds, bed supply, and the competitive position of the venture being financed. Realistic definitions of target markets are critical: doing analyses of resident origins and determining where and from how far most originate; considering geographic and sociological barriers; traffic flow, and drive times. Demand for beds depends on good demographic information: numbers of age-qualified and income-qualified and frailty-qualified households, as well as income-qualified adult children. Then, these raw "data" must be correlated with the number of occupied beds in the market, to determine the depth of demand for additional beds—all of this greatly aided, and only recently, by the penetration measures generated from NIC's MAP data.

In determining existing and on-coming supply, underwriters are advised to investigate all relevant competition; to use directories of industry supply and planned starts (again, the ability to do this has been hugely augmented by the ability to reference NIC MAP's quarterly compilations of both existing and on-coming supply); telephone books, state directories of licensed facilities, and the U.S. Department of Health and Human Services' CMS "Nursing Home Compare" database.

The likelihood of the property to be financed being able to attract sufficient demand is influenced, in addition to supply/demand imbalances, by the services offered, by the venture's location (its accessibility, convenience, visibility, attractiveness, proximity to shopping and medical services); the physical appearance of the community, and its reputation (if it already exists) for care quality.

Underwriting based on the characteristics of the residence (the property) itself is aided by a site inspection; analysis of the design and floor plan; the quality of construction; and (if the building already exists) the amount of maintenance that has been deferred. Capital providers' underwriting based on credit issues involves examining the borrower's liquidity (will cash flow be available to repay the capital provider?); his net worth; access to additional capital; and credit references based on past borrowings. Capital providers' underwriting based on the regulatory environment involves examining the status of the borrower's certificate of need (if required) and its ability to create barriers to further entry of supply; its licensure (is it in compliance?) and the economic impact of the Medicare and Medicaid reimbursement environments.

APPENDIX 3. FUTURE STATE OF THE ART: UNDERWRITING CAPITAL INVESTMENT IN THE SENIOR HOUSING AND CARE SECTOR

The state of this "art" (which is becoming more science than art, based on the types of data now available about demand, supply, rents and occupancy, and the use of such data in underwriting analysis as detailed above) will take a quantum leap forward when reasonable and comparable information about *expense* levels, *profit margins,* and *profitability* becomes available to the industry, rather than having to estimate these crucial measures of the numerator—the "return"—in the quantity "return on investment."

The availability of such information, however, is not just a pipe dream. The ASHA has started to compile such information and NIC has targeted the provision of such line-item expense data, and resulting profitability from revenues, as its next major area of research; and a pilot program displaying such data may be expected in the near future.

REFERENCES

American Seniors Housing Association. 2004. *Seniors housing statistical handbook.* 4th ed. Washington, DC: American Seniors Housing Association.
American Seniors Housing Association. 2005. *Seniors housing construction report, 2005.* Washington, DC: American Seniors Housing Association.
Buttar, A., Blaum, C., & Fries, B. 2005. Clinical characteristics and six-month out-

comes of nursing home residents with low activities of daily living dependency. *Research in Nursing and Health 28* (3), 660–665.

Claritas Demographics. 2006. *Population and household estimates.* San Diego: Claritas Demographics. www.Claritas.com.

Centers for Medicare and Medicaid Services, U.S. Department of Health and Human Services. 2005. *OSCAR (Online Survey, Certification and Reporting) database reports, current survey data: Patient characteristics and operational characteristics.* Washington, DC: Department of Health and Human Services. www .AHCA.org.

Howard, E. 2002. Reducing operating costs as a means to affordable assisted living: Is it feasible? *Seniors Housing and Care Journal 10* (1), 65–75.

Insurance Information Institute. *U.S. group disability sales survey, 2003.* www.iii .org/media/facts/statsbyissue/disability.

Jenkens, R., Carder, P., & Maher, L. 2004. The Coming Home Program: Creating a state road map for affordable assisted living policy. *Journal of Housing for the Elderly 18* (3/4), 179–201.

Mollica, R. L. 2002. *State assisted living policy, 2002.* Portland, ME: National Association for State Health Policy.

Mullen, A. J. 2003. Why is the occupancy rate down for independent living properties? Potential causes and solutions. *Seniors Housing and Care Journal 11* (1), 31–40.

National Investment Center. 2000a. *NIC national supply estimate of seniors housing and care properties.* Annapolis, MD: National Investment Center for the Seniors Housing and Care Industries.

National Investment Center. 2000b. *NIC national survey of adult children: How they influence their parents' housing and care.* Annapolis, MD: National Investment Center for the Seniors Housing and Care Industries.

National Investment Center. 2001. *NIC national housing survey of adults age 60+: Opinions, attitudes, perceptions, and behaviors.* Annapolis, MD: National Investment Center for the Seniors Housing and Care Industries.

National Investment Center. 2003. *2003 Lender survey: Preferences in financing seniors housing and long term care properties.* Annapolis, MD: National Investment Center for the Seniors Housing and Care Industries.

National Investment Center. 2006a. *Key financial indicators.* Annapolis, MD: National Investment Center for the Seniors Housing and Care Industry, Inc. www.NIC.org.

National Investment Center. 2006b. *NIC market area profiles: Data from the thirty largest metropolitan statistical areas.* Annapolis, MD: National Investment Center for the Seniors Housing and Care Industry, Inc. www.NICMAP.org.

National Investment Conference. 1998. *National survey of assisted living residents: Who is the customer?* Annapolis, MD: National Investment Conference for the Senior Living and Long Term Care Industries.

U.S. Census Bureau. 2001. *Household net worth and asset ownership: 1995.* Current Population Reports, P70-71. Washington, DC: Government Printing Office.

U.S. Census Bureau. 2003. *Survey of income and program participation, 1996 panel and asset ownership of households, 2000*. Table 5. www.census.gov/hhes/www/wealth/1998_2000/wlth00-5.html.

U.S. Census Bureau. 2006. *Current population survey, annual social and economic supplement*. www.census.gov/hhes/www/income/histinc/h10ar.html.

van der Walde, L. 2003. *CMS health care industry market update: Nursing facilities*. Washington, DC: Centers for Medicare and Medicaid Services.

PART III

PUBLIC-SECTOR INFLUENCES ON TOMORROW'S ASSISTED LIVING RESIDENCES

The Influence of Public and Private Financing on Assisted Living and Nursing Home Care

The Past, the Present, and Possible Futures

PAMELA DOTY, PH.D.

Private-pay market forces and the availability of public financing have significantly influenced the evolution of both nursing homes and assisted living. In this chapter, I offer some insights into why, after 20 years, assisted living is a private market success story whereas Medicaid remains only marginally involved in paying for this type of residential care. I draw on historical trends, survey research findings, and my personal experience as a policy analyst in the federal government to make some predictions about the future of both assisted living and nursing homes in the United States.

A Historical Overview of Residential Eldercare

A hundred years ago, residential elder care was available almost exclusively in municipal and county homes for the aged (some of which were still called almshouses or poor farms), church- or charity-run old age homes, or state mental hospitals (Haber, 1983). Facilities run by local governments were, by definition, homes for the destitute because extreme poverty was a prerequisite for admission. Indeed, institutions—quaintly termed "indoor relief"—were the only form of public assistance or welfare available. In contrast, church- or other charity-run homes for the aged were more likely to be residences for the genteel poor (typically childless widows or maiden aunts who had outlived their inheritances). Although costs were subsidized by churches or charitable organizations, residents were generally expected to sign over any income or savings they had on admission. Finally, state mental hospitals housed elders who had dementia, especially those who had behavioral problems that made it difficult for their families to manage them at home or for other public and charitable institutions to accommodate them. Census data indicate that in 1910 approximately 2 percent of elderly Americans resided in these settings (Assistant Secretary for Planning and Evaluation, U.S. Department of Health and Human Services [ASPE], 1981).

The Emergence of Nursing Homes in the 1930s

In the first several decades of the twentieth century, directors of public old age homes began to ask policy makers to increase public funding for "nursing" (by which they meant what we now call aide services, not professional nursing). Many of the more reform-minded among them supported the idea that indigent elders who were not sick or disabled should be eligible for financial assistance and that local homes for the aged should be reserved for elders too physically disabled or too cognitively impaired to live on their own in the community.

Municipal and county homes for the aged began to disappear in the 1930s. Federal and state social security legislation that established old age cash assistance payments ("outdoor relief") explicitly prohibited payments to residents of institutions. Reformers who favored "outdoor" over "indoor" relief targeted these homes for closure and thought they needed to get rid of institutions to carry the day. Size determined which settings were considered institutions. To be eligible for cash assistance, elders unable to live alone moved into small, privately run board-and-care homes. As these evolved into "nursing homes," regulators upped the permissible bed size so these settings could be economically viable without becoming ineligible for funding as "institutions" (Thomas, 1969). Nursing homes have been characterized as modern descendants of almshouses and poor farms (Moss & Halamandaris, 1977). This is not merely unflattering, but also not entirely true. Whereas all of the residents of such institutions had been dependent on public charity, private nursing homes catered to a mixed clientele of public and private pay patients, which suggests that the emergence of this new type of residential elder care was, to some extent, driven by market demand and not wholly by public policy decisions.

Federal Funding for Nursing Homes in the Late 1950s and Early 1960s

The fastest growth in use of nursing home care occurred between 1950 and 1955 and later between 1965 and 1975, because of the dramatic increase in the survival rates of elders 85 and older (the age cohort at greatest risk of developing age-related disabilities and of being admitted to a nursing home). These higher rates can be linked to advances in medicine, especially in the treatment of pneumonia and other infectious diseases (Russell, 1981).

Before World War II, the now familiar phenomenon of "spend down" seems to have been virtually unknown. By the late 1950s, though, politicians were becoming acutely aware that elderly Americans who were not poor by traditional standards were experiencing more difficulty paying for their medical care, especially in inpatient settings, including nursing homes. In 1960, for the first time, the Kerr-Mills program (a precursor to Medicaid) created a separate category of matching grants to states to pay medical care providers serving elderly persons who were considered poor enough to need assistance to cover the costs of medical care, although they were not poor enough to qualify for cash assistance welfare. Under the Kerr-Mills program, payments to vendors for nursing home care rose from $47 million in 1960 to $449 million in 1965 (Stevens and Stevens, 1974). Payments for nursing home care accounted for nearly one-third (32 percent) of the total vendor payments made during the final year before Kerr-Mills was replaced by Medicaid. This is remarkably similar to the percentage of Medicaid expenditures that have consistently gone to pay for long-term care. Since Representative Wilbur Mills authored both programs, present-day claims that one sometimes hears that Congress "never intended" for Medicaid to have so large a role in funding nursing homes or long-term care are not credible.

Medicaid and the Nursing Home Building Boom: 1965 through the 1970s

In historical perspective, the passage of Medicaid in 1965 looks to have been as much a response to as a stimulus of rising demand for nursing home care. Elderly Americans were entering nursing and personal care homes as private payers and then running out of money to pay for care. Residents, their families, and facility owners wanted a solution to the problem. Before Medicaid, states allowed elders who were unable to pay for hospital or nursing home care to apply for public assistance but, in return for granting such assistance, placed a lien on the elder's home, even if a well spouse was still residing in it. Kerr-Mills prohibited states from applying such liens but allowed states to refuse financial assistance until after the state had attempted to collect unpaid medical bills from the in-digent elder's adult children. Medicaid eliminated family responsibility for such debts for all relatives other than spouses and parents of minor children.

Medicaid did not create nursing homes, but, by providing a dependable funding source for nursing home care for chronically disabled elders who could not afford to pay out of pocket and by establishing regulatory "con-ditions of participation" for providers, the program came to define this residential care setting and made it the dominant one. Would-be providers had a strong financial motive to come into compliance to qualify for reim-bursement but often found it easier to build and staff new physical plants than to attempt to remodel existing buildings. Thus, Medicaid's provider standards sparked a building boom.

Although Medicaid increased the share of public funding for nursing home care, private financing continued to play a major role. In 1965 out-of-pocket payments for nursing home care by residents and their families accounted for nearly two-thirds (64.5 percent) of total national expendi-tures on nursing home care (Gibson, 1980). By the 1970s, the public share of funding had increased, but in 1975 private payment still accounted for 49 percent of total expenditures and 42 percent in 1979. The 1976 Survey of Institutionalized Persons (SIP) found that fewer than one in four (22.2 percent) elders who had spent more than 30 days in a long-term care facil-ity (the great majority of which were certified nursing facilities) depended entirely or primarily on Medicaid or other public assistance to pay for their care. Almost 30 percent of residents paid for their nursing home care from exclusively private sources; 48 percent relied on a combination of public and private funding. SIP data also reveal two distinctly different categories of private pay nursing home residents. The 7.2 percent of nursing home residents who relied on pension income alone to pay for their care were disproportionately male and either separated or divorced; they were also less functionally disabled than other residents—nearly 30 percent of this group reported no impairments in basic activities of daily living, or ADLs (need for assistance with bathing, dressing, transferring, toileting, eating), whereas only 16 percent of other residents reported no ADL impairments. These attributes suggested that many in this group elected to live in nursing homes more for social than medical reasons. The other, much larger category of exclusively private pay nursing facility residents was significantly more impaired than public or mixed public-private pay residents (more likely to have four or five ADL impairments).

The Role of Private Payment in Nursing Homes: 1980 to the Present

If we fast forward to the late 1990s and early 2000s, we find that in 1998 private payments accounted for 39.6 percent of total nursing home expenditures, down from 46 percent in 1980 (Cowan et al., 1999). By 2001, the share of private payments had further decreased to 38 percent of nursing home care (Levit et al., 2001). Experts credited two factors: the increased use of nursing homes to provide short-term postacute "skilled nursing facility" care that was Medicare-funded and a growing preference among private payer consumers for assisted living.

The Rise of Assisted Living

Indeed, by the late 1990s, the era in which long-term residential care for elderly people was virtually synonymous with nursing homes had ended. By 1997, nearly a quarter of all residential elder care was no longer in nursing home settings, with an estimated 500,000–600,000 beds in congregate settings (11 or more beds) that were not certified or licensed as nursing homes compared to approximately 1.7 million nursing home beds (Hawes et al., 2000).

The relative share of assisted living compared to nursing homes had increased still further by the early years of the twenty-first century. The most recent estimate, based on the 1999 National Long-Term Care Survey and the 2002 Medicare Current Beneficiary Survey, is that between 6.4 and 6.5 percent of Americans 65 or older reside in nursing homes and other residential settings, of whom 4.2 percent reside in nursing homes, with the remaining 2.2–2.3 percent living in alternative residential care settings, which are increasingly referred to as "assisted living" (Spillman & Black, 2005). Thus, close to one-third of all elders in residential care are now in assisted living rather than nursing homes.

Although assisted living may substitute for nursing homes for some segment of the elderly population, the two settings are not equivalent (Waidman, 2003; Spillman & Black, 2005). Elders who moved into nursing homes were, on average, both older and more impaired with respect to basic ADLs than those who moved into assisted living. Controlling for health-related factors, nursing home residents are also more likely to have lower incomes. Residential elder care settings offering the lowest level of medical/health services and supervision had the highest percentages of occupants with low levels of disability and incomes of $20,000 or more (53 percent) versus 38 percent of the occupants in residential care settings that offered more medical/health supervision, and 25 percent of nursing home beds (Spillman & Black, 2005). That less disabled elders not eligible for Medicaid are moving into assisted living (where they risk spending down their assets) is important because it contradicts conventional wisdom that older Americans would choose to stay in their own homes were it not for what critics decry as Medicaid's "institutional bias." Medicaid policy may limit the options of those eligible for Medicaid but cannot be held responsible for the care choices that elders make as private payers.

Phase-Out of Intermediate-Care Nursing Homes

The emergence of new residential alternatives to nursing homes that began in the late 1980s coincided with the passage of legislation that reformed nursing home regulations to eliminate the distinction between skilled nursing and intermediate care facilities. Medicaid originally only covered care in skilled nursing facilities. Before coverage for intermediate care facilities was added to Medicaid in 1972, residents in these facilities had to rely on cash assistance payments—federal Supplemental Security Income (SSI) and (where available) state supplemental payments (SSP).

Rather than increase SSP funding as the cost of care in intermediate care facilities increased, states petitioned Congress to cover this level of residential care under Medicaid. States argued that otherwise the availability of federal matching funds under Medicaid would lead them to expand capacity in the more expensive skilled nursing homes meant for residents who needed a higher level of care.

By the late 1980s, however, federal analyses of nursing home survey and certification reports (conducted internally and never published) indicated that residents of intermediate care facilities were not necessarily less disabled or less in need of medical and nursing care than residents of skilled nursing facilities. Authorizing most Medicaid residents for intermediate care was a popular cost containment strategy for state Medicaid programs (but often not a reliable measure of case mix) in certain regions of the country.

Nationally, freestanding intermediate care facilities were becoming less common. Nursing facilities increasingly accepted both residents certified at skilled nursing care or intermediate care payment levels in all beds and staffed to the higher standard. In other words, most nursing home operators had already come to the pragmatic conclusion that to meet residents' needs they had to staff at the minimum level mandated for a skilled nursing facility. As states moved to more sophisticated case-mix reimbursement methods, making a regulatory distinction between intermediate and skilled nursing facilities became less important for cost containment. Federal Medicaid officials thus concluded that moving to a single regulatory standard mandating at least one registered nurse in charge on the day shift, seven days per week would not dramatically increase Medicaid costs because this would ratify a practice standard already conformed to by most of the nursing home industry. The minority could be given ample time to come into compliance. Accordingly, the 1987 Omnibus Budget Reconciliation Act abolished the distinction between intermediate and skilled nursing facilities.

It is probably not entirely coincidental that assisted living emerged at much the same time. A former deputy administrator of the Health Care Financing Administration, who later served as executive director of a nursing home trade association and subsequently as executive director of an assisted living trade association, liked to quip that assisted living was nothing more than an intermediate care nursing home with a chandelier. However, with the elimination of what many regarded as the social model of care represented by intermediate care facilities that did not have to have registered nurses in favor of the medical model (i.e., facilities that were required to employ registered nurses), only a handful of state Medicaid officials initially showed interest in finding ways to pay for care in assisted living (see chapters 14 and 15).

Third-Party Financing for Assisted Living

The third-party financing available for assisted living is different from that available to nursing homes. Private long-term care insurance emerged as a potential source of third-party financing for long-term care at the same time that assisted living began to be an attractive alternative to nursing homes for private payers. Although the early private long-term care policies covered care in licensed nursing homes only or offered care "at home" as the only alternative to nursing home coverage, most insurers soon decided to permit claimants to use their policies to pay for assisted living and newer policies explicitly cover assisted living. Private policies will cover all assisted living costs up to the policy's daily limits. If the daily limit for nursing home care is greater than for home care, insurers typically pay up to the nursing home limit for assisted living. In contrast, Medicaid programs are prohibited under federal law from covering the "room-and-board" component of assisted living and can cover only the services provided in these residential settings. Thus, to cover the entire cost of assisted living, low income Medicaid eligibles must pay for room and board with SSI (and any SSP their state may also offer) or from personal income (Social Security, private pensions). Typically, however, SSI/SSP or personal monthly income that does not exceed Medicaid means-tested limits is insufficient to cover room and board costs in assisted living. Moreover, other housing subsidies have limited availability, such as from the Department of Housing and Urban Development (HUD; see chapters 5 and 12).

Private Long-Term Care Insurance
Prevalence and Use

Before the mid-1980s, private long-term care insurance barely existed, but in the mid-1980s several large, reputable companies decided that long-term care was an insurable risk and presented a new business opportunity. Sales of private long-term care insurance grew, on average, 18 percent per year between 1987 and 2002. Over this period, 9.16 million policies were sold. In 2002, 104 companies sold more than 900,000 policies, the largest number ever sold in a single year to date (America's Health Insurance Plans, 2004). Data from the National Association of Insurance Commissioners indicated that by 2003, approximately 16 percent of elderly Americans with annual incomes of $20,000 or higher had private long-term care insurance coverage (Long-Term Care Financing Strategy Group, 2003).

Nevertheless, private long-term care insurance is not yet a major source of financing for long-term care services. Whether it will become so in the future remains to be seen, but if it does, it will likely favor assisted living. A 1998 study of claims for private long-term care insurance among eight major insurers (covering an estimated 80 percent of all private long-term care insurance policies then in force) found that more than a quarter (28 percent) of the claimants who were using their policies to pay for residential elder care were in assisted living rather than nursing homes (Cohen & Miller, 2000).

This study found few differences in the socioeconomic profiles of nursing home and assisted living claimants but that claimants in assisted living residences tended to have fewer disabilities, averaging 2.8 ADL dependencies as compared to 4.7 for claimants in nursing homes. Privately insured residents in assisted living, however, were more disabled than other assisted living residents, who averaged only 1.7 ADL dependencies and were also about half as likely to be cognitively impaired.

This study also found that on average private long-term care insurance covered a little more than two-thirds of the cost of care for claimants in nursing homes and most (88 percent) of the cost for claimants in assisted living. Nursing home residents with private long-term care insurance paid an estimated 10–20 percent more than residents with other payment sources; while privately insured claimants in assisted living paid 1.3–1.8 times more than other assisted living residents.

A more recent (still ongoing) study of policy holders who were just beginning to file claims under their private long-term care insurance plans found that claimants are currently more likely to use their insurance payments to purchase assisted living than nursing home care. Among first-time claimants interviewed for the study (who held policies with 10 major private insurers), 37 percent of initial claims were for home care, 23 percent for assisted living, and 14 percent for nursing home care. Twenty-six percent of claimants had not yet decided which mode of care they planned to use. Claimants in assisted living were slightly older, more likely to be female, less likely to be married or college educated, and had lower incomes than either nursing home or home care claimants. Claimants in assisted living had fewer ADL impairments than claimants in nursing homes or receiving home care. Approximately two-thirds of claimants in nursing homes and assisted living had significant cognitive impairments as compared to slightly more than a fourth of claimants receiving home care (Miller & Cohen, 2006).

This study questioned respondents about why they had chosen home care, assisted living, or nursing home care and whether they had explored other options. Not all who chose home care explored residential care alternatives, but the great majority of those in nursing homes had explored home care and assisted living alternatives, and, similarly, most assisted living residents had considered home care and nursing homes. Most nursing home residents (who were more severely disabled than claimants in other settings) said that they needed to be in this setting to get the amount and type of care they needed. Assisted living residents typically cited "safety" as the main reason for their choice, coupled with a determination that they could get the required level and type of help. The "safety" concerns reported by claimants in assisted living appeared to reflect their older age, their high likelihood of living alone (if they had remained at home), and their much greater prevalence of cognitive impairments than among claimants who used home care. At the same time, claimants in assisted living reported less need for help with basic ADLs than both home care and nursing home claimants, which appears to be why they felt that the type and amount of assistance available in assisted living was sufficient. It is interesting to note that home care claimants were more likely to report that they did not get all the help they required, but—probably because most had no cognitive impairment and lived with family members who provided informal help—they could make do without feeling unsafe or that their assistance was seriously inadequate.

More Choice

Private long-term care insurance permits choices that are not available to either disabled elders who are poor enough to qualify for Medicaid home care or non-privately insured elders whose incomes and resources are such that they can only get Medicaid coverage by "spending down" in a nursing home. Many states have lengthy waiting lists for Medicaid covered home care and personal care limits that make home care coverage inadequate unless considerable informal family care is available.

To date, there has been little evidence of elders entering assisted living as private payers, running out of money, and having to move to nursing homes to get on Medicaid. It is not clear why medical indigence has not emerged as a serious issue for assisted living residents in the same way that it did for nursing home residents, but we can speculate. In their national study of assisted living facilities, Hawes and colleagues (2000) noted that, on average, residents did not have—or just barely had—enough income to cover monthly charges. A majority of older Americans, however, own their own homes and many low- to moderate-income elders have accumulated modest wealth in the form of home equity even if they lack much in the way of other savings. Thus, the most likely explanation is that for many residents, assisted living is affordable only if they are willing to use the proceeds from the sale of their former homes to help pay for it.

It is an intriguing notion that assisted living residents who pay out of pocket for assisted living are voluntarily doing so by cashing in their home equity, given that an individual's home (his or her principal place of residence) has protected status in means testing for Medicaid or cash assistance. One of the most unpopular aspects of public assistance for medically indigent elders before the enactment of Medicaid was the application of liens to enable states to recover costs of care from the estates of deceased recipients of assistance. For the first several decades after enactment of Medicaid, only a handful of states made serious efforts to recoup from the estates of deceased nursing home residents and most of these exempted home equity from their recovery efforts. This was partly a matter of politics (that is, the strong feelings aroused by liens) and partly a matter of pragmatism. Because most homes were passed to heirs outside of probate, home equity would likely not be included in recovery from the estate unless the state was willing to apply a lien on the home before the resident's death.

The special protection accorded the home has, however, been reduced over time. Since 1993, federal Medicaid law has required states to engage in efforts to recover costs from the estates of deceased beneficiaries. Although nursing home residents who own a home can still qualify financially for Medicaid coverage—if its value does not exceed $500,000—the home is no longer exempt from prohibitions on transferring assets and will become a target of estate recovery after the nursing home resident dies (unless a spouse or other qualifying relative is still residing there, in which case estate recovery is only supposed to be postponed, not waived.) States do vary greatly, however, in how strictly or thoroughly they enforce these rules. Recently enacted legislation (Deficit Reduction Act of 2006) will close several of the remaining loopholes.

There is disagreement about the prevalence of Medicaid estate planning (i.e., individuals' efforts to divest their assets by transferring them to family members or other third parties to qualify financially for Medicaid) and its financial impact on Medicaid (Waidmann & Liu, 2006). Whatever the truth may be, stricter prohibitions on Medicaid estate planning will level the playing field for assisted living relative to nursing home care by discouraging elders from choosing a nursing home over assisted living in hopes of passing their homes to their heirs.

Private long-term care insurance may make it possible for elders who are not eligible for Medicaid to have their cake and eat it, too; that is, to afford care in their preferred setting while also preserving an estate for their heirs. Cohen (2002) estimated that having private long-term care insurance coverage reduces by 66 percent a disabled elder's chances of having to spend down his or her income and assets to the point of impoverishment and eligibility for Medicaid. He found that the average reduction in out-of-pocket costs for nursing home residents with private long-term care insurance coverage at between $60,000 and $75,000, while reductions for residents in assisted living rose to $100,000 and higher.

Medicaid as a Source of Funding for Assisted Living

With the notable exception of Oregon, where developer Keren Brown Wilson and the state's director of Senior and Disabled Services, Dick Ladd, pioneered Medicaid-affordable assisted living in the late 1980s and early 1990s, Medicaid has been a Johnny-come-lately with respect to funding newer forms of assisted living. Only a handful of state Medicaid programs (e.g., North Carolina) have a long history of using the optional personal care services benefit under the state plan to reimburse traditional (smaller, mom-and-pop-owned) board-and-care facilities, which can offer little privacy and few amenities and serve primarily low-income elders who are eligible for federal SSI and state SSP welfare payments (see chapter 5). Medicaid funds enable such facilities to provide some personal care in addition to housing and meals. State officials and facility operators may feel that it improves the image of these facilities to relabel them "assisted living for low-income elders," but this is not the type of assisted living that attracts many private payers.

According to Mollica and Johnson-Lamarche (2005), the number of Medicaid-financed residents in "assisted living"—by their definition, any residential setting that is not licensed or certified as a nursing home—has increased rapidly in recent years, from an estimated 40,000 in 1998 to an estimated 109,000 in 2003 and 121,000 in 2004. In 2004, states reported a total of 937,601 units or beds in 36,451 state-licensed non-nursing-home residential care facilities of all types, which would indicate that approximately 13 percent of residents are Medicaid beneficiaries. It is important to recognize, however, that a substantial percentage of the "assisted living" settings occupied by Medicaid recipients resemble traditional board and care rather than the kind of assisted living that is being marketed to private payers. Half of these Meidcaid-funded "assisted living" beds were in North Carolina, Missouri, and New York, where the residents reside mainly in settings intended to serve predominantly SSI-eligible elders. This is further evidence that Medicaid residents in assisted living tend to be segregated in low-income settings rather than mixed in with private payers as has more often been the case in nursing homes (see chapter 5).

In states that have attempted to expand access to assisted living for Medicaid beneficiaries, officials grapple with restrictions that allow them to cover room and board *only* in nursing homes. States have tried a variety of strategies to make the room and board costs of assisted living affordable to low-income Medicaid beneficiaries, but all are problematic in one way or another. Rather than attempt to summarize the excellent technical information that is already available about the problems state officials face in trying to promote Medicaid affordable assisted living (O'Keeffe et al., 2003; Mollica & Johnson-Lamarche, 2005), I want to draw on my experience over a 25-year career in the federal government to offer a personal historical perspective on these questions.

Housing with Services: Making the Link between HUD and Medicaid Funding
The Potential for Innovation

A much-discussed strategy for expanding the availability of assisted living to low-income elders is to finance the housing component with monies from HUD, principally Section 202 housing for the elderly and Section 8 rental vouchers, and to cover the cost of the long-term care services through Medicaid. I first heard this idea in 1985 when a group of developers who specialized in low-income housing for the elderly asked to meet with the Health Care Financing Administration (now the Centers for Medicare and Medicaid), where I then worked. We were mystified why these housing guys wanted to talk to us about Medicaid.

The developers had already built or renovated a number of buildings in several western states to create model low-income housing for seniors. They foresaw that, over time, aging tenants would need long-term care services that neither the tenants themselves nor the buildings' managers could pay for. They pointed out that, unless appropriate services could be arranged, HUD rules would require managers to evict tenants who came to need such care. They believed, however, that the types of senior housing they were building could accommodate elders with disabilities if there were a way to finance the service component without requiring the buildings themselves to transform themselves into licensed nursing homes (see chapter 12).

These developers described the architectural innovations and features they designed into their buildings and grounds to make their housing projects not just accessible and user-friendly to individuals with disabilities in all sorts of unobtrusive ways (e.g., safe wandering paths for the cognitively impaired) but also visually appealing. They went on to speak of emerging possibilities in assistive technology and robotics, information technology, and the engineering of "smart" buildings, as well as new ways of managing and staffing. In short, they laid out most of the ideas associated with the pioneers of assisted living without putting that label on their vision.

The developers' purpose in asking to meet with Centers for Medicare and Medicaid Services (CMS) officials was not to seek funding for any particular project but rather to sell a vision of affordable, Medicaid-funded assisted living or housing with services that would allow elders to age in place (though they did not use these now familiar terms). They were deal makers and "big picture" guys who thought that once high-level policy makers at HUD and the Department of Health and Human Services (HHS) understood what could be gained from coordinating HUD housing subsidies with Medicaid funding for home and community-based long-term care, the details of an interdepartmental partnership could easily and quickly be worked out at lower levels by career staff (such as me). Their leader was politically very well connected and was among the original coiners (and exemplars) of the term "compassionate conservative." This got them a polite hearing, period.

I was excited by their ideas and leaped at the opportunity to visit their most recent project, which also involved a Native American corporation (a key element in obtaining HUD financing in a highly competitive environment) and the Catholic Sisters of Providence. This building, like another on the same campus that had been constructed earlier, had some highly innovative architectural features. Both were very beautiful, in a subtle, low-key way that blended well with the natural setting. I toured the project with others, including the state Medicaid director, who looked around and commented dryly that Medicaid's philosophy was, "Why pay for a Hyatt Regency when a Holiday Inn will do?"

That remark could be the subject of an entire essay by itself. Suffice it to say here that, among other things, he was expressing skepticism that the capital cost component of a state's Medicaid rate-setting methodology would support paying off the construction loans for a building that looked so upscale. The Medicaid director knew that this was *low-income* housing and had been built with a creative combination of HUD and private financing, the details of which none of us were privy to. The developers had already told me that through intelligent choice of architects and building materials and good project management, they were convinced that it was possible to build housing with services to a much higher standard than was typical of either low-income public housing or nursing homes and to do so economically. By "higher standard," they specifically meant private units (which for many proponents is the key quality-of-life feature that distinguishes an assisted living residence from a nursing home).

But what does building to a higher standard mean in terms of a dollars-and-cents comparison of assisted living and nursing home costs? On the one hand, did the developers mean that they could literally build their kind of building for no more than the average nursing home developer would spend to build a much less attractive, double-occupancy facility? On the other hand, did their understanding of "economical" mean that by spending—say, 20 percent more—it would be possible to obtain 50 or even 100 percent more value? That's a big difference from a Medicaid perspective, because, since the early 1980s the world of Medicaid has been ruled by a philosophy of no-frills cost containment that seeks to pay providers enough to meet regulatory requirements but provides little if any financial incentive or reward to surpass those minimum standards.

The Stark Reality

In the years that I stayed in touch with these developers (I lost track of them in the early 1990s), they complained that it was becoming increasingly difficult to cobble together the necessary financing and that they were burning out. Each of their projects was unique, and each was individually financed. Nonetheless, there were some common themes. For example, each project reflected in some interesting way the geographical area where it was built in terms of its relationship to the natural or urban landscape, local history, or aspects of regional or ethnic cultures.

Also, the developers always seemed to have minority partners. The HUD funding they sought typically required or favored minority businesses, but the minority partners they chose also brought investment funds to the table—and it may have been this funding, rather than the government funding that specifically financed the most innovative and distinctive design features. This method of financing projects puts a premium on innovation because that is what it takes to compete successfully for government and foundation grants and for the attention of well-heeled investors from minority groups who are looking not just for a good return on investment but also to give something back to their community. This is very different from attempting to win government business by being the lowest bidder capable of meeting the minimum specifications for a product or service set by the government.

Other grant-funded innovators have done much the same. Examples include On Lok, a program emphasizing day care for low-income, disabled Chinese immigrant elders begun in San Francisco's Chinatown in the 1970s with philanthropic support from affluent Chinese Americans. This was subsequently expanded with CMS grant funding and the PACE program (Program of All-Inclusive Care for the Elderly) it inspired, which later obtained legislative authority for joint Medicare/Medicaid funding. Another private philanthropic example is the Robert Wood Johnson Foundation's "Coming Home" partnership with the NCB Development Corporation.

The upside of this approach is high quality; the downside is low volume. As of April 2006, 14 years after it was launched, the Coming Home initiative had in operation or under development 96 assisted living projects providing 3,445 affordable units (www.rwjf.org/reports/npreports/

cominghome.htm). NCB Development Corporation's 2005 Annual Report lists 40 projects in operation with a total of 944 units (www.ncbdc.org) When nursing homes serve an estimated 1.2 million Medicaid users annually, I will let the reader speculate whether, or how long it will be before, these kinds of "artisanal," grant-funded initiatives can provide a real alternative for low-income elders.

The problem of building enough high-quality assisted living to constitute a real alternative to nursing homes goes well beyond a shortage of grant funding to seed development and construction costs, however. With the exception of federal SSI payments ($623 per month cash assistance in 2007, to which only the poorest old and disabled individuals are entitled), the public financing available to fund operating costs of assisted living is *discretionary* funding, not a mandated entitlement. Indeed, most proponents of affordable assisted living look to a discretionary funding source—Medicaid's 1915(c) waivers for home and community-based services (HCBS)—as the preferred mechanism for non-nursing-home residential care. But while there has been rapid growth in HCBS funding via the 1915(c) waivers over the past 25 years, two-thirds of those expenditures are for services for people with mental retardation/developmental disabilities, not elderly people. Also, whereas some states do operate HCBS waiver programs as if they were entitlements, nationwide there are as many Medicaid-eligible individuals on waiting lists for HCBS services as there are enrollees being served (Kitchener et al., 2004).

Title III of the Older Americans Act (OOA) is another discretionary funding source that is often used to finance the board component of room and board for residents of non–nursing home facilities, as well as transportation services to enable them to do some local shopping, get to and from medical appointments, and attend senior centers and other group activities. A colleague has aptly described pulling these three funding sources—HUD monies, HCBS waivers, and Title III funds—together to support assisted living as akin to crafting a three-legged stool at least one of whose legs is nearly always wobbly and not reliably capable of supporting its share of the weight.

Since 1985, I have periodically participated in meetings between HHS and HUD to explore interagency partnering around assisted living or senior housing with services. Toward the end of the Clinton administration, HUD sponsored a small grant program to encourage conversion of older Section 202 senior housing to assisted living. This grant program had fewer applicants than expected for reasons that illustrate some of the structural in-compatibilities of HUD and Medicaid funding. HUD wanted state Medi-caid programs to guarantee occupancy assistance, but Medicaid program participants are required by law to have free choice of providers. The institutional and programmatic obstacles are so daunting that strong com-mitment at the highest executive levels and from Congress would be re-quired to overcome them.

Probably the fundamental reason the political will to assure affordable assisted living has never materialized is that discretionary funding (as distinct from funding for entitlements such as Medicare, Medicaid, and Social Security) has been progressively squeezed out of both federal and state budgets. This process was already under way in 1985 and has only become more obvious since. Two reports on senior housing prepared by the American Association of Retired Persons have noted that federal fund-ing for senior housing was at its zenith in the 1950s; that in recent years HUD 202 funding has been "flat lined"; and that the 2005 budget ($741 million) was below the funded levels of the 1970s (Bright, 2005; Redfoot, 2001). President Bush's proposed FY 2007 budget calls for a 26 percent reduction in 202 funding for low-income senior housing.

Epilogue—Recently, I decided to find out what had become of the proj-ect I visited in 1985. I was surprised to discover that there is no assisted living or housing with services on the site. One building operates as a nursing home. The low-income senior housing complex across the street maintains a referral list to Medicaid home- and community-based ser-vices providers but does not provide, arrange, or coordinate services for tenants. The developers' original vision of covering "rent" with HUD sub-sidies and paying for services with Medicaid was not realized in either building.

Market-Driven Affordable Assisted Living

Another often-recommended approach to promoting Medicaid-afford-able assisted living is to piggyback on projects built to appeal to a pre-dominantly private pay market. In 1990 (now a staff member of the Office of the Assistant Secretary for Planning and Evaluation, or ASPE), I trav-eled to see two new programs being developed in Washington and Oregon. In Seattle, the Sisters of Providence had just built a facility (the developers I had met five years before had no role in this project); it was so new that it was still a week away from welcoming its first residents. In Oregon, Keren Brown Wilson had recently opened an assisted living residence in a suburb of Portland.

The Sisters of Providence Seattle Assisted Living Residence

The health care corporation of the Sisters of Providence (founded in the nineteenth century by a missionary nun from Quebec) includes acute medical facilities, nursing homes, assisted living residences, and home care. I was impressed with the combination of traditional religious charity and shrewd business sense that characterized the Sisters' operation. At their new assisted living residence, I learned the advantages of unbundling services that in a nursing home would be included in a single per diem rate so that payers other than Medicaid (or the resident) would cover or subsidize the cost of some discrete services. These other payers could include Medicare, the OOA, other building tenants and other service users not residing in the assisted living property.

The Sisters owned the entire building, of which the assisted living residence only occupied a portion. The building's other tenants were medical providers, including physicians and an outpatient rehabilitation center. The close proximity of these other providers—especially the rehabilitation center—enabled the assisted living residence to minimize the number of on-staff medical personnel. If residents got sick, they could walk or roll their wheelchairs across the hall for a Medicare-covered physician visit and if they needed physical or other rehabilitation therapies, they could similarly walk or roll across the hall to the rehabilitation center and receive these Medicare-covered outpatient services. In addition, the building was in an extremely desirable location, which allowed for lucrative rental income that could have helped subsidize the assisted living residence (see chapter 1).

The Sisters could have implemented other unbundling strategies to lower the basic per diem assisted living rates. For example, they might have attracted a senior center funded by the OAA to the building to avoid the expense of an activity program within the assisted living. If the senior center was also an OAA congregate meal site, assisted living residents could choose to purchase lunch from the assisted living residence (as an extra, not part of the daily rate) or pay much less for a subsidized lunch at the senior center.

The director of this assisted living residence (a lay professional) told me that she had previously been the administrator of a Medicaid-certified intermediate care facility. I was curious to learn more about the decision to open an assisted living property rather than a nursing home. How important was the freedom to unbundle services and get more payers to share the costs? I could see that costs might appear "low" to each payer, although total costs might not be lower and might even be higher than the bundled daily nursing home rate. Although the administrator insisted that assisted living care was better because it was "home and community based," whereas nursing homes were "institutions," it was hard to pin her down about just how Medicaid regulations made nursing homes institutional whereas freedom from those rules made assisted living something entirely different. Unlike some assisted living residences, this one planned to have registered nurses on staff, so it did not exemplify the oft-mentioned difference between a social or medical model. When I asked the director which Medicaid nursing facility requirements could not be met by her assisted living facility or others without compromising the assisted living philosophy, the only requirement she could specifically point to was that the corridors in her building would need to be wider.

Keren Brown Wilson's Portland, Oregon, Assisted Living Residence
Assisted Living, Seattle Style

In Portland, Oregon, Dick Ladd, then director of Oregon Senior and Disabled Services, and Keren Brown Wilson personally guided us through an assisted living residence that she had opened in 1989. Wilson said things very similar to what I had heard five years before from the developers promoting senior housing with services—for example, with intelligent choice of materials it was possible to build all private units with private baths and it was not necessary to build to a double occupancy standard just to keep construction costs down. I noticed that her building was pleasant and attractive but not beautiful. It passed the test set by the Medicaid director I had met touring the HUD financed building five years earlier of looking more like a Holiday Inn than a Hyatt Regency (see chapter 5).

Wilson explained that she built for a moderate-income private pay market, which was also a standard that Oregon Medicaid considered affordable. The accommodations were mostly efficiency apartments. They were quite small and reminded me of single-occupancy college dorm rooms (although, unlike most dorm rooms, they did have private bathrooms). For safety reasons, the kitchenettes were rudimentary, consisting only of a shelf holding a small refrigerator, a microwave oven, and an electric kettle (with automatic turn-off). Wilson pointed out that a full "common" kitchen was available elsewhere, if they or their visitors wanted to cook a full-fledged, family-style meal. Facilities were also available for residents or their family to do their own laundry if they preferred to avoid paying an extra fee for laundry service (another example of an unbundled service that Medicaid requires nursing facilities to cover in the basic per diem).

Wilson explained that the assisted living residence had a subcontract with a Medicare/Medicaid-certified home health agency to provide personal care and other services—again, an example of unbundling because it meant that Medicare home health benefits could finance some of these services. This helped lower both what Medicaid and moderate income private payers had to pay; however, when I asked whether assisted living tenants could make their own service arrangements instead of receiving services from her subcontractor, Wilson said no. I understood her rationale, which included lower costs because of economies of scale. Although I understood why Wilson preferred to refer to the assisted living residents as "tenants," I felt that most people would agree that when your landlord also provides or arranges your health or personal care, you are in a specialized care setting of some sort, not a tenant in rental housing.

I also asked how her assisted living differed from a "nursing home." I realized, of course, that her decision not to have nurses on staff meant that her setting could not meet Medicaid nursing home requirements. But what I was really getting at was how Wilson thought her residence would be perceived by an ordinary consumer looking for care. In my experience, the average person readily perceives the difference between a disabled elder's "own home" (house or apartment) and a specialized congregate care setting for disabled elders; however, such people often use the labels "rest home," "retirement home," "nursing home," and "assisted living" imprecisely and interchangeably. If persons lacking a background in long-term care and government regulations responded favorably to Wilson's facility, would they see it as a new type of "home- and community-based care" totally different from a nursing home or would they simply judge it to be a "good" as opposed to a "bad" nursing home. Ladd almost seemed to find such questions offensive (or perhaps heretical). Wilson just smiled, shrugged, and said that based on her own personal experience with her mother she had developed strong opinions about how she wanted her assisted living residences to be different from the typical nursing home. To be able to call her residences assisted living, coupled with Oregon's willingness to write regulations specifically for assisted living, made it easier for her to do things her way.

Expanding Nationally

Within a year or two of my visit to Oregon, Wall Street became bullish about the growth and profit potential of assisted living. Keren Brown Wilson decided to expand, not only by building more assisted living residences in Oregon but also by moving into other states. To obtain the necessary capital, she took her company (Assisted Living Concepts) public in 1994.

Arguably, in contemporary American society only for-profit corporations are capable anymore of making available a sufficient supply of alternative residential eldercare to challenge the dominance of the nursing home industry. Nevertheless, launching a public company with such a goal in mind was a bold and risky move for someone without an extensive business background. In 1995, Wilson told *Forbes* magazine, "We have been called the Wal-Mart of assisted living. I don't have a problem with that" (Barrett & Walth, 2001).

Others were less optimistic about the prospects for assisted living for low- to moderate-income elders. In 1996, ASPE commissioned a report about trends and barriers to further development of assisted living based on interviews with assisted living developers (Manard & Cameron, 1997). The consensus of the 29 developers interviewed (Wilson was not among them) was that the market for high-end assisted living was becoming saturated, that there was a need for more affordable assisted living, but that meeting this need would be a major challenge to the industry. A majority of the developers thought costs could be reduced, as well as profit margins, but were wary of becoming involved in Medicaid-financed assisted living because they questioned Medicaid's willingness to reimburse adequately. Indeed, almost all said that their companies would not do so until Medicaid offered better rates. They also expressed concerns that Medicaid officials might impose unrealistic regulations or make questionable trade-offs of quality for affordability and warned that Medicaid could attract "shoddy operators" (see chapter 4).

By the late 1990s, Wilson and ALC had become a lightening rod for criticism of assisted living by regulators and the media (Barnett & Walth, 2001), though the concerns they raised about the quality of care in some of her residences or about the company's financial accounting practices were scarcely unique to ALC. There were some possible reasons for the greater scrutiny: ALC's schedule for building or acquiring assisted living residences was more ambitious than most; Wilson's history of involvement with Oregon Medicaid, whereas other companies mostly stayed away from Medicaid; and Wilson's willingness to speak candidly to the press. In July 2001, for example, she was quoted in the *Oregonian* as saying, "Sometimes, your systems don't stay up with your growth, and that happened to us. There was never any conscious decision to ignore quality. In fact, just the opposite" (Barnett & Walth, 2001).

ALC addressed the quality issues, settled a shareholder lawsuit, and survived. The company, having gone through many changes, is currently thriving. Wilson, who left in 2000 to run a private foundation, teach, and do research, continues to speak out candidly about the challenges facing assisted living (Wilson, 2003) and was honored by the Gerontological Society of America with the 2005 Maxell Pollock Award for her pioneering role in assisted living. The late 1990s and early 2000s, however, were a difficult "trial by fire." Wall Street grew disenchanted with assisted living and expansion slowed industry-wide—2002 was an especially troubled year for the assisted living industry. Some companies that had never even taken on the extra challenge of developing affordable assisted living found themselves struggling to stave off bankruptcy (e.g., Alterra Healthcare Corp.) or left the business (e.g., Marriott decided the hotel business was its strength and sold its assisted living residences to Sunrise) (*Provider*, 2003).

In 2005, ALC was acquired by Extendicare, a health care corporation based in Canada that operates nursing homes, assisted living residences, and subacute and rehabilitation facilities in the United States and Canada and that provides home care services in Canada. As of December 2005, Extendicare had recovered ALC's position as sixth largest among assisted living chains (*Provider*, June 2006); it had earlier dropped to eighth position. In a June 7, 2006, press release (www.Extendicare.com/news), Extendicare announced plans for ALC to be spun off as a separate, publicly traded company, at which point it was projected to rank as the fifth largest assisted living company in the United States. This spinoff occurred in November 2006, and almost immediately the company announced that it would be getting out of the Medicaid business. In July 2007, Laurie Bebo, president and chief executive officer of Assisted Living Concepts, issued the following statement (www.marketwatch.com/news/story/assisted-living-concepts-inc-reports/story):

> During the second quarter of 2007 we completed the accelerated phase of our exit from traditional Medicaid programs primarily due to the initiation of the managed Medicaid system in Texas. This enables us to continue forward with our overall strategy of growing private pay occupancy. Revenue gains of $0.7 million from private pay occupancy combined with $0.4 million from rate increases and $0.6 million from an extra day in the quarter offset Medicaid revenue reductions of $1.8 million. In the second quarter of 2007, revenues from private pay residents as a percent of overall revenues increased to 84.4% from 78.8% in the quarter ended June 30, 2006. Our team members did a fantastic job assisting Medicaid residents with their transition to new accommodations and will now turn their focus towards filling the vacated units with private pay residents.

Conclusions and Implications for the Future

The evidence is clear that when elders who can afford to pay for assisted living privately (whether out of pocket or through long-term care insurance) vote with their wallets, they are increasingly choosing assisted living. Low-income elders, on the other hand, currently have very limited ability to choose assisted living. Sometimes Medicaid does not cover assisted living at all. Perhaps more often, however, Medicaid does not cover enough of the total cost of assisted living to make affordable assisted living readily available, or there are waiting lists for the Medicaid HCBS waivers that finance the services component. Many observers—particularly researchers and other expert consultants and professional advocates for the elderly—believe that public policy needs to be reformed to give low-income elders the option to choose assisted living.

Several experts have described the difficulties that state officials and assisted living developers face when they try to bring multiple public funding streams together to make assisted living accessible to low-income elders, but describing these problems does not explain *why* they persist and do not appear likely to be resolved any time soon. If assisted living is truly a less expensive substitute for nursing home care, why not amend Medicaid to cover its room and board component along with its services?

I am not one who thinks the political clout of the nursing home lobby is the explanation, especially because so many nursing home providers now also offer assisted living. I think the reason is that the privately paying consumers who have driven the growth of assisted living are looking for and finding something different from what Medicaid is willing to reimburse. This is partly a question of amenities. It is clear that Medicaid is unwilling and should not be expected to pay for the high-end assisted living that is often mockingly equated with chandeliers, atriums, and the like—the Hyatt Regency version of residential care. Proponents of affordable assisted living have long debated, even agonized, over the extent to which it is possible to offer the so-called essential amenities of assisted living (e.g., private accommodations) at a cost that Medicaid will tolerate. The answer to that question seems to vary from state to state, but Wilson certainly proved many years ago that it *can* be done.

The crux of the affordable assisted living conundrum lies elsewhere. That is, elders who pay privately for residential care do not necessarily substitute assisted living for nursing home care; rather, they often prefer assisted living to home care. We know this because private consumers often enter assisted living with low levels of need for medical, nursing, or aide services. Their emotional attachment to staying at home is clearly much weaker than conventional wisdom would have us believe. Many private consumers who choose assisted living want to escape from burdens of homeownership and home maintenance, especially when their dwellings are aging and in need of ongoing maintenance (Golant, 2003). More important, many private pay consumers are seeking an alternative to—and are willing to pay good money to be free from—dependency on informal family care. Research on private long-term care insurance purchase behavior has found avoiding dependency on family care to be a major motivating factor; indeed, this motive, along with—and perhaps even more than—estate protection is among the reasons for the emergence of this insurance market (Cohen et al., 1992; HIAA, 2000).

Medicaid policy, however, is now evolving in the opposite direction. Medicaid's top priority is cost containment. Legislation just enacted in the Deficit Reduction Act of 2006 will allow states to offer home- and community-based care alternatives to individuals who are eligible for Medicaid but do not meet the medical or functional need criteria for nursing home care. Under this new provision, states will be permitted to cover services, but not room and board in assisted living. The intent is to not to expand access to assisted living but to allow states to make coverage criteria for nursing homes more restrictive without having to deny any coverage to those who are less impaired. Policy makers argue that Medicaid should enable and encourage elders to stay at home, where they prefer to be, but a main reason why Medicaid home care coverage is so much more attractive as a policy option is that its benefits are designed to supplement informal family care and are therefore much less costly than either nursing home or assisted living care. For most disabled elders living at home, Medicaid's home care coverage by itself would be inadequate to meet their needs; the family members' substantial care commitment (in-kind contribution) is crucial.

In sum, the prospects for *large-scale* expansion of Medicaid-financed assisted living do not appear promising. Except under very limited circumstances—for example, when SSI-eligible elders lack close family and therefore have almost no informal support available to them at home and may not even be able to afford the cost of housing and food that is not publicly subsidized—promoting Medicaid-affordable assisted living is not consistent with the goals that most federal and state policy makers currently have for cost containment. Even if, in individual cases, assisted living substitutes for Medicaid-funded nursing home care, total public costs may be greater when the combined total of Medicaid HCBS, HUD housing subsidies, SSI/SSP benefits, and increased use of Medicare outpatient services are taken into account.

An alternative to swimming against the stream of policy makers' resistance to expanding Medicaid coverage for assisted living is to commit to improving the quality of nursing homes that are increasingly serving the most severely disabled elders—who need more care than can be provided at home by unpaid family members even supplemented by Medicaid-financed formal services. Thus, it might be better to pursue a strategy of "deinstitutionalizing" nursing homes instead of nursing home residents. The powerful financial leverage that Medicaid has vis-à-vis nursing homes could be used to motivate nursing home owners and operators to adopt as much as possible, assisted living's social model of care. It must be conceded, however, that many nursing home operators report diversifying into private pay assisted living because Medicaid's low nursing home reimbursement otherwise endangers their business survival (*Provider*, August 2005).

Nevertheless, what is being called a culture change in the nursing home world is, in fact, already under way (see chapter 3). The building I visited in 1985, envisioned as a HUD-subsidized, low-income senior housing complex with Medicaid-funded service available to residents with disabilities, is now operated by the Sisters of Providence as a nursing home. It proudly advertises itself as an "Edenized" nursing home. The early pioneers of the assisted living movement mostly built and operated freestanding residences. Increasingly, however, the trend appears to be for assisted living residences to be owned and operated by large systems (nonprofit as well as for-profit) that also own and operate hospitals, subacute and rehabilitation facilities, nursing homes, and home health/home care agencies. Assisted living is also being increasingly co-located on campuses that include nursing facilities, residential care for elders with dementia, and independent living apartments for seniors. I hope—though I'm not sure I dare to predict—that these trends will facilitate the growth of a culture of shared values that is no longer considered unique to assisted living but has diffused across the entire spectrum of long-term care services and settings.

NOTE

This chapter represents the author's own perspective and professional experience and does not in any way express the views or policies of the U.S. Department of Health and Human Services.

REFERENCES

America's Health Insurance Plans. 2004. *Long-term care insurance in 2002*. Washington, DC: America's Health Insurance Plans.

Assistant Secretary for Planning and Evaluation, U.S. Department of Health and Human Services. 1981. *Working papers on long-term care: 1980 Under Secretary's Task Force on Long-Term Care*. Washington, DC: U.S. Department of Health and Human Services, Office of the Assistant Secretary for Planning and Evaluation.

Barnett, E. H., & Walth, B. 2001. Assisted living pioneer sees dream fall short. *Oregonian,* June 24. www.oregonlive.com.

Bright, K. 2005. *Section 202 supportive housing for the elderly: Research report.* Washington, DC: AARP Public Policy Institute.

Cohen, M., Kumar, N., & Wallack, S. 1992. Who buys long-term care insurance? *Health Affairs 11,* 208–223.

Cohen, M. 2002. *Benefits of long-term care insurance: Enhanced care for disabled elders, improved quality of life for caregivers and savings to Medicare and Medicaid.* Washington, DC: Health Insurance Association of America.

Cohen, M. A., & Miller, J. 2000, April. *The use of nursing home and assisted living facilities among privately insured and non-privately insured disabled elders.* Washington, DC: Assistant Secretary for Planning and Evaluation, U.S. Department of Health and Human Services. http://aspe.hhs.gov/_/index.cfm.

Cowan, C., Lazenby, H. C., Martin, A. B., McDonnell, P. A., Sensenig, A. L., Stiller, J. M., Whittle, L. S. Kotova, K. A. Zezza, M. A., Donham, C. S., Long, A.M., & Stewart, M. W. 1999. National health expenditures, 1998. *Health Care Financing Review 21* (2), 210.

Gibson, R. 1980. National health expenditures, 1979. *Health Care Financing Review 2* (1), 1–36.

Golant, S. M. 2003. Government-assisted rental accommodations: Should they accommodate homeowners with unmet needs? *Maine Policy Review 12* (2), 36–57.

Gold, M. F. 2005. Redefining the long term care landscape. *Provider* (August), 25–38.

Haber, C. 1983. *Beyond sixty-five: The dilemma of old age in America's past.* Cambridge: Cambridge University Press.

Hawes, C., Phillips, C.D., & Rose, M. 2000. *A national study of assisted living for the frail elderly: Final report.* Washington, DC: Office of the Assistant Secretary for Planning and Evalution, U.S. Department of Health and Human Services. http://aspe.hhs.gov/_/index.cfm.

Health Care Financing Administration. 1981. *Long term care: Background and future directions.* HCFA-81-20047. Washington, DC: Health Care Financing Administration, U.S. Department of Health and Human Services.

Health Insurance Institute of America. 2000. *Who buys long-term care insurance in 2000? A decade of study of buyers and non-buyers.* Washington, DC: Health Insurance Institute of America.

Kitchener, M, Ng, T., & Harrington, C. 2004. Medicaid 1915 (c) home and community based services waivers: A national survey of eligibility criteria, caps, and waiting lists. *Home Health Services Quarterly 23* (2), 55–69.

Levit, K., Smith, C., Cowan, C., Lazenby, H., Sensenig, A., & Catlin, A. 2003. Trends in U.S. health care spending, 2001. *Health Affairs 22* (1), 154–164.

Liu, K., & Mossey, J. 1980. The role of payment source in differentiating nursing home residents: Services and payments. *Health Care Financing Review 2* (summer), 51–62.

Long-Term Care Financing Strategy Group. 2003. New index: 85 percent in America uninsured against long-term care risk. Press Release, Matz, Blancato & Associates and DJC Communications, Washington, DC, May 22.

Manard, B. L., & Cameron, R. 1997. *A national study of assisted living for the frail elderly: Report on in-depth interviews with developers.* Washington, DC: Assistant Secretary for Planning and Evaluation, U.S. Department of Health and Human Services. http://aspe.hhs.gov/_/index.cfm.

Moss, F. E., & Halamandaris, V. J. 1977. *Too old, too sick, too bad: Nursing homes in America.* Germantown, MD: Aspen Publications.

Miller, J., & Cohen, M. 2006. *Service use and transitions: Decisions, choices, and care management among an admissions cohort of privately insured disabled elders, baseline interview results.* Washington, DC: Assistant Secretary for Planning and Evaluation, U.S. Department of Health and Human Services. http://aspe.hhs.gov/_/index.cfm.

Mollica, R., & Johnson-Lamarche, H. 2005. *Residential care and assisted living compendium, 2004.* Research Triangle Park, NC: RTI International.

O'Keeffe, J., O'Keeffe, C., & Bernard, S. 2003, December. *Using Medicaid to cover services for elderly persons in residential care settings: State policy maker and stakeholder views in six states.* Research Triangle, NC: RTI International.

Provider. 2003. Top 30 assisted living chains, economically troubled year for assisted living. August, 33–35.

Provider. 2006. Top 40 assisted living chains. June, 41–53.

Russell, L. B. 1981. An aging population and the use of medical care. *Medical Care* 19, no. 6 (June), 633–642.

Spillman, B. C., & Black, K. J. 2005. *The size of the long-term care population in residential care.* Washington, DC: Assistant Secretary for Planning and Evaluation, U.S. Department of Health and Human Services. http://aspe.hhs.gov/_/index.cfm.

Spillman, B. C., Liu, K., & McGilliard, C. 2002. *Trends in residential long-term Care: Use of nursing homes and assisted living and characteristics of facilities and residents.* Washington, DC: Assistant Secretary for Planning and Evaluation, U.S. Department of Health and Human Services. http://aspe.hhs.gov/_/index.cfm.

Redfoot, D. L. 2001. *In brief: The 1999 national survey of section 202 elderly housing, research report.* Washington, DC: AARP Public Policy Institute.

Stevens, R., & Stevens, R. 1974. *Welfare medicine in America: A case study of Medicaid.* New York: Free Press.

Thomas, W. C. Jr. 1969. *Nursing homes and public policy: Drift and decision in New York state.* Ithaca, NY: Cornell University Press.

Waidman, T. A. 2003. *Estimates of the risk of long-term care: Assisted living and nursing home facilities.* Washington, DC: Assistant Secretary for Planning and Evaluation, U.S. Department of Health and Human Services. http://aspe.hhs.gov/_/index.cfm.

Waidmann, T., & Liu, K. 2006. *Asset transfer and nursing home use: Empirical*

evidence and policy significance. Washington, DC: Kaiser Commission on Medicaid and the Uninsured, Kaiser Family Foundation.

Wilson, K. B. 2003. Testimony before the Federal Trade Commission, June 11, Washington, DC. www.ftc.gov/ogc/healthcarehearings/docs/030611wilson.pdf.

CHAPTER 12

Expanding Affordable Housing with Services for Older Adults

Challenges and Potential

ROBYN I. STONE, DR.P.H.
MARY HARAHAN, M.A.
ALISHA SANDERS, M.P.AFF.

Home- and community-based services during the past 25 years have made it increasingly possible for older adults with disabilities to remain in their own homes rather than having to move to a nursing home. Today, however, the goal of "aging in place" is increasingly beyond the means of many older adults with low or modest incomes. This is true for those whose "home" is either a private dwelling that they no longer can afford or easily maintain or a publicly subsidized apartment where they have lived for many years. The challenge is to create efficient and effective community- and dwelling-based supportive and health-related services for both these groups of individuals.

This chapter explores the various issues connected with creating affordable housing with service options to meet the needs of both these current and future low- and modest-income older adults to enable them to remain in the community. Linking affordable housing and services is currently a relatively small part of the larger universe of home- and community-based services, but there is great potential to expand these options. We need, however, to understand the current demand for affordable housing with services and the range of existing options. We must also identify and address policy and operational barriers to replicating existing models and developing new ones. We begin by defining what we mean by "affordable housing with services" and examine briefly the rationale for public and policy support for them.

What Is Affordable Housing with Services?

Among federal, state, and local entities, as well as in the private sector, we can find a variety of different residential arrangements in which the older occupants have access to health-related and supportive services. These include "congregate housing," "supportive housing," "assisted living," and "naturally occurring retirement communities." To emphasize our focus on affordability, we will broadly encompass these various arrangements under the category of "affordable housing with services."

Overall, these arrangements are characterized by a low-cost or subsidized residential setting, a significant proportion of frail or disabled elders among the resident population, and access to a coordinated program of health-related and supportive services. The residential component provides permanent, independent, largely multiple-unit housing to older adults with low or moderate incomes. The housing is owned or subsidized by government entities, or is otherwise affordable to seniors whose incomes could make them eligible for government subsidies (e.g., selected mobile or manufactured home parks and communities, limited equity cooperatives, shared housing, and some spontaneously created or naturally occurring retirement communities, where once younger occupants have become old). Health-related and supportive services are available as a result of a purposeful collaboration among the housing sponsor or individual property, residents and their families, aging services agencies, and state or local programs. Residents are free to accept or reject services.

The Case for Affordable Housing with Services

There are a number of reasons why the various stakeholders in the low-income housing arena should support these options. Like their wealthier counterparts, most elderly persons with low or modest incomes want to remain in their own homes even in the face of health and functional decline. They want to maintain their networks of neighbors and friends, choose where and from whom they receive services, and avoid the trauma of relocating to a relative's home or a nursing home.

Other lower- and modest-income older persons who are experiencing increased disability and currently reside in low-income housing will not be able to afford most private-pay options, most notably assisted living and its high accommodation costs.

Policy makers in the fields of aging services and housing also have a stake in the expansion of affordable housing with services. In light of the burden that nursing homes and, more recently, assisted living have placed on Medicaid budgets, states are looking for less costly and more efficient ways to deliver home- and community-based services. Multi-unit, low-income housing offers potential economies of scale and increased efficiency in service delivery that could help states stretch their long-term care dollars. A strategy for affordable housing with services also provides the opportunity to use existing housing stock creatively instead of making capital investments to build new assisted living facilities (see chapter 10). A recent study by the Government Accountability Office (2005b) noted that older residents in public housing developments for the elderly and persons with disabilities must often move out of their apartments because of a lack of social services. Thus, formally linking services with housing may help to avoid or delay the need for tenant relocation.

In service-rich communities, targeting low-income residents who have long-term care needs offers the chance to serve a larger population at low marginal costs. In addition, anecdotal evidence suggests that offering health screening and chronic care management to groups of residents in low-income housing may help save Medicare and Medicaid dollars by reducing emergency room use, hospital days, and nursing home placement (see chapter 11). For local policy makers, the expansion of affordable housing with services may help support community and economic development, including creating new job opportunities and fostering formal partnerships among local hospitals, clinics, and other service providers to offer free or discounted services in return for new sources of referrals.

Finally, those who provide low-income senior housing also stand to benefit tremendously from linkages between housing and services as their residents age. The availability of supportive and health-related services can help to mitigate health and safety problems experienced by both disabled residents and others living in the housing complex. They may also reduce building maintenance problems related to poor housekeeping by frail elderly tenants and thus delay the deterioration of the physical plant. Service linkages can also reduce the pressure on property managers to respond to off-hour emergency calls and to engage in crisis intervention. A housing-with-services strategy, furthermore, may reduce the potential for evictions and unnecessary tenant turnover by helping residents—even those with cognitive impairments—to remain safely in their own apartments.

Current Demand for Affordable Housing with Services

Demand for affordable housing with services is a function of the number of older individuals who require financial assistance to secure affordable housing and the extent to which they experience disabilities that threaten their ability to live independently.

Affordable Rental Housing Options

Complete and accurate data on the number of older persons who live in publicly subsidized housing or receive help with their rent are not available. This is due, in large part, to the wide range of subsidy systems and routes to the creation of low-income or affordable housing serving an elderly population and variation in how the number and type of residents are documented.

Wilden and Redfoot (2002) estimated that almost 1.8 million older adults, mostly low-income single women in their mid-seventies to early eighties, live in federally assisted multi-unit rental housing, more than the number who live in nursing homes. Researchers at the Housing Research Foundation (2002) indicate that between 600,000 and 700,000 seniors live in public housing, with fully half residing in "seniors only" developments. The American Association of Retired Person's (AARP) Public Policy Institute found that the number of elderly households (as opposed to individuals) served by federal housing programs in 1999 included 350,000 in public housing, 213,000 in properties receiving tenant-based subsidies (Section 8 certificates or vouchers), 319,000 in Section 202 Supportive Housing for the Elderly properties, 108,000 in Low Income Housing Tax Credit properties, and 191,000 in Section 515 Rural Rental Housing properties.

The Section 202 program is the only federal financing source specifically designated as senior housing. Today's Section 202 program provides nonprofit entities with interest-free capital advances to help finance construction and rental assistance to subsidize resident rents. Qualified tenants generally must be at least 62 years old and have incomes less than 50 percent of their locality's median income. Low-income housing tax credits administered by state governments provide equity capital to help finance the development of affordable housing. The credits are competitively awarded to housing project sponsors who then sell the credits to investors to offset their federal tax liability. Projects are required to target a minimum of number of units to residents with incomes less than 50 or 60 percent of their locality's median income. The Section 515 program provides direct loans to finance affordable rental housing in rural areas for low-income families, elderly people, and persons with disabilities. Properties financed by all these programs may also have Section 8 rental assistance (certificates or vouchers) attached to them. Section 8 assistance pays landlords the difference between 30 percent of the household income and an established fair market rent for the area.

An unknown number of seniors live in rental properties subsidized through state and municipal programs. There are also no national estimates of the number of poor and near-poor older adults who live in affordable private sector housing (e.g., housing cooperatives, mobile home parks and manufactured housing communities, shared and accessory housing, and single room occupancy hotels).

National data indicate that nearly one-third of all senior households and two-thirds of low-income elderly renters spend more than 30 percent of their income on housing costs (GAO, 2005a). Almost 40 percent of low-income elderly homeowners face similar problems (GAO, 2005a). Because 46 percent of elderly homeowners are older than 75 and 9 percent are older than 85 (U.S. Census Bureau 2000) (and at greater risk for disability), it is likely that a large proportion of these individuals would be candidates for affordable housing with services. The Commission on Affordable Senior Housing report (2002) estimated that 11 million older adults will have difficulty paying for housing or will live in substandard housing by 2020; many of these individuals will also need supportive and health-related services to maximize their potential for aging in place.

Impaired Older Adults

Level of disability or need is the second factor defining demand for housing with services. Studies of senior residents living in publicly assisted housing report that they experience more than twice the disability as their homeowner counterparts. Redfoot and Kochera (2004), for example, analyzed data from the 2002 American Communities Survey and found that almost two-thirds of subsidized renters experienced long-term limitations in daily activities, whereas slightly more than one-third (37 percent) of older homeowners (62 years and older) had similar disabilities. Other estimates prepared for the Commission on Affordable Housing and Health Facility Needs for Seniors in the 21st Century (2002) show that one third of subsidized renters have physical disabilities or limitations that result in some difficulty with routine activities of daily living and 12 percent have a mental or cognitive disability that interferes with everyday activities (see chapter 2). Similarly, a 1999 survey of subsidized housing properties in Florida found that between 14 and 17 percent of residents were perceived by housing managers as having trouble remaining responsible for themselves or their apartments, and between 11 and 17 percent were perceived to be confused, depressed, or abusive. This survey also found that only 37 percent of the low-income tenants interviewed believed there was someone they could rely on for help for as long as needed, should they became sick or disabled (Golant, 1999). Moreover, managers of Section 202 housing estimated that approximately 30 percent of their residents ultimately are transferred to nursing homes (Heumann and Nelson, 2001).

Surveys of low-income senior housing properties funded by the U.S. Department of Housing and Urban Development (HUD) also show that the average age of older residents is increasing. For example, in the past decade, the population aged 85 and older has become the fastest-growing segment of residents in Section 202 senior housing properties built before 1975 (Heumann and Nelson, 2001). Although there are few data to confirm what happens to these poor and near-poor elderly tenants, the risk of disability and frailty increases significantly with age (Stone, 2006). Overall, then, what data we have regarding the number of older persons who need or could benefit from both affordable housing and health-related or supportive services indicate significant demand for these arrangements unaddressed by current public programs.

Current Ways We Provide Affordable Housing with Services

A number of creative programs and strategies scattered throughout the country link affordable senior housing with services. They range from those that offer minimal information and referral to those offering personal assistance, chronic care management, and other health-related services. Some have been purposefully developed through federal, state, or local government programs. Most, however, have been cobbled together by housing providers who have recognized that a growing proportion of their aging residents need services in addition to a roof over their heads.

The inventory of affordable housing with services projects can be divided into two broad categories of housing: privately financed and publicly subsidized. Privately financed housing refers to multi-unit owner and rental housing that is privately funded and receives no public subsidies but is still affordable to low- and moderate-income older adults. It may also include neighborhoods of single-family homes with large concentrations of senior households. Publicly subsidized housing refers to multiple-unit rental housing that is subsidized by government entities at the federal, state, or local level. It may be owned and operated by a public entity, such as a housing authority, or a private entity, such as a nonprofit organization or real estate syndicate. It is not surprising that formal service linkages are much more prevalent in publicly assisted housing.

Affordable Private Housing with Services

One strategy found primarily in densely populated urban areas in which a large proportion of seniors with modest incomes have aged over time is the "limited equity housing cooperative." In this model, residents own an apartment-type unit through a cooperative corporation in which they own stock and are actively involved in management and programming decisions. The affordability of a cooperative is typically achieved by capping the resale price. Services are provided both informally through mutual support developed among the residents themselves, and formally through the joint purchase of supportive services or a coordinated and managed services program staffed by community agencies or by personnel employed by the cooperative. Several mature programs offer an extensive array of services including assessment and care planning, personal and home care, counseling benefits and entitlement assistance, financial management, crisis intervention, and home-delivered meals.

Penn South in New York City, for example, is a limited-equity cooperative built in 1961 with 6,200 residents. As Penn South's residents began to age, the co-op set up a collaborative program with community agencies to provide supportive services. The program, now a separate nonprofit agency, Penn South Social Services, Inc., offers cultural and educational programs, case management, day care, home care services, primary health care and wellness services, personal care, and a variety of supportive services to residents of the cooperative.

Other examples of limited equity housing cooperatives include low- or modest-income housing cooperatives created in mobile home parks or manufactured home communities where elderly residents own and control the park. In addition to the usual shared amenities, such as social and recreational activities, several communities, such as Leisureville Mobile Home Park in Woodland, California, have created informal help networks and are exploring strategies for attracting service providers who wish to capitalize on the park's group purchasing capabilities.

Publicly Assisted Housing with Services

Because housing providers themselves typically have few resources to invest in extra amenities or resident services, a low-cost alternative for those committed to helping residents to age in place is to work informally with community groups and service providers to encourage them to locate supportive services either in or near the housing property. The most common service programs are the meals sites and senior centers supported by Title III of the Older Americans Act. Community agencies may also offer limited services at no cost to residents, such as scheduled transportation, housekeeping, shopping, and other community-based activities. There are currently a variety of linkage models.

Congregate Housing

In 1975 HUD created the Congregate Housing Services Program to help elderly or younger people who reside in federally subsidized housing and who have limitations in three or more activities of living to live independently. Grants to state and local governments, public housing authorities, tribally designated housing entities, and nonprofit housing sponsors through this program provide funding for at least one daily congregate meal and other supportive services, such as housekeeping, personal care, transportation, and service coordination. HUD funds as much as 40 percent of the program costs, while grantees pay at least 50 percent of the costs (through cash or in-kind staff support) and participants cover the remainder. (Participant fees cannot exceed 20 percent of the resident's adjusted income.)

Although HUD has not funded any new grants since 1995, it continues to extend expiring grants on an annual basis. One interesting example is the Housing Authority of Portland, Oregon's congregate housing services program that operates in cooperation with the Multnomah County Department of Aging and Disability Services at four senior housing sites. This program provides service coordination, evening meals, housekeeping assistance, personal care, medication management, senior companions, transportation, and health and wellness programs. HUD funding is supplemented with matching funds from the Medicaid home and community-based waiver program, the Older Americans Act, and participant fees (see chapter 11).

Coordinating Services

Most low-income senior housing is not part of the Congregate Housing Services Program. To facilitate linkages among formal services, many property managers or housing sponsors employ a full- or part-time service coordinator whose role is to help residents identify needs, link them to community service providers, and monitor and assist residents with accessing needed services. Service coordinators typically are social workers whose primary focus is on identifying the supportive services needs of residents and creating appropriate service linkages. A few housing providers/sponsors have recognized the increasing health-related needs of their aging residents and have hired nurses as service coordinators. These individuals are also able to perform functional assessments, monitor health, and offer health education.

To support such efforts, HUD offers competitive grants to fund service coordinators in federally assisted multiple-family housing that is designated for occupancy by seniors or persons with disabilities. The grants support salaries, benefits, training, and administrative expenses. Service coordinators can also be paid for through the property's operating budget, if the funds are available. According to a 1999 survey of Section 202 properties, 37 percent had an on-site service coordinator (Heumann & Nelson, 2001).

Some service-coordination programs are far more extensive. They offer older residents who are aging in place or those who are particularly frail at entry a formal, structured assessment of their functioning, health status, and services needs. Residents who are found to be frail or disabled and who have unmet needs are offered a formal services plan that is then coordinated and monitored by property staff in collaboration with community services agencies and providers. Services that typically include 24-hour staffing, personal response systems, personal care, medication management, and housekeeping may be provided through formal contracts between the housing property and community services agencies or by in-house staff as a result of ownership of a home health agency. These services are often bundled into different level-of-care packages and are funded through a variety of sources, including the Medicaid home and community-based waiver and personal care programs, the Older Americans Act, municipal and philanthropic funds, property refinancing, and out of pocket. Peter Sanborn Place, in Redding, Massachusetts, and the housing strategy employed by the Osceola County Council on Aging, in Kissimmee, Florida, provide examples of these kinds of formalized service coordination and enriched service programs.

Comprehensive Service Programs

A number of organizations have developed more comprehensive, integrated programs of supportive and health-related services linked to publicly assisted housing. This integration is achieved through formal, purposeful collaboration among one or more low-income housing properties, neighborhood health care providers, and aging services agencies. In some cases the range of available services may approximate what is available to residents of a continuing care retirement community. The availability of adult day health care either co-located on or in proximity to the housing property, is often a key resource for making this strategy workable. Access to primary care and wellness services may be achieved by locating a community health center on the property or nearby.

Presentation Senior Housing is a collaboration between Mercy Housing California and North and South Market Adult Day Health that integrates affordable housing with on-site adult day health services. Residents participating in the day health program have access to a variety of services such as nurse care, social work services, physical, occupational and speech therapy, podiatry services, mental health support, case management, transportation, and a daily meal. Operating as a separate day health program and independent living apartments allows the project to avoid state licensing as an assisted living residence while providing roughly the same level of services to residents.

Some sponsors of low-income senior housing have been able to help their residents gain access to the full range of primary, acute, and long-term care services by encouraging them to enroll in the Program for All Inclusive Care for the Elderly (PACE). PACE providers receive monthly Medicare and Medicaid capitation payments for each enrollee. Providers assume full financial risk for participants' care and may not limit the amount, duration, or scope of services. To participate in the PACE program, a person must be at least 55 years old, live in the PACE service area, and be certified by the state as eligible for nursing home care. An interdisciplinary team that usually includes physicians, nurses, physical, occupational and recreational therapists, social workers, personal care attendants, dieticians, and drivers, assesses each participant's needs, develops a care plan, and delivers all services. Social and medical services are generally provided in an adult day health center and are supplemented by in-home or specialty referral services as needed. PACE programs have strong incentives to keep their enrollees out of nursing homes and hospitals because they are responsible for covering and coordinating those services by their capitation revenues.

Most of the housing sponsors who rely on PACE have partnered with the PACE provider either through co-location of the adult day health center or through close proximity to the PACE site. Mable Howard Apartments in Oakland, California, for example, has collaborated with a federally qualified health center (Over 60 Health Center) and a PACE program (Center for Elders Independence) to provide an assisted living level of care without special licensing or funding. The health center serves healthy and moderately disabled seniors, providing primary care, mental health services, adult day care, podiatry, dental care, and other services. PACE serves nursing home eligible residents with a full spectrum of primary, acute, and long-term care services.

Several *state initiatives* have produced affordable housing with services programs for older adults. Connecticut and Massachusetts have developed formal supportive service programs linked to publicly subsidized housing through collaboration between the state housing agency, state health and aging agencies, and individual properties. The explicit goal is to reduce Medicaid nursing home costs by maintaining older adults in independent housing for a longer period, thus delaying institutionalization. A state agency selects one or more licensed service providers to deliver a range of personal care and supportive services to participating housing properties and the housing property, a designated state agency, or both provide care coordination. Participating providers may also organize their own enriched services programs to wrap around the state program to ensure a wider range of services and to cover individuals who may not be eligible for state funded services (Mollica & Morris, 2005).

In the past decade, a number of naturally occurring retirement communities (NORCs) of lower- and modest-income older adults have developed formal service programs to address a range of social, personal care, and health-related needs. The term "NORC" refers to a geographic area—a neighborhood or large building—in which a large proportion of individuals have "aged in place." Typically, the residents collaborate with property managers and community service providers to develop specific programs targeted to the aging tenants or community residents. Services, including assessment and case management, wellness programs, housekeeping, and personal care, are paid for out of pocket by individual residents; supported with federal, state, local, and philanthropic funds; or provided through the in-kind efforts of volunteers. New York City has a unique program earmarked specifically for supportive services programs targeted to NORC residents in designated public housing and housing cooperatives (Vladeck, 2004).

Innovative collaborations between housing and health care providers offer yet another approach. In a number of communities across the country, local health systems or hospitals, community development organizations, and sponsors of low-income housing have partnered to expand affordable housing with services for older adults. The partnership between Mercy Health Systems and Mercy Housing in seven U.S. communities, for example, was instrumental in developing low-income senior housing properties as well as coordinating some care for the residents provided by Mercy hospital staff. Another partnership between the MedStar Health System's Housecalls Program and several low-income senior housing properties in Washington, DC, provides comprehensive chronic care management and primary care to frail, disabled elderly residents who have difficulty getting to a doctor's office. (See www.npr.org, December 19, 2005.) The incentives for these partnerships include the desire of many nonprofit organizations, particularly those that are faith based, to honor their mission and to meet the social accountability requirements associated with their tax-exempt status. Other incentives include tax benefits derived from the partnership, opportunities for creating new uses for defunct community hospitals, and the expansion of their markets by encouraging referrals of elderly residents to their health systems in return for services.

Affordable Assisted Living within Subsidized Housing

Most of the examples of housing with services described above involve housing properties that are not licensed by their states as assisted living residences or some equivalent category. Recent efforts to develop an affordable assisted living market have included rehabilitating or reconfiguring existing facilities or adding supportive services to the current stock of subsidized housing. In most cases, in order for a housing property to provide its own assisted living services, it must be licensed. An early example of this type of program was developed in 1999 at the Helen Sawyer Plaza, in Miami, owned by the Miami Dade Housing Authority and the first licensed assisted living program in public housing. The housing authority used public housing funding to renovate and modify the existing structure and received a special state Medicaid waiver allocation to pay for personal care, medication supervision, and other supportive services that were provided primarily by on-site staff.

In 2000 HUD instituted the Assisted Living Conversion Program, providing grants to owners of Section 202 and other federally subsidized senior housing projects to physically retrofit their properties and become licensed as assisted living residences. HUD funds may not be used for services, and applicants must demonstrate commitments from other funding sources, such as Medicaid waivers, to support services. The take-up rate for this program has been much lower than expected. Between 2000 and 2005, this program had supported the conversion of only 2,318 units in publicly subsidized properties. This has been due primarily to the perceived or real difficulties in obtaining Medicaid waiver funds, and reluctance on the part of many housing providers to become licensed as assisted living residences.

A very different example is the partnership established in 1999 between the local area agency on aging, a local provider of private senior housing, and the Michigan State Housing Development Authority that created the Affordable Assisted Housing Project pilot. In this case, a certain number of Section 8 rental assistance vouchers were set aside to subsidize housing at the facility for low-income seniors who were receiving care management (primarily through the area agency on aging) and personal care services under the Medicaid waiver program.

Several states have programs that explicitly recognize or license the assisted living services that are provided in publicly subsidized housing for older adults. In Minnesota, for example, housing properties registered as "housing with services establishments" may contract with a licensed home care agency or operate their own licensed agency. New Jersey has developed a statewide strategy for providing personal care and other supportive services in subsidized housing by licensing the service program rather than the property itself. This permits assisted living services to be provided in HUD-subsidized public housing for older persons without requiring expensive retrofitting to meet state-assisted living building standards.

A number of organizations that operate both low-income senior housing properties and assisted living (on a campus or in close proximity) share services across the settings to assist their low-income residents in the independent living property who have experienced a decline in their health or functional status. For example, case managers at the assisted living residence assess the status of the residents of the independent living property and develop care plans for them where appropriate. The assisted living and independent living properties may also share other services, such as medication management, 24-hour staffing, and after-hours care. The assisted living services are funded through the Medicaid program, and residents not eligible for Medicaid pay for some services out of pocket.

Barriers to Integrating Housing and Services

Maintaining older adults at home and enabling them to age in place in the face of increased disability and declining health is a well-accepted goal of aging policy. There is a large body of knowledge and experience about how to organize, implement, and fund home- and community-based services for disabled older adults living in their own homes to prevent unnecessary use of higher levels of more expensive care.

For elders living in subsidized housing, however, the story is different. Several scholars have explored the question of barriers to affordable housing with services (Pynoos, Feldman, & Ahrens, 2004; Golant, 2003; Wilden & Redfoot, 2002; Lawler, 2001). In brief, lack of coordinated policy making; agencies at the federal, state, and local levels that operate in "silos"; and the availability or lack of services in local communities can all impede progress in assuring that those who need it have access to affordable housing with services.

Policy governing publicly assisted housing has historically been disconnected from policies regarding health, long-term care, and related aging services. With a few exceptions, federal housing funds may not be used to pay for health or supportive services. Similarly, the primary sources of funds for health and supportive services—Medicaid, the Older Americans Act, and the Social Services Block Grant—cannot be used to supplement an individual's rent, even though adequate, affordable housing may be so critical to an older person's ability to obtain needed services outside an institution.

Housing providers and residents may find funding for services difficult to leverage. First, the availability of public funds for health-related and supportive services varies greatly across communities. Second, funding streams are fragmented, and federal and state regulatory and administrative program rules may be in conflict with the needs of low-income residents. Medicaid, for example, allows states wide discretion in its design and implementation. Medicaid eligibility requirements, however, are often obstacles to the use of these dollars (e.g., waivered services are available only to persons needing a nursing home level of care). In contrast, depending on their state of residence, low-income persons with higher levels of functioning may be eligible for Medicaid personal care benefits (O'Keefe & Weiner, 2004). These rules are very confusing to residents and housing providers (see chapter 1).

The structure and organization of federal, state, and local housing and aging services bureaucracies; program eligibility rules and regulations; the budget process; and resource allocation approaches all separate the worlds of housing and services—and there is little incentive to foster cooperation and collaboration. The public agencies responsible for financing, managing, and regulating low-income housing and those responsible for health and supportive services programs are separate entities with separate missions. They measure performance and success in different ways. Although long-term care policy tends to focus on maintaining people with significant disabilities in the least restrictive setting, the culture, rules, and "bricks and mortar" mentality that influence publicly assisted housing can work in opposition, making it difficult or impossible to bring in needed services that might delay or prevent institutionalization. Providers of housing and aging services often mirror the silo thinking of their funders.

In many cases, the residents of affordable housing arrangements are financially and functionally eligible for a wide range of home- and community-based services that could be accessed at no cost to the housing providers, but the services themselves are not available in a particular community. Where they are, community service providers are often not aware of the needs of low-income housing residents and may incorrectly believe that the housing property is able on its own to provide necessary services (Golant, 1999)

Housing managers are often concerned about their liability for tenants with cognitive impairments who might forget the stove is on, leave a cigarette burning, or injure themselves or others. Fear of litigation and the desire to remain under the regulatory "radar screen" have kept many housing providers from even coordinating supportive services for their aging residents. (Our own informal focus groups with housing operators and service coordinators indicate a belief among many providers that under no circumstances are they allowed to ask residents to respond to questions that would help determine the need for services.) Finally, many housing and community service providers simply lack experience in working together to meet the changing needs of aging residents in ways that are economically and programmatically feasible.

Older residents of affordable housing may also face some unique barriers to obtaining needed services and supports. They are less likely than older homeowners to have families on whom they can rely for direct support or care management. When families are available, they may face great difficulty in finding willing service providers to arrange appropriate services, particularly in high-risk, high-crime communities. Other tenants may pressure management to evict residents they perceive to be particularly physically frail or cognitively impaired.

Perhaps the major barrier to the expansion of programs, however, is lack of public awareness and political will to invest in affordable housing with services. Unlike the homeless, who have found their voice through a very proactive coalition, low- and modest-income older adults who are living in publicly subsidized housing, are on waiting lists, or who need both housing and services, are almost invisible. There is very little consumer advocacy in this area.

Conclusions and Implications for the Future
Affordable Housing with Services: The Ideal

In light of the continued decline in the federal investment in low-income senior housing throughout the past few years, one could argue that the future of affordable housing with services is not very bright. On the other hand, we know that the demand for affordable options that link housing with services is going to grow as the population of baby boomers ages. As the federal and state governments continue to struggle with the burden that long-term care places on Medicare and Medicaid budgets, they will be looking for lower cost solutions to help disabled elderly individuals remain in the community for as long as possible.

A viable system of affordable housing with services that allows older people to age in place for as long as they choose would look considerably different from what most aging residents living in publicly assisted housing or private-sector affordable housing communities now encounter. As we see it, an ideal housing with services program would incorporate at least the following elements as an organizing framework:

- A shared commitment—among residents and their families, the housing property, and the community—to "do what it takes" to help lower-income older adults age in place;
- Resident access to a full spectrum of primary, preventive, and chronic care, as well as supportive and personal care services;
- Protection of resident choice and privacy to assure that decisions to accept or decline services are voluntary;
- Optimal use of existing resources from all sources, including the resident and family, the housing community, and the neighborhood and community at large, as well as municipal, state, and federal governments; and

- Deliberate use of the economies of scale created by congregate apartment settings or the high concentrations of elderly persons living in the community, to create service delivery efficiencies and stretch existing resources.

Achieving a system that exhibits these features will require taking advantage of existing options as well as designing new ones, assuring the quality of care and safety, developing a solid base of evidence to demonstrate need and potential, and, finally, achieving a new vision of what constitutes the healthy aging in community.

Taking Advantage of Existing Approaches

To address the needs of a geographically and culturally diverse population of low- and modest-income elders will require a range of approaches. The first step is for policy makers and providers of aging services and housing to take fuller advantage of the existing stock of subsidized housing and community-based services in communities across the country. They must develop a better understanding of funding sources, the distribution of services in a particular community, and strategies for coordinating with the most appropriate organizations and individuals.

They must also address many programmatic issues. If policy makers are interested in formalizing programs that have currently been patched together by providers in a primarily idiosyncratic fashion, they will need to make decisions about the range of services to be included within a service package, how these services will be organized, and how and by whom they will be delivered. Most of the publicly subsidized programs, furthermore, meet the needs only of very low-income elderly people. Older adults who are near poor but whose incomes are too high to qualify for public programs and elderly individuals of very modest means have no available options. The real challenge is how to develop affordable market-rate housing with services programs that address the needs of modest-income elders.

Quality Oversight

Policy makers must address the issue of quality oversight and the balance between resident autonomy and safety. Concerns about safety and the potential for resident abuse were major factors in the growth of state regulation of assisted living. Fear of litigation has been a potent deterrent for many housing providers. The development of formal policies and programs linking affordable housing with services will require policy makers to construct a regulatory framework that maximizes quality outcomes and cost-effectiveness without creating disincentives for housing providers. Achieving the delicate balance between recognizing that affordable housing with services is still an individual's home and ensuring appropriate safeguards will be a significant challenge to expanding the options of affordable housing with services.

A New Vision for Aging Communities

Ultimately, the expansion of affordable housing with services will require a new vision for the future of healthy aging communities. We must acknowledge that we are facing an affordable housing crisis in this country from which neither current nor future elderly cohorts are immune. We must also recognize that the needs for housing and services are co-equal (Stone, 2005). In fact, some have argued that housing itself is just one form of essential service and support that elderly individuals need if they are to remain in the community.

We must also insist that policy makers and providers address the future of health, long-term care, and housing policy as a whole, including how public and private resources can be best used to create viable options for low- and modest-income older adults. The goal must be to create coherent policy for housing with services that meets the needs of all. This discussion must explore mechanisms for redistributing Medicaid and Medicare housing and service dollars to facilitate the development of community-based options.

In recent years, policy staff at HUD and in the Department of Health and Human Services have shown a glimmer of interest in this issue. The agencies have jointly supported the development of a typology of housing with service models and sponsored four regional stakeholder workshops to explore the barriers to and opportunities for expanding affordable housing with services programs for older adults. The Centers for Medicare and Medicaid (2005) also focused on this issue as part of their Systems Change initiative to foster home- and community-based alternatives in the states.

The examples highlighted earlier in this chapter reflect a broad range of strategies, but these programs represent only a fraction of what is possible to achieve within current policy and operational boundaries. Strategies that link older persons who live (or want to live) in affordable housing to health-related and supportive services deserve a systematic look. Before policy makers and providers are likely to support widespread replication and expansion of affordable housing with services strategies, the need—and potential—must be clearly demonstrated. We know from our own research (Harahan, Sanders, & Stone, 2006) and the work of others (Lawler, 2001; Wilden & Redfoot, 2002; Golant, 2003; Pynoos, et al., 2004) that affordable housing with services already play a role in meeting some of the needs of low- and modest-income older adults. As we have seen, however, we do not have accurate estimates of the number of elderly individuals currently living in publicly assisted or privately financed affordable housing arrangements. We have little information about their characteristics, including their health and functional status, the types and volume of services they use, and how these services are obtained and financed. And we do not know how long individuals remain in independent housing and where they relocate, either voluntarily or involuntarily.

Policy makers and providers of aging services and housing also need information that documents the characteristics of various strategies and how they actually work, including how different approaches affect residents' access to services and their quality of life and care, and what they cost.

It is time, therefore, to invest in creating the evidence base that will enable policy makers and assisted living providers to assess the value of current programs. We especially need information that compares the costs and outcomes for residents of various strategies to each other and to facility-based care, such as assisted living and nursing homes. At the same time, government and private funders should be encouraged to support the development, implementation, and evaluation of new models of affordable housing with services to help meet current and future needs (see chapter 15).

One key question that remains to be addressed is how affordable senior housing linked with services relates to the development of assisted living policy and expansion of the assisted living market. As noted above, the private assisted living market is, for the most part, only accessible to elderly individuals who are relatively secure financially. One might argue, therefore, that programs linking housing for low- and modest-income elders with supportive and health-related services could become the *poor person's* assisted living option in the future. We believe that the concept of assisted living should be critically examined within the larger context of an overarching agenda for affordable senior housing with services. This would encompass strategies that help elderly individuals who prefer to age in their own homes and their own communities gain access to supportive and health-related services that run the gamut from wellness and social integration to chronic care management, palliative care, and hospice.

REFERENCES

Centers for Medicare and Medicaid Services. 2005. *Coordinating and leveraging long-term supports with affordable and accessible housing.* Report from the State Leadership Symposium, Washington, DC, November 15–16.

Commission on Affordable Housing and Health Facility Needs for Seniors in the 21st Century. 2002. *A quiet crisis in America: A report to Congress.* Washington, DC: Government Printing Office.

Golant, S. 1999. *The CASERA Project: Tallahassee, FL.* Stephen Golant and Margaret Dugger and Associates. www.geog.ufl.edu/faculty/golant/CASERAREPORT FINAL.pdf.

Golant, S. 2003. Political and organizational barriers to satisfying low-income U.S seniors need for affordable rental housing with supportive services. *Journal of Aging and Social Policy 15,* 21–47.

Harahan, M., Sanders, A., & Stone, R. 2006. *Creating new long-term care choices for older adults: A synthesis of findings from a study of affordable housing plus services linkages.* Prepared for the Office of the Assistant Secretary for Planning and Evaluation, U.S. Department of Health and Human Services, Washington, DC.

Housing Research Foundation. 2002. *Public housing for seniors: Past, present and future.* Washington, DC: Housing Research Foundation. www.housingresearch .org.

Heumann, L., & Nelson, K. 2001. *The 1999 national survey of section 202 elderly housing.* Washington, DC: American Association of Retired Persons.

Lawler, K. 2001. *Aging in place: Coordinating housing and health care provision of America's growing elderly population.* Cambridge, MA: Harvard Joint Center on Housing Studies.

Mollica, R., & Morris, M. 2005. *State policy in practice: Massachusetts supportive housing program.* New Brunswick, NJ: Rutgers Center for State Health Policy.

O'Keeffe, J., & Weiner, J. 2004. Public funding for long-term care services for older people in residential care settings. *Journal of Housing for the Elderly 18,* 51–79.

Pynoos, J., Liebig, P., Alley, D., & Nishita, C. M. 2004. Homes of choice: Toward more effective linkages between housing and services. *Journal of Housing for the Elderly 18,* 5–49.

Pynoos, J., Feldman, P. D., & Ahrens, J. (Eds.). 2004. *Linking housing and services for older adults: Obstacles, options and opportunities.* New York: Haworth Press.

Redfoot, D., & Kochera, A. 2004. Targeting services to those most at risk: Characteristics of residents in federally subsidized housing. *Journal of Housing for the Elderly 18,* 137–163.

Stone, R.I. 2006. Emerging issues in long-term care. In R. H. Binstock & L. K. George (Eds.), *Handbook of aging and the social sciences.* 6th ed. (pp. 397–418). Amsterdam: Elsevier.

U.S. Census Bureau. *HCT8. Tenure by age of householder: 2000.* http://factfinder. census.gov/servlet/DTTable?_bm=y&-geo_id=01000US&-reg=DEC_2000_SF2_ U_HCT008:001&-ds_name=DEC_2000_SF2_U&-_lang=en&-mt_ name=DEC_2000_SF2_U_HCT008&-format=&-CONTEXT=dt

U.S. Government Accountability Office. 2005a. *Elderly housing programs that offer assistance for the elderly.* GAO-05-074, Washington, DC: Government Printing Office.

U.S. Government Accountability Office. 2005b. *Public housing: Distressed conditions in developments for the elderly and persons with disabilities and strategies used for improvement.* GAO-06-163, Washington, DC: Government Printing Office.

Vladeck, F. 2004. *A good place to grow old: New York's model for NORC supportive service programs.* New York: United Hospital Fund.

Wilden, R., & Redfoot, D. 2002. *Adding assisted living services to subsidized housing: Serving frail older persons with low incomes.* Washington, DC: American Association of Retired Persons.

CHAPTER 13

State and Federal Policies and Regulations

Intended and Unintended Consequences

ROBERT NEWCOMER, PH.D.
CRISTINA FLORES, PH.D., R.N.
MAURO HERNANDEZ, PH.D.

In the interest of protecting consumer rights over the past two decades, the press and federal agencies alike have criticized the quality of care offered by the residential care or assisted living industry (e.g., U.S. General Accounting Office, 1989, 1999, 2004; U.S. Department of Health and Human Services, 1982). With the criticisms have come demands for improvement in state oversight. Predictably, there have also been industry concerns that the nascent federal policy in this area could evolve to emulate federal regulation in the nursing home industry (Assisted Living Workgroup, 2003). Even with these ongoing debates over appropriate policies and jurisdiction, state governments have continued to execute their regulatory responsibilities by addressing such concerns as setting minimum standards with respect to the levels of care to be licensed as assisted living, measuring the quality of care, defining minimum staffing, and setting standards for medications management.

In their efforts to change the management behavior and operations of providers, and thereby improve the living environment of assisted living, these policy changes have intended consequences. These changes also, however, often increase the cost of providing services and thus in turn can have unintended consequences. For example, if costs of operation (and rents) rise faster than the consumer's ability to purchase assistance, the results may include a reduction in the supply of services or in more limited access to occupancy by lower-income elders. In turn, restricted access or availability of assisted living may have the additional consequence that some of the demand for the level of care offered in assisted living is shifted to alternative programs. These shifts may be intended as well as unintended, but they can have expense implications for other state and federally funded programs. Changes in other public programs, such as in Medicaid home- and community-based care or income eligibility, while not explicitly directed to assisted living, in turn can have consequences for this industry, by influencing those who might seek this level of care.

In short, policies affecting the assisted living industry come in many forms and can have effects both on the supportive housing industry itself and on other service-related sectors of government and industry (see chapters 11 and 12). In this chapter, we examine two broad effects of policy: the availability of assisted living residences and residents' ability to afford the types of services they offer. We adapt an economic framework of Paringer (1985) to help organize the presentation and consider the host of potential policy effects. The chapter's discussion begins with an outline of the conceptual framework and then progresses through a sequence of the policy domains. In each of these subsections, we describe illustrative policies and some of the intended and unintended consequences that have been experienced (or might be expected) by assisted living providers and older consumers.

Policy and Its Effects on Service Supply and Demand

Our adaptation of Paringer's work assumes that the use of long-term care services is a function of the interaction between service supply and consumer demand. Demand, in this context, refers to the number of people who wish to purchase a service at a given price. Demand may be different from the number of people who are using a service and from the number of those assessed as having a "need" for it within the population.

As Table 13.1 shows, we have categorized policies into four major domains based on the issues they address: financing and reimbursement,

TABLE 13.1
*A Framework for Classifying the Effects of Policy on
Assisted Living Residences*

Category	Supply	Demand
Financing and reimbursement:		
Loans, bonds, tax incentives	X	
Zoning/moratoria/certificate of need	X	
Reimbursement rate	X	X
Program eligibility critera		X
Level-of-care requirements:		
Admission/retention requirements	X	X
Negotiated risk/rental agreements	X	X
Staffing standards	X	
Staff training	X	
Unit size and amenity requirements	X	X
Other operational requirements:		
Occupancy limits	X	X
Health benefits	X	X
Liability insurance	X	X
Workers compensation	X	X
Fire codes/standards	X	X
Competition:		
Other assisted living beds supply	X	X
Nursing home beds supply		X
Controls of use of nursing homes		X
Home care supply	X	X
Payments for home care	X	X

level of care requirements, other operational requirements, and competition. Under financing and reimbursement, we examine the impact of broad
mechanisms, such as loans, bonds, and Medicaid reimbursement, on the
availability of and consumer access to assisted living. The examples in this
domain include both federal and state policies. Next, we explore the effects
of regulations specifically focused on the assisted living sector, including
level of care requirements, licensing, and quality assurance. Currently this
domain consists solely of state policies.

Operational requirements encompass public policies with broad safety
and consumer protection goals. These can have significant consequences
for the operating costs of assisted living residences. Here we examine the
impact of insurance requirements and local ordinances, such as fire and
building codes, on assisted living. The examples in this domain include
both state and local policies. Finally, we consider how a variety of state
and federal policies directed at the supply and distribution of long-term
care over the past two decades have shaped the environment in which
assisted living operates and competes with other forms of housing with

services. In the short term, competition is a constant environmental feature, but perceptions of the types and strengths of competition can influence change in assisted living supply and consumer demand over time.

Although some policies affect only supply or demand, many affect both. For example, policies that have an effect on operating costs usually have consequences for both provider willingness (supply) and consumer preferences and prices (demand). Similarly, easing admission and retention requirements for assisted living may increase the pool of eligible residents (with the intention of reducing the use of nursing homes), but operators must be willing (and able) to assume associated service responsibilities. Willingness may be tied to organizational, local, or state factors, such as staffing requirements and building design, competition or fire codes, or reimbursement or negotiated risk policies.

In completing this discussion of our economic framework, we reiterate two underlying notions and introduce a third one. First, the intended effect of any given policy can be expressed as an influence on either service supply or consumer demand. Second, not all the consequences arising from a policy are those that were intended. Finally, and perhaps less obvious, the effect of a policy may be influenced by the balance between supply and demand in the communities governed by that policy. For example, when there is "market equilibrium"—that is, when demand equals supply—policies intended to shift use by increasing demand for a substitute service will not be effective unless there is an increase in the supply of those services. The excess demand created by this policy example may eventually stimulate new supply, but the changes may be lagged. Similarly, policies that increase supply, when supply already exceeds demand, may not increase use unless the price of the service becomes low enough to increase demand.

In the discussion to follow, we provide selected examples of policy effects on supply and demand, and in some cases we illustrate how these effects may vary under conditions of market equilibrium and disequilibrium. We also attempt to distinguish intended from unintended consequences.

Financing and Reimbursement

In 2004, the licensed resident capacity in assisted living was 1,027,000 beds (Harrington et al., 2005). When we consider the comparable 1983 estimates of 410,000 (Stone & Newcomer, 1985), it appears that the resident capacity has more than doubled in 20 years. A variety of financial instruments and consumer demand has stimulated this growth (see chapter 10). Loans, bonds, government-sponsored mortgage insurance, tax incentives, and grants affect the availability of capital; zoning ordinances and building codes partly determine where services are located; and public reimbursement programs significantly influence who has access to assisted living. One intention of policy is to increase supply, but additional questions are whether this supply is located where it is needed and which groups of consumers are gaining access to it.

Loans, Bonds, Insurance, Tax Incentives, and Grants

Low-interest loans, tax-exempt bonds, mortgage insurance, and tax incentives directly facilitate the construction, acquisition, renovation, or conversion of assisted living supply. Several states have adopted such financing policies with the intention of increasing the supply of affordable assisted living. These financial policies have at least two main effects: to provide access to capital and to reduce operating expenses via lower mortgage payments. Secondarily, lower costs are expected to result in lower rents and more consumer "demand."

Such policies, however, have differential effects. Not all providers have equal access to loans and other financial resources. The size of a facility and its nonprofit status, for example, may be very important.

Small buildings (e.g., resident capacity less than 10) often have limited access to investor capital, such as long-term, unsecured credit from a bank—that is, not secured by the business's value. Banks may be willing to make loans secured by the individual's assets, but prospective service providers may be unwilling or unable to finance acquisition and construction under these terms. Moreover, with the exception of some bonds and low-interest loans intended to enable renovation to comply with relevant codes, public funds are usually not available to small assisted living residences either (see chapter 5).

Constraints on small residences' access to financing should be a public policy concern, but this is not the case. Mostly family owned and operated (Eckert, Cox & Morgan, 1999), these residences tend to have higher proportions of residents with dementia and functional limitations than do larger assisted living buildings (Morgan, Gruber-Baldini, & Magaziner, 2001;

Newcomer, Breuer & Zhang, 1994). Also, small residences are usually more accessible to individuals with low or moderate incomes (Eckert et al., 1999; Morgan, Eckert & Lyon, 1995), and to racial or ethnic minorities (Howard et al., 2002). Without access to low-interest loans or grants for code compliance or needed renovation, there is likely to be limited growth or upgrading in the small assisted living sector.

Assisted living residences operated by religious or civic organizations may qualify to operate as a nonprofit entity. This is a legal classification, not a description of whether the facility actually makes money. Among the advantages of nonprofit status is that property taxes may be exempted. There are disadvantages, too. Among them, nonprofits have limited access to investor capital, but they are better able to obtain loans than other comparably sized projects. Nonprofits also have access to governmental funds. For example, some financial institutions provide loans for the construction of moderate income housing for the elderly, including assisted living. Programs operated by the U.S. Housing and Urban Development, such as Section 223f and 232 can also be used to subsidize loans (see chapter 12). Nonprofit organizations also have access to state and municipal bonds, when there is local and state support and investors are willing to purchase them. A limiting problem, especially with federal funds, is that the terms of the loans may place restrictions on the projects such as limiting unit sizes and public area amenities. Such design restrictions may affect both provider interest and consumer demand. Somewhat offsetting these problems is that nonprofits can engage in community fundraising to subsidize operating costs, renovations, and even new construction. This advantages smaller projects.

Larger for-profit assisted living providers, particularly national corporations, have access to conventional sources of loans (see chapter 10). During the 1990s, this then newly emerging housing sector also had extraordinary access to investor capital. For example, there were 15 public stock offerings totaling $1.4 billion and $8.8 billion in private investment and lending for assisted living companies in 1997 alone (Vickery, 1998). These monies enabled rapid growth in the construction of new buildings and acquisition of existing ones. The explosive growth of some companies stimulated state and public attention to the supportive housing industry and may have obscured the static trends among other sectors. The growth among these larger, for-profit providers was targeted primarily to higher-income consumers who could afford market rate housing prices—not those with low and moderate incomes. Investor funds also were not available either to the small or to nonprofit providers. To introduce an issue to be addressed later, it is important to note that none of these financial polices was inherently intended to foster development of assisted living in specific locations or to direct attention to underserved populations.

Zoning, Building Codes, and Licensing

Through its building codes and zoning regulations, local government can influence an assisted living building's design features and location, even though, like financial policies, these codes have not been designed specifically to promote development of assisted living in underserved areas. They are more typically engaged only when a sponsor or operator applies for approval—*after* the project location has been determined.

State and local governments also influence development through their ability to grant building permits or to license assisted living. In particular, moratoria (a policy generally intended to control overbuilding) on building permits or on the issuance of new licenses can effectively discourage development of assisted living in specific locations. A secondary consequence of moratoria, if they succeed in capping the service supply, is to protect existing providers from having to compete with new providers. Where demand for market rate housing exceeds the available supply of this housing, providers have no incentive to ensure that they offer services to those who are unable to pay market rates.

Unless public agencies implement zoning laws, building permits, and licensing regulations to encourage assisted living development for low-income populations—or public programs are willing and able to subsidize market rate rents—the supply of assisted living available to Medicaid-eligible and other low-income residents may decrease even as the supply of this housing grows for the rest of the population. Some evidence in support of this concern shows that market forces are not yet working to distribute assisted living effectively. This is seen in the state-level ratios of assisted living and nursing home capacity per 1,000 elderly (Table 13.2). The resident capacity of assisted living approached or exceeded that of nursing homes in only 15 states. The inequity in supply is even more dramatic at the community level. For example, a five-state study found that most counties had less than one licensed assisted living "bed" for every four nursing home beds (Swan & Newcomer, 2000); no counties

TABLE 13.2
Assisted Living Bed Supply and Medicaid Personal Care Participation

State	No. of AL[a] beds	Medicaid[a] Participants	Participants/ AL Beds (%)	AL/1000 Aged[b]	NH/1000 Aged[c]
Alabama	9,876	0	0.0	16.6	38.5
Alaska	1,650	632	38.3	39.2	16.3
Arkansas	4,644	2,205	47.5	12.3	62.6
Arizona	24,500	3,076	12.6	33.0	18.3
California	154,830	0	0.0	40.5	31.5
Colorado	13,799	3,804	27.6	30.9	42.4
Connecticut[d]	9,479	65	0.7	19.9	53.4
Delaware[d]	2,772	14	0.5	25.6	37.0
Distict of Columbia	1,866	0	0.0	28.9	47.5
Florida[d]	78,564	18,355	23.4	26.5	25.8
Georgia	25,434	2,851	11.2	30.3	42.8
Hawaii	3,890	0	0.0	23.2	15.3
Idaho	6,160	1,870	30.4	39.6	35.6
Illinois	14,406	1,602	11.1	9.5	61.5
Indiana	11,767	71	0.6	15.4	60.0
Iowa	5,220	126	2.4	12.0	73.0
Kansas	7,971	769	9.6	22.3	65.4
Kentucky[d]	7,673	0	0.0	14.9	47.8
Louisana	4,443	60	1.4	8.3	69.6
Maine	9,022	3,762	41.7	47.3	36.5
Maryland	17,148	1,823	10.6	27.1	40.2
Massachusetts	10,585	1,120	10.6	12.4	55.6
Michigan	47,503	14,138	29.8	38.4	37.2
Minnesota[d]	20,192	6,442	31.9	33.1	57.1
Mississippi	4,197	68	1.6	11.9	45.8
Missouri	21,797	8,125	37.3	28.5	61.9
Montana	3,730	475	12.7	29.3	53.2
Nebraska	9,187	1,500	16.3	39.5	63.2
Nevada	4,021	222	5.5	15.7	18.2
New Hampshire	4,013	176	4.4	25.8	45.0
New Jersey	16,084	2,195	13.6	14.2	42.6
New Mexico[d]	5,558	189	3.4	23.8	25.3
New York	43,601	3,315	7.6	17.5	44.6
North Carolina	39,942	24,000	60.1	39.1	40.0
North Dakota	2,851	31	1.1	30.4	69.0
Ohio	41,921	0	0.0	27.6	55.6
Oklahoma	9,666	0	0.0	21.0	56.1
Oregon[d]	28,469	4,858	17.1	64.0	27.5
Pennsylvania	76,385	0	0.0	40.3	44.9
Rhode Island	3,676	230	6.3	24.4	51.9
South Carolina	16,641	600	3.6	32.1	29.3
South Dakota	3,360	727	21.6	30.8	58.5
Tennessee	13,929	0	0.0	18.9	49.8
Texas	42,245	2,851	6.7	19.0	49.5
Utah	4,478	380	8.5	22.1	32.5
Vermont	2,410	644	26.7	29.8	38.8
Virginia	34,598	0	0.0	40.7	33.4
Washington	24,498	5,735	23.4	35.4	31.5
West Virginia[d]	3,697	150	4.1	13.3	32.8
Wisconsin	27,375	3,956	14.5	38.2	54.1
Wyoming	1,285	100	7.8	20.7	46.5
Total	983,008	123,312	12.5	27.1	43.4

Note: AL refers to assisted living residences.

[a]Compiled from Appendix 3, pages 3-1 to 3-367 (Mollica et al., 2005).

[b]U.S. Bureau of the Census (2005).

[c]Harrington, Carillo & Mercado-Scott (2005).

[d]Indicates that the state did not report data or reported incomplete AL data in 2004 to Mollica et al. (2005). 2002 AL bed supply data were substituted, using Table 2, pages 275–277 (Harrington et al., 2005).

approached a 1:1 ratio. Similar findings were reported in a study in Florida. This work was able to identify assisted living residences that are affordable for low-income residents and for this group found that the supply per 1,000 population is inadequate relative to the low-income frail older population (Golant & Salmon 2004). Some Florida counties lacked any assisted living residences serving publicly financed residents.

If assisted living is to be an alternative for nursing homes for persons with low incomes, there must be a sufficient capacity. Studies such as the two mentioned suggest wide gaps between supply and demand from community to community. Although state and local policies potentially can influence the location of assisted living residences, there is little evidence that they have as yet been used to proactively influence where the assisted living supply is located.

Reimbursement Rates and Program Eligibility Criteria

The predominant source of payment for all forms of assisted living is private pay. The most widespread public income subsidy programs available are the federal supplemental security income (SSI) program and state supplemental payments (SSP) to SSI. SSI/SSP essentially provides a rent voucher for low-income persons but at a level well below what the private market typically charges for assisted living. This has had the potentially dual effect of limiting access to assisted living for low-income individuals when providers are able to fill their units with private pay clients or of necessitating that many low-income persons accept shared rooms. For example, an SSI/SSP payment of $900 a month ($30/day) would be expected to cover room, meals, housekeeping, and some personal care services for assisted living residents. In most states, however, combined SSI/SSP payments do not reach even $800 per month. This contrasts with private-pay rates for assisted living. Nationwide, base monthly rates averaged $2,969 per month in 2007 ($99/day) (MetLife, 2007). These expenses are adjusted upward depending on the level of care needs of residents. States recognize that SSI/SSP payments are not sufficient to cover extensive levels of personal care assistance and, as we soon discuss, many use the Medicaid program to finance additional services.

Income Eligibility and Access to Housing

States have a financial interest in keeping SSI/SSP income levels low because these are also categorical criteria of eligibility for Medicaid. Recognizing this constraint, states have adopted other means of addressing access to assisted living for low-income persons. One common policy response is to permit shared room occupancy by unrelated individuals. Another approach, used in 21 states, allows families to supplement SSI payments for rent and other living expenses (Mollica et al., 2005). The remaining 29 states either expressly prohibit this practice or do not address family supplementation. Prohibiting families from subsidizing a resident's SSI income may have the unintended consequence of shifting costs to private pay residents, and that in turn could affect how quickly families spend assets used to supplement personal income. Whether allowing families to subsidize income has improved access to assisted living, influenced the rate of spend down by older persons making them eligible for Medicaid, or reduced the use of nursing homes is not known.

Medicaid Reimbursement for Assisted Living

Most states (41 in 2004) have adopted programs to address the problem of inadequate funding for assisted living services by allowing eligible individuals to use their SSI/SSP or pay privately to cover room and board while Medicaid covers personal care expenses (Mollica et al., 2005). Medicaid home- and community-based services (HCBS) waivers are the mechanisms most widely used for this purpose (32 states and the District of Columbia in 2004). Another resource is the optional personal care services program under the Medicaid state plan (11 states used this approach in 2004). Assisted living services are also covered under capitated Medicaid long-term care programs in three states, and by some PACE (Program in All-Inclusive Care for the Elderly) sites. States may use various combinations of these options. Personal care under any of these programs includes assistance with activities of daily living, or ADLs (e.g., bathing, dressing, toileting, transferring, and eating) and with instrumental activities of daily living, or IADLs (e.g., shopping, meal preparation, ambulation, housekeeping, medication supervision).

A state's decision to use an HCBS waiver has both advantages and disadvantages. On the positive side, a waiver may allow a state to use less stringent income criteria to determine Medicaid eligibility than under a "state plan," thus facilitating access to assisted living services for a larger share of its nursing home eligible population. Specifically, in states using an HCBS income eligibility standard that is 300 percent of the federal SSI benefit ($1,869 per month for an aged individual in 2007), a larger proportion of lower-income residents may access assisted living.

Because the number of recipients an HCBS waiver may grant is fixed, and because recipients must meet greater impairment criteria to be eligible, states can use these mechanisms to control overall use of services and in principle reduce the use of nursing homes. This may be unfavorable to consumers who apply after a state's HCBS waiver slots have been used up or who do not meet the more restrictive nursing home level of care criteria. In comparison to the HCBS waiver program, the Personal Care Option services are less restrictive for recipients. These programs are statewide, recipients need not be as functionally impaired, and they cannot be put on a state waiting list. On the other hand, income eligibility may be less generous. Many states set eligibility at 100 percent of SSI ($623 in 2007). Because states have less ability to control or cap expenditures under this state plan program, they have been reluctant to make this benefit available to assisted living residents.

Medicaid Assisted Living Program Enrollment

Nationally, in 2004 Medicaid subsidized about 123,300 assisted living residents (Mollica et al., 2005). This is about 13 percent of the total assisted living capacity nationwide. By comparison, in the same year Medicaid was the primary payment source for almost two-thirds of nursing home residents (Harrington et al., 2005). Although these comparative figures are not particularly encouraging, they reflect a doubling of Medicaid-subsidized residents in assisted living between 2000 and 2004 (Mollica, 2000; Mollica et al., 2005). This growth has received positive attention, but as Table 13.2 shows there are vast differences among states. Three states account for about half of all Medicaid-subsidized residents nationally, while most states have programs with fewer than 2,000 participants. States have moved slowly in expanding benefits and eligibility, reflecting perhaps the limited evidence to date that assisted living residence reduces or avoids nursing home stays. Another contributing factor is that providers may not always be available who are willing to accept the payment levels even when the benefit is offered. Data are not available to indicate how many low-income persons would be interested in assisted living settings if they could use Medicaid benefits to subsidize the cost of such facilities (see chapter 11).

Level of Care Requirements

Policy provisions that define the level of care a provider must or may offer also have significant consequences for the availability of and demand for assisted living. Assisted living residences, both licensed and unlicensed, offer hotel services (e.g., housekeeping, laundry, and meals) and assistance with securing needed medical and social services. Licensed residences assume the additional responsibility of providing hands-on personal care and such health-related services as medication supervision. Across the assisted living industry, levels of care are thought to be rising; licensed residences are permitted to accept residents with more acute needs and greater physical and cognitive dependency than previously. Currently, all states permit (through a license or regulatory waivers) residents to remain in supportive housing with such special needs as being semiambulatory, using oxygen, having substantial cognitive impairments, or receiving hospice care (Mollica et al., 2005). The most consistently used regulatory distinction remaining between a nursing home resident and an assisted living resident is the need for 24-hour skilled nursing care. Even so, all states permit assisted living residents to receive short-term or intermittent skilled nursing care from a home health agency. States vary with respect to how they define "short-term" care (in number of days) and the particular health conditions for which such care may be provided.

Typically, when regulation allows assisted living to provide more services, additional requirements are created to ensure residents' health and safety. This can produce potentially contradictory results. On one hand, permitting more services may increase supply and demand, while on the other, requiring additional protections may reduce supply or increase cost and reduce demand. For example, most states require that residences serving those with dementia meet higher admission or discharge criteria and more stringent standards for staffing, training, activities, environment, and security, all of which increase operating costs significantly. Similarly, when residents need intermittent skilled nursing care, such as injections and wound care, regulations may allow short-term care to be provided by home health agencies under a resident's Medicare benefits but require the presence of a licensed nurse if care must be provided long term (see chapter 15).

Setting Standards: State-Determined Criteria versus Resident Agreements

A fundamental policy question concerning assisted living properties is the extent to which they should be permitted to define what services they will provide and to determine what level of care their residents need. How much discretion in defining entry and exit criteria should be given to the provider? Who assumes the risk and responsibility if care is not appropriate? Should properties be permitted to negotiate with their residents how much risk each party will assume? And if contracts do apportion risk between resident and property, will such agreements be recognized by the courts?

There is a continuum of perspectives on these issues among the states. At one end is an idealized system in which the specifics of who should reside in a particular property are determined on a resident-by-resident basis, based largely on a contract between the property and the resident. In practice, few states defer completely to individual contracts. At the other end of the continuum, states require that properties provide certain services and define which conditions disqualify an individual from becoming or remaining a resident in assisted living. In most states, providers are given the discretion to set the maximum level of care for which they will assume responsibility.

States differ more in their role relative to publicly subsidized residents versus private pay residents. For Medicaid residents (or those likely to become Medicaid eligible), the state (or its designee) assesses the needs of applicants and continuing residents and determines whether they are eligible for benefits. This may mean specifying the services and the amount of services a property provides and/or establishing the amount of funding that will be made available for the beneficiary. For private-pay residents, the state's role in evaluating the fit between needs and the level of care is commonly limited to assuring that the provider has disclosed what it is able and willing to do and that the property complies with its resident agreements and other licensing provisions.

The ideal of contracts specifically negotiated between providers and individual residents and the imposition by the state of uniform standards across properties reflect often competing concerns among advocates, providers, and consumers. More particularly, these ends of the oversight continuum reflect the tension between the value of allowing residents to say how they wish to live and what will support a good quality of life for them and the need to protect their interests and well-being. On one hand, there is the desire to enable a resident to "age in place." On the other, there are concerns about the kind of oversight, staffing, and property design needed for an appropriate level of care. These concerns reflect the realization that even the best run assisted living residences may encounter difficulties from time to time in meeting resident and state expectations for the quality and appropriateness of care.

Beyond the issue of standards is that of enforcement. All states have policies assuring that they will respond to resident complaints, but standards of appropriate care are usually enforced retroactively. For example, a doctor's evaluation of a resident's appropriateness for admission and a continued stay, along with resident records about incidents and changes in status are used as basis to evaluate the appropriateness of care. This is done retrospectively during periodic licensing recertification visits. Whether pre-admission screening criteria and admission or discharge criteria specified in rental agreements have effects on service supply, demand, quality and appropriateness of care, and "aging in place" independent of the enforcement of these standards remains undetermined.

Standards for Staffing and Training

In addition to entry and exit criteria and standards for level of care, public policy often addresses questions of appropriate levels of staffing and appropriate competencies for staff. Staffing-related regulations set forth the minimum number of staff to be awake or on site, the qualifications of those who perform certain tasks, pre-employment procedures (such as criminal background checks), and initial and ongoing training. Personnel costs account for 40–60 percent of provider expenses (Sterns & Morgan, 2001). Staffing requirements directly affect operating costs; if rents cannot be adjusted to cover these expenses, they also affect housing supply. Hiring and training requirements also affect the pool of eligible labor and the levels of care that can be supported. Smaller properties may have fewer resources to finance the training of staff or to pay competitive wages for those with training and experience.

In general, state staffing regulations have been cautious in asserting stringent standards. All states require properties to maintain "sufficient staff" to meet residents' needs for 24-hour service, but most (86 percent) do not specify staff-to-resident ratios that are adjusted by level of care needed by residents (resident acuity) or time of day. Requirements for staff training are generally low and vary considerably with respect to initial orientation and regular in-service education (Mollica et al., 2005). Required training, as reported in surveys, includes such topics as first aid, providing personal care, caring for patients with Alzheimer disease, responding to challenging behaviors, resident rights, and medication management (Hawes & Phillips, 2000).

Some believe that staffing standards, such as requiring a nurse on site, may lag behind actual property practice. In 2002, 17 states required the larger assisted living properties to have either a registered nurse (RN) or licensed practical nurse (LPN) on staff or available on-call (Mollica, 2002). Assisted living residences that have more than 10 beds, however, generally exceed these standards. For example, a 1998 study found that 71 percent of these residences employed an RN or LPN on a full- or part-time basis (Hawes et al., 1999). An additional 10 percent of properties reported that nursing services were arranged "as needed." There are no comparable data for properties with fewer than 10 beds. Having a nurse on staff is thought to be helpful for residents who have more complex health care needs. Findings from the few studies of nurse staffing in assisted living are mixed relative to staffing impact on reducing hospitalizations and avoiding a nursing home transfer (Phillips et al., 2003; Zimmerman et al., 2005; Newcomer & Preston, 1994).

Standards for Unit Size, Design, and Amenities

Expansion of permitted levels of care is often paralleled by changes to standards related to property features and amenities (e.g., single apartment units with kitchenette and private bathrooms). Such standards are thought to support higher levels and quality of care and to enrich the living situation for many residents (see chapter 4). Compliance with such standards has implications for both the cost of operations and the number of providers available in the community. While amenities may increase consumer interest, such features increase prices and in the absence of public or insurance subsidies narrow the effective demand for (and access to) assisted living.

Access to Care and State Costs

One rationale underlying state support for assisted living has been the expectation that residents will be able to "age in place," with these individuals either being able to avoid a nursing home placement or to have fewer lifetime days in a nursing facility. Any such reductions would result in lower private nursing home expenditures and ultimately in lower Medicaid nursing home expenditures. The effectiveness of such efforts has remained largely unexamined. Any Medicaid savings realized, however, are contingent on whether those likely to spend down to Medicaid eligibility have access to assisted living. To the extent that assisted living is available only to persons in the upper quartiles of incomes and assets (who would never spend down to Medicaid eligibility), the likelihood of Medicaid savings is reduced. Currently, low- and moderate-income persons are more likely to be able to afford smaller and older properties than nonprofit or new, investor-owned assisted living residences. The newer properties in turn are the ones most likely to feature expanded amenities. While the expansion of market rate assisted living bed supply has few cost implications for the state (e.g., regulatory oversight), there remains the possible irony that this resource is unavailable for the low and moderate income population. To the extent that such access is limited, apartment style assisted living will have little effect on nursing home use and expenditures among the low- or moderate-income population.

Provider Participation

Certain restrictions on provider participation may also affect who uses which kinds of properties. For example, standards for minimum property size (often excluding small properties), square footage allocated per resident (even if in a shared room), and number of persons sharing a bathroom may all determine whether a property can participate under a publicly financed program such as a Medicaid assisted living waiver (Mollica et al., 2005). Privacy standards with respect to whether residents have a choice in sharing a room are also relevant in this regard. Unit size and privacy standards (e.g., private room, private bath) have direct implications for monthly rental charges (independent of personal care and meals), and thus for the number of properties available at the rents that can be afforded by the private-pay and Medicaid markets.

In 2004, 13 states required that properties licensed specifically as "assisted living" properties provide apartment-like units to qualify for Medicaid. Among these, Oregon and Washington restricted the maximum number of unrelated occupants to one person per unit. All states also licensed other types of supportive housing under titles like "residential care," "adult foster care," and "sheltered care" properties but imposed less restrictive size and privacy standards. Most states set maximum occupancy at two persons per unit, with about half permitting double occupancy by resident choice, though this choice may be exercised by a family member such as in situations involving dementia care.

Setting such criteria for Medicaid participation has both advantages and disadvantages for states. One advantage of higher standards is that these limit the supply of eligible housing units and thus cap a state's financial risk by limiting the number of persons who might receive subsidized care in an entitlement program. A disadvantage is that public subsidies have to be sufficient to cover the added rental costs. Imposing less restrictive standards for unit size and occupancy also has a mix of advantages and disadvantages. On the negative side, this approach is not responsive to consumer preferences and may narrow demand for such accommodations. On the other hand, such standards may increase supply (by increasing the number of available capacity even if the number of rooms is unchanged) and allow properties to charge lower rents (by permitting residents to share rooms). This may increase effective demand.

In general, data systems that compile information on licensed housing do not document whether the growth in service supply in recent years (particularly that available to low income persons) has favored apartment-like supply or other types of units. Oregon offers an illustrative exception, providing data about housing in all state licensing classifications. Between 1990 and 2004, the state offered a higher payment for apartment-style assisted living properties than for other types of supportive housing. In 2004, assisted living comprised 30 percent of the state's supply of licensed long-term care, compared to 19 percent for adult foster care homes (private residences licensed to provide care for up to 5 residents), 21 percent for residential care properties (licensed for 6 or more residents in non-apartment-style units, which may be semiprivate), and 30 percent for nursing homes. Ninety percent of Oregon's assisted living properties were accepting Medicaid recipients, compared to 69 percent of residential care properties (Hernandez, 2005).

Absent definitive studies demonstrating that apartment-like settings provide better resident outcomes (e.g., greater length of stay, less use of health care, avoidance of admission to a nursing home), most states appear to be less likely than Oregon to expand access to apartment-style accommodations for low-income persons by subsidizing rental costs, judging by the Medicaid participants in assisted living (see Table 13.2).

Other Operational Requirements

Beyond policies that address financing and reimbursement mechanisms or standards for care, a wide range of regulations, licensing standards, and other requirements affect assisted living operations and the costs of doing business. These range from explicit standards of practice to those of private sector influences, such as the cost of insurance (Table 13.1). States could be helpful in working with the industry either to alleviate these costs or by changing reimbursement rates so that these costs are affordable to the providers when receiving public program payment. Some examples illustrate the potential consequences for both assisted living supply and consumer demand.

Occupancy or Size Limits

Where Medicaid restrictions exclude smaller properties, this may reflect the presumed difficulties such properties have in meeting the requirements for highly frail residents (e.g., staff available and awake 24 hours a day). The majority of properties that have fewer than nine beds have no staff beyond the owner-operators and their families (Hawes et al., 1995; Newcomer et al., 1994). Consideration of the other tasks (e.g., meals, laundry, and housework) that must be performed for even a few more functionally disabled residents raises questions about how much personal care such properties can provide without hiring additional staff. If supplemental staff are added, there is also the question of the scale (number of rent-paying residents) needed to sustain a financially viable operation.

When states effectively exclude small properties from waiver or other reimbursement programs there are several potentially adverse consequences for consumers and for service supply. One of these is associated with the unknown demand for supportive housing among nonwhite residents who comprised 4 percent of assisted living Medicare beneficiaries in 1998 (compared to 14 percent of nursing home) (Spillman et al., 2002). Minority residents also disproportionately reside in smaller properties (Howard et al., 2002; Newcomer et al., 1994). Does this reflect racial or ethnic preferences for smaller properties, the location of small properties in minority neighborhoods, operator practices among larger properties that are not responsive to the preferences of minority populations, prejudice on the part of white residents in larger properties, or simply lower income and the inability of minority populations to afford the larger properties (see chapter 5)? Data that might answer these questions are limited because small properties have not been included in recent national studies of assisted living (e.g., Hawes et al., 1999; Zimmerman et al., 2005).

Employee Benefits, Liability Insurance, and Worker's Compensation

Most employees in government and the private sector expect to receive benefits from their employers in the form of health insurance, sick days, vacation days, and retirement savings contributions. Yet these are among the operating costs that owners of assisted living properties have been able to reduce or eliminate (Hawes et al., 1995, 1999; Newcomer et al., 1994). One means of doing so is the use of part-time employees, for whom these benefits are not mandated. Such practices stand in contrast to the benefits usually available to hospital and nursing home workers. The extent to which the absence or limited availability of health insurance and other fringe benefits contributes to worker turnover in assisted living has not been documented. Worker turnover is thought to affect the quality of care for residents, but this may not have a substantial effect on service supply or consumer demand.

Two other insurance issues directly affect providers and service supply, neither of which a property can avoid by using only part-time staff. One of these is the rising cost of general and professional liability insurance. Large increases in premiums for providers are passed along to residents in the form of rent increases. These increases are attributable in part to litigation outcomes and legislative changes (American Seniors Housing Association, 2004) and in part to growth in the assisted living industry and changing levels of care. Larger assisted living residences have been able to lower liability costs through risk management strategies, such as negotiating risk agreements with residents or restricting what residents the property will accept and retain and by purchasing high-deductible (as high as $1,000,000) insurance. Many smaller properties cannot afford the insurance, even with high deductibles. If they cannot raise rents, they face the choice of operating without liability insurance or going out of business.

Research has yet documented the extent to which supply and access to higher levels of care have been affected by liability insurance and the strategies properties have adopted to lower these costs, but these effects may be substantial. States have responded to these issues by allowing properties wide discretion in writing admission and retention agreements (Carlson, 2005). Consumer advocates, attorneys, and the federal government have taken issue with these state practices but have done little to reduce insurance costs.

Worker's compensation insurance is another rapidly rising cost. These expenditures vary from state to state, but they amount to almost 5 percent of hourly wages. In setting rates for assisted living, insurance companies use the experience basis of nursing homes, for which there are relatively well-developed data systems for reporting occupational injury (Bureau of Labor Statistics, 2005). Whether the use of injury rates for nursing home workers is equitable for assisted living is unknown. Assisted living properties are not readily identifiable in data available from the Bureau of Labor Statistics, and there is substantial variation in the level of care and in staff training among assisted living properties. We seem to need more systematic compilation of injury reporting and injury prevention efforts.

Fire Codes/Standards

Tragic stories of elderly persons suffering fire and fire-related injury in homes that care for the elderly have made fire protection a prominent concern. The International Association of Fire Chiefs (2004) proposed a number of life safety features for assisted living, notably the use of fire-suppression systems. The life-saving benefits of such systems have been amply demonstrated (Rohr, 2003; Dewar, 2004; Hall, 2004) and provide strong grounds for states to require automatic suppression systems in long-term care properties, especially those occupied by nonambulatory, frail, or cognitively impaired individuals. Newer, purpose-built properties are likely to be required by building codes to include fire sprinklers, but the cost of retrofitting may be prohibitive for many older properties. Grants, low-interest loans, and tax incentives are potential ways to address this problem but are not widely available.

Competition for and Alternatives to Assisted Living

Assisted living operates in a complex environment. On one hand, this level of care is seen and used as an alternative to nursing home care. On the other hand, assisted living is an option when other forms of community based care are not viable. This combination of factors affects the supply of assisted living (including the levels of care provided) and demand (including the levels of care being sought and the case mix or levels of frailty among residents).

In the past 20 years, multiple state and federal government efforts have been implemented to reduce "unnecessary" nursing home placements and days. Policies have attempted to constrain nursing home bed supply and to alter demand. Supply-directed policies include limits on the number of new beds licensed, incentives for closing or converting nursing home beds to lower levels of care, and case-mix adjusted payments for nursing home residents. Policies intended to affect "consumer" demand include preadmission screening and postadmission utilization review, this with the intention of reducing inappropriate admissions.

To the extent that these programs have been successful in reducing nursing home use, they have permitted individuals to remain in community settings. This in turn has necessitated an expansion of community-based personal care programs. The most extensive of these are the Medicaid state plan personal care services and HCBS waiver programs discussed earlier. Access to and demand for assisted living, especially among individuals eligible for Medicaid, is directly influenced by the combination of constraints on admission to nursing homes, the home care alternatives available, and the relative subsidies available for assisted living.

Home care offers several advantages over assisted living for states. Among these are that for many recipients living expenses and task assistance can be shared with or provided by family members at no cost to the state. This reduces upward pressure on SSI/SSP payments or other subsidies that might be needed to cover the expenses of assisted living, and it may reduce the amount of personal care assistance that is paid. Assisted living is an alternative for the subset of the population who do not have family members or for whom instrumental task needs (e.g., shopping, cooking, and transportation) or personal care tasks (e.g., bathing, transferring, medication management) cannot be met in independent housing (see chapter 7).

The effect that community-based personal care programs and constraints on nursing home use have had on consumer behavior—for example, on the age and frailty level associated with the decision to move into assisted living—has not been studied extensively or with representative samples. Nevertheless, the consensus from available studies is that age of entry and average frailty levels of residents in assisted living have been increasing. For example, in the 10 years between 1983 and 1993 residents residing in assisted living became older (64 percent in 1993 were 75 and older, compared to 38 percent in 1983); were more cognitively impaired (40 percent versus 30 percent); more often incontinent (23 percent versus 7 percent); were more likely to be wheelchair dependent (15 percent versus 3 percent); and required greater assistance with bathing (45 percent versus 27 percent) and taking medications (75 percent versus 43 percent) (Hawes et al., 1995). Such changes have both supply and demand implications for levels of care, and operating expenses.

Another source of competition for assisted living is the practice initiated in some states to combine the personal care program with low-income housing to "create" a supply of unlicensed housing as an alternative to income-subsidized assisted living. Such policies couple rent subsidies available through various federal and state programs (see chapter 12), the provision of personal care services financed through Medicaid, and a relaxing of local fire and safety regulations that might otherwise require that cognitively impaired or physically disabled residents be relocated to assisted living or nursing home properties. The size of the low-income population served (or potentially served) in this manner is not known, but this approach is consistent with the notion of allowing individuals to age in place and receive care in the least restrictive setting. If it proves cost effective and easily replicated and no major evidence of inadequate care emerges, this approach will likely grow and could emerge as the most viable of approaches for assisted living for those with low or moderate income.

Conclusions and Implications for the Future

The preceding review of how public policies affect the supply of and demand for assisted living has brought to light problematic gaps between their intended and actual outcomes. We have suggested (and where possible documented) some of the intended and unintended consequences that arise from sometimes competing policies. Examples of these policies and their effects are summarized in Table 13.3, but we recognize that there are many gaps in knowledge. Notably, we have seen that there is sometimes a tension between the policy goal of improving quality and policy makers' willingness to provide sufficient funding to ensure that individuals who could benefit have access to assisted living. Complicating matters is the fact that decision making and accountability are sometimes fragmented among multiple units and levels of government. This is particularly evident in policies affecting program income eligibility, and policies affecting service alternatives with the long-term care continuum.

How might public policy be developed and implemented to more effectively assure that assisted living is more widely available, especially for lower-income populations? One possible answer to this fundamental question is to take better advantage of the experience among and within states. These practices provide a naturally occurring experiment for evaluating the effects of policies and regulations on service supply and demand; and perhaps for testing the efficacy of various approaches to providing assisted living services. Among the efficacy issues that have not been fully tested are the connection between levels of staffing, case mix, and resident outcomes; the extent to which assisted living reduces lifetime days in nursing homes; and the extent to which assisted living (compared to other community-based care) prevents avoidable health care use (e.g., ambulance, emergency room, hospitalization). The unanswered questions stand in marked contrast to the information available from ongoing data systems. To date, reports are available that track policy changes, but only a handful of studies have attempted to link policy and regulations to system outcomes, such as service supply, demand, quality of care, and resident outcomes. Most such studies focus on a single year, rather than looking at effects over time; and, where comparisons are made by states, they draw on aggregated data. Intrastate longitudinal comparisons are virtually non-

TABLE 13.3
Intended and Unintended Consequences of
State and Federal Policies and Regulations

Policy/Program Change	Intended Consequence	(Possible) Unintended Consequence
Financing and Reimbursement		
Loans, bonds, and tax incentives	Facilitate increased supply by providing capital and reducing expenses; lower rents and increase consumer demand.	Poor accessibility by smaller homes and nonprofits. Limits growth among smaller non-apartment-style assisted living and the low- to moderate-income, racial/ethnic minorities, dementia, and high-need residents they serve.
Zoning and moratoria	Control overbuilding of assisted living facilities by discouraging development in particular areas.	Reduces competition and increases prices in selected markets over time. May decrease supply of beds available to lower-income and Medicaid residents.
Reimbursement	Provide subsidy to lower-income residents and improve accessibility to assisted living for these residents.	Low payments limit access to AL availability to lower income residents over time when private pay clients are in demand of assisted living supply.
Program eligibility	Facilitate access to assisted living for more nursing home eligible residents by using less restrictive income eligibility criteria.	Decreases access to residents with needs below nursing home eligibility threshold.
Level-of-Care Requirements		
Admission/retention requirements	Define the extent to which assisted living facilities can determine services provided and level of care needs of their residents.	Variable and confusing requirements lead to unclear expectations regarding level of care and services. Assisted living facility assumes increasing risk and liability. Risk concerns for facilities in conflict with protection of consumer rights.
Negotiated risk/rental agreements	Ensure that services safely meet the need levels of residents and promote aging in place.	
Staffing standards and training	Reduce problems of quality of care and improve ability of assisted living to retain high care clients by setting higher standards; reduce hospitalizations and nursing home discharges.	Increased operating costs affect supply of assisted living when rents cannot be adjusted (small homes most affected). Standards and oversight often inadequate to ensure high quality of care.

TABLE 13.3
(continued)

Level-of-Care Requirements		
Unit size and amenities requirements	Enrich residents' living situation by supporting higher levels and quality of care.	Increased cost of operations, increased prices and less accessibility for lower income residents (small homes unable to meet requirements).

Other Operational Requirements		
Occupancy limits	Ensure that facilities will be able to meet the needs of highly frail residents.	Exclusion of smaller homes decreases availability to low-/moderate-income residents, racial/ethnic minorities and residents with dementia and high levels of need.
Insurance	Protection for consumers, staff, and facilities.	Increases operating costs. Affects supply of assisted living (especially small facilities) if rents not adjusted.
Fire codes/standards	Protect vulnerable elderly from fire-related injury and death.	Increases rent and operating costs. Affects supply of assisted living (especially small facilities) if rents not adjusted.

Competition		
Other supplies of assisted living and nursing home beds; controls on use of nursing homes; home care payments and supply	Reduce nursing home placements and days. Expand community-based personal care programs. Meet consumer demand and reduce costs for states.	May affect quality of care and safety as highly frail residents remain in assisted living facilities.

existent. Studies testing cost effectiveness and other performance outcomes relative to particular policies or standards are also very limited.

Policy development is not dependent on data, but it might benefit from objective information that tracks consequences after a policy's implementation. State governments have the infrastructure in place to record changes in property and staffing characteristics but usually have not taken advantage of this capability to produce either monitoring systems or consumer-oriented databases. As these resources begin to be effectively used, it will be important that policy makers are explicit about the consequences sought from changes in regulations, service financing, and other policies; and for states to share information on their experiences.

REFERENCES

American Seniors Housing Association. 2004. *2004: Seniors housing liability insurance report.* Washington, DC: American Seniors Housing Association.

Assisted Living Workgroup. 2003. *Assuring quality in assisted living: guidelines for federal and state policy, state regulation and operations: A report to the U.S. Senate Special Committee on Aging.* Washington, DC: Government Printing Office.

Bureau of Labor Statistics. 2005. *Table 1. Incidence rates of nonfatal occupational injuries and illnesses by industry and case types, 2003.* www.bls.gov/iif/osh/os/ostb13555.pdf.

Carlson, E. 2005. *Critical issues in assisted living: Who's in, who's out and who's providing the care.* Washington DC: National Senior Citizen's Law Center.

Dewar, B. 2001. *Residential fire sprinklers for life safety: An economic and insurance perspective.* Patterson, NY: National Fire Sprinkler Association. www.nfsa.org/info/residential/econsprinklers.pdf.

Eckert, J. K., Cox, D., & Morgan, L. 1999. The meaning of family-like care among operators of small board and care homes. *Journal of Aging Studies 13* (3), 333–347.

Golant, S. M., & Salmon, J. R. 2004. The unequal availability of affordable assisted living units in Florida's counties. *Journal of Applied Gerontology 23* (4), 349–369.

Hall, J. R., Jr. 2004. *The total cost of fire in the United States.* Patterson, NY: National Fire Protection Association. www.nfpa.org/catalog/services/ customer/download memberonlypdf.asp?pdfname=totalcost%2Epdf&src=nfpa.

Harrington, C., Carrillo, H., & Mercado-Scott, C. 2005. *Nursing facilities, staffing, residents, and facility deficiencies, 1998 through 2004.* San Francisco: University of California.

Harrington, C., Chapman, S., Miller, E., Miller, N., and Newcomer, R. 2005. Trends in the supply of long-term-care facilities and beds in the United States. *Journal of Applied Gerontology 24* (4), 265–282.

Hawes, C., Mor, V., Wildfire, J., Iannacchione, V., Lux, L., Green, R., Greene A., Wilcox, V., Spore, D., & Phillips, C. 1995. *Executive summary: Analysis of the effect of regulation on the quality of care in board and care homes.* Washington, DC: U.S. Department of Health and Human Services.

Hawes, C., & Phillips, C. 2000. *A national study of assisted living for the frail elderly: Final summary report.* Washington, DC: U.S. Department of Health and Human Services.

Hawes, C., Phillips, C., & Rose, M. 1999. *A national study of assisted living for the frail elderly: Results of a national survey of facilities.* Washington, DC: U.S. Department of Health and Human Services.

Hernandez, M. 2005. Residential LTC in Oregon: Policy and supply trends across provider types and regions, 1986 to 2004. Paper presented at the Gerontological Society of America, Orlando, FL.

Howard, D. L., Sloane, P. D., Zimmerman, S., Eckert, J. K., Walsh, J. F., Buie, V. C., Taylor, P. J., & Koch, G. G. 2002. Distribution of African Americans in residential care/assisted living and nursing homes: More evidence of racial disparity? *American Journal of Public Health 92* (8),1272–1277.

International Association of Fire Chiefs. 2004. *Healthcare fire safety: Roundtable report*. Washington, DC: International Association of Fire Chiefs.

MetLife. 2007. *The MetLife market survey of nursing home and assisted living costs*. Westport, CT: MetLife Mature Market Institute.

Mollica, R. 2000. *State assisted living policy, 2000*. Portland, ME: National Academy for State Health Policy.

Mollica, R. 2002. *State Assisted Living Policy, 2002*. Portland, ME. National Academy for State Health Policy.

Mollica, R., Johnson-Lamarche, H., & O'Keeffe, J. 2005. *Residential care and assisted living compendium, 2004*. Washington, DC: Department of Health and Human Services, Office of Assistant Secretary for Planning and Evaluation.

Morgan, L. A., Eckert, J. K., & Lyon, S. L. 1995. *Small board-and-care homes: Residential care in transition*. Baltimore: Johns Hopkins University Press.

Morgan, L., Gruber-Baldini, A., & Magaziner, J. 2001. Resident characteristics. In S. Zimmerman, P. D. Sloane, & J. K. Eckert (Eds.). *Assisted living: Needs, practices and policies in residential care for the elderly* (pp. 144–172). Baltimore: Johns Hopkins University Press.

Newcomer, R. J., Breuer, W., & Zhang, X. 1994. *Residents and the appropriateness of placement in residential care for the elderly: a 1993 survey of California RCFE operators and residents*. San Francisco: University of California–San Francisco.

Newcomer, R., & S. Preston. 1994. Relationship between acute care and nursing home unit use in two continuing care retirement communities. *Research on Aging 16* (3), 149–167.

Newcomer, R., Preston, S., & Roderick, S. 1996. Assisted living and nursing unit use among continuing care retirement community residents. *Research on Aging 17* (2), 149–167

Paringer, L. 1985. Medicaid policy changes in long term care: a framework for impact assessment. In C. Harrington, R. Newcomer, & C. Estes (Eds.). *Long term care for the elderly: Public policy issue* (pp. 233–250). Thousand Oaks, CA: Sage.

Phillips, C., Munoz, Y., Sherman, M., Rose, M., Spector, W., & Hawes, C. 2003. Effects of facility characteristics on departures from assisted living: Results from a national study. *Gerontologist 43* (5), 690–696.

Rohr, K. 2003. *U.S. experience with sprinklers*. Patterson, NY: National Fire Protection Association. www.nfpa.org/catalog/services/customer/downloadmember onlypdf.asp?pdfname=OS.sprinkler01.pdf&src=nfpa.

Schuetz, J. 2003. *Affordable assisted living: Surveying the possibilities.* Cambridge, MA: Joint Center for Housing Studies of Harvard University and Volunteers of America.

Spillman, B., & Black, K. 2005. *The size of the long term care population in residential care: A review of estimates and methodology.* Washington, DC: U.S. Department of Health and Human Services.

Sterns, S., & Morgan, L. 2001. Economics and financing. In S. Zimmerman, P. D. Sloane, & J. K. Eckert (Eds.). *Assisted living: Needs, practices and policies in residential care for the elderly* (pp. 271–291). Baltimore: Johns Hopkins University Press.

Stone, R., & Newcomer, R. 1985. The state role in board and care housing. In C. Harrington, R. Newcomer, & C. L. Estes & Associates (Eds.). *Long term care for the elderly: Public policy issues* (pp.177–195). Beverly Hills, CA: Sage.

Swan, J., & Newcomer, R. 2000. Residential care supply, nursing home licensing and case mix in four states. *Health Care Financing Review 21* (3), 203–230.

U.S. Bureau of the Census. 2005. *Interim state population projections.* www.census.gov/population/www/projections/projectionsagesex.html.

U.S. Department of Health and Human Services, Office of the Inspector General. 1982. *Board and care homes: A study of federal and state actions to safeguard the health and safety of board and care home residents.* Washington, DC: U.S. Department of Health and Human Services.

U.S. General Accounting Office. 1989. *Board and care: Insufficient assurances that residents' needs are identified and met.* GAO/HRD-89-50. Washington, DC: U.S. General Accounting Office.

U.S. General Accounting Office. 1999. *Assisted living: Quality of care and consumer protection issues.* GAO/T-HEHS-99-111. Washington, DC: U.S. General Accounting Office.

U.S. General Accounting Office. 2004. *Assisted living: Examples of state efforts to improve consumer protections.* (GAO-04-684). Washington, DC: U.S. General Accounting Office.

Vickery, K. 1998. While stocks dry up, new financing options emerge for assisted living companies. *Provider 24* (11), 31, 33–34.

Zimmerman, S., Sloane, P. D., Eckert, J. K., Gruber-Baldini, A. L., Morgan, L. A., Hebel, J. R., Magaziner, J., Stearns, S. C., & Chen, C. K. 2005. How good is assisted living? Findings and implications from an outcomes study. *Journals of Gerontology B Psychological Sciences and Social Science 60* (4), S195–120.

CHAPTER 14

Tomorrow's Assisted Living

Inseparable from the Looming Financial Crisis in Long-term Care

KEREN BROWN WILSON, PH.D.

When it first emerged, assisted living was a beacon, a model for long-term care that would be more desirable to consumers, cost less, and offer greater quality of life than traditional nursing homes. Assisted living, however, has turned out to be susceptible to many of the challenges faced by other forms of long-term care. In addition, assisted living faces two unique issues of its own: (1) its failure to be clearly defined and (2) the absence of public funding that can make this option affordable to lower-income older adults. Together, these two issues intersect in ways that create a looming crisis in long-term care, putting quality of care and quality of life at risk for America's older adults. This crisis, with its attendant opportunities and challenges, may be a dark cloud or a silver lining for the entire system of long-term care in the United States.

This chapter posits four possible scenarios through which the looming crisis in financing assisted living might be resolved. Some of these scenarios would reinforce the worst aspects of long-term care as we know it today, whereas others could help solve the problems it is facing.

The Emergence of Assisted Living

In the late 1970s and early 1980s, consumers began rebelling against traditional forms of long-term care as media exposés and research reports documented squalid living conditions and poor quality of care for many nursing home residents. Congressional hearings ultimately led to reform and stricter regulation, such as the Nursing Home Reform Act of 1987. Consumer discontent was also fueled in part by advocacy organizations actively promoting consumer choice and consumer-directed care as central to quality long-term care (see chapter 9). But perhaps the most significant impetus for change was the maturation of a cohort, the baby boomers, who suddenly were key decision makers in the lives of parents who needed care. Taken together with the improved economic condition of many older adults, the stage was set for revolution (Wilson, 2005) (see chapter 1).

One of the most notable features of assisted living is the impact it has had on consumer expectations for long-term care (Barton, 2003). In many ways, it has transformed the look and the feel of long-term care options with their accessible, attractive, and well-designed private living areas where residents have greater autonomy (Wilson, 2003; Assisted Living Work Group 2003; Kane & Wilson 2001; Kane & Kane 2001). Indeed, much of the current debate is whether settings that do not have these features are and should be called "assisted living" (see chapter 15).

Assisted living residences also distinguished themselves because, for the most part, they were designed to appeal not so much to its current users as to their adult children. The Great Depression and World War II were the defining periods in the lives of the majority of the older residents now in assisted living. When they were growing up, delaying personal gratification was the norm. They came to adulthood when going to college was a distant dream for the majority and home ownership came only because of GI loans.

Their children are quite different. Today, most of the "baby boom" generation is in midlife. They are typically an active older adult group. Most are still working, although some are already leading busy lives in "retirement." The first generation to benefit from union wages, fully funded pension plans, and great advances in the management of chronic diseases, their expectations are markedly higher than those of their parents. And as the chief negotiators for their parents when assistance is needed, baby boomers often substitute their own expectations for those of their parents when it comes to long-term care. They ask about such concrete things as healthier meals, meaningful individual activities, and more proactive management of individual health status (see chapter 6).

Consumers and families vote with their feet and their pocketbooks. Although the percentage of those who need long-term care has remained fairly constant, where they live and what assistance they receive radically changed between 1990 and 2000. The profile of nursing home use shows declining length of stay as residents enter nursing homes closer to the end of their lives or for short stays to receive skilled specialized care (Decker, 2006; Commission on Health Care Facilities in the 21st Century, 2006).

So where are the older adults who would once have been nursing home residents? Many are in assisted living settings. This is true despite the fact that early Cinderella stories about assisted living have sometimes given way to episodes of bad publicity. In recent years, reports have chronicled consumer complaints of deception, poor care, and inadequate oversight not unlike those heard earlier about nursing homes (for examples, see *Consumer Reports* 2004; Ziemba 2004; Finkelstein 2001; Trapps 2001; and Branigin 2000). Consumers continue to seek out assisted living because they hope it will still be better than a nursing home. They go, albeit reluctantly, hoping for more a more familiar lifestyle. They go seeking continuity, purpose, and relevance. They also go betting they will die without moving again. Even though it is often less like "home" than they want, and a third or more will have to move again, assisted living at its best offers the possibility of something approaching a normal life (see chapter 4).

The Growing Challenge of Private Payment

Two serious issues are very likely to affect aging baby boomers and their parents, both immediately and in the longer term: the shortfalls in some retirees' pension plans, retirement accounts, and the shrinking safety net of services (Institute of Medicine, 2000; Norton & Lipson, 1998; Weiner, Sullivan, & Skaggs, 1997).

The pending collapse of many pension plans is a cause of special concern. In 2005 the Pension Benefit Guaranty Corporation, the federal government's pension insurance agency and watchdog, reported that more than 1,100 plans currently show a shortfall of $50 million or more, each for a total of as much as $450 billion (Diamond & Orszag, 2005; Dus, Maurer, & Mitchell, 2005). Taken on top of the financial "haircut" that many Americans got in the market downturn of 2001–2002, their unparalleled use of home equity credit lines to pay for such large ticket items as college tuition, and the slump in the housing market, retirement nest eggs are shrinking. At this point, a credible case can be made for rising poverty rates among individuals born between 1945 and 1960 because they have little time to adjust to a changing retirement environment. Dealing with the cost of shelter, let alone any care they may need, is a significant challenge, particularly for older adults who do not have equity in a home that can be used to generate assets to help finance a move to another living arrangement (whether assisted living or something else).

At the same time that older adults come to need greater assistance in activities of daily living (ADLs) or other care, they also come to need greater assistance in managing other aspects of their lives and gradually cede control to others. Assistance with money is one of the first indicators of shifting power between the elder and another person, frequently an adult child. Often this assistance begins in the form of a joint bank account. It usually ends with the child or other third party actually managing the elder's money and, when necessary, finding ways to pay for whatever services are needed, regardless of where the elder is living. In many cases, funds are obtained by liquidating assets, such as a home, supplemented by cash support from children if necessary. How much money is coming from which source is often difficult to determine, given that this is often a time when assets are being transferred as a part of estate planning, no matter the size of the estate. Studies conducted by the senior housing industry provide some insight into the extent to which families are already financially involved (Pew Research Center, 2005; ProMatura, 1998). Their findings indicate that the majority of those living in assisted living and paying privately are relying either on asset use or on others, such as children to help to pay their monthly fees.

Diminishing Government Support

Even as financial responsibility for long-term care is increasingly being pushed onto adult children and other relatives because of the harsh realities of retirement planning, we are witnessing a deterioration in the availability of what can be called "early intervention" or "safety net" services (see chapter 7). Many services for older persons, previously funded from state or federal sources, have vanished in the past decade. At one time, programs such as home repair to build wheelchair ramps, chore services for housekeeping, laundry, and meal preparation, and escorted transportation were available to anyone at no cost or on a sliding scale. Indeed, there used to be "outreach" workers whose job it was to find older persons and enroll them in services. Today, what were once dedicated "senior centers" are becoming "multipurpose centers" where access to a variety of services is coordinated not just for seniors but also for younger populations. And there has been a significant shift to a narrow focus on services for those frail and vulnerable older adults who are at imminent risk for institutional placement: day health programs, in-home health, and door-to-door health-related transportation. Similarly, case management services, both private and public, are increasingly being used to keep seniors in independent settings.

Funding for community services, at least in part, reflects the response of politicians to their constituency groups. After the terrorist attacks in 2001, significant resources in the United States have been redirected toward security related activities and a series of natural disasters have pulled more resources away from regularly provided community services. Moreover, this has been coupled with a period of dissatisfaction with various government-supported interventions believed by some to be less "efficient" because of the inflated program enrollment and higher costs that result from lax enforcement of client eligibility and poor oversight of provider billing. While the experts and advocates are hailing innovative programs like the "cash and counseling" for their effectiveness, it does not seem likely that state governments will support such wholesale empowerment of frail, lower income seniors any time soon. This effort was funded for three years starting in October 2004 by a joint effort of the Robert Wood Johnson Foundation and the Office of the Assistant Secretary of Planning and Evaluation, Department of Health and Human Services, to develop programs in approximately 14 states. Cash and Counseling is a program that gives a monthly cash allowance directly to Medicaid clients eligible to receive personal care and community-based services. Clients use these funds to arrange and pay themselves for their own services.

Assisted living is potentially a neater "package" of services that could be more easily overseen while still allowing states to claim that they are funding noninstitutional alternatives. To meet this governmental preference for ease of oversight, however, assisted living would likely need to conform to a standardized definition, even as it now operates and is regulated very differently in the 50 states. Not surprisingly, mindful of the fate of nursing homes, assisted living providers have resisted the kind of uniform definition that would make it more compatible with government structures (see chapter 15).

Defining "Assisted Living": Implications for Public Policy

If public policy is to address the growing challenge of paying for the support older adults need, one of the key tasks facing leaders is to settle just what qualifies as "assisted living." Without an agreed-on definition that is consistently employed at both the state and federal level, it will not be politically feasible to ensure that those who need such care have access to it. The problem of defining assisted living has at least two aspects: (1) the extent to which the housing component of assisted living is central to its definition and services and (2) the question of what services and environmental features minimally define assisted living as a "covered service," distinct from other non-nursing-home long-term care services.

Housing with Services, or Housing and Services?

The answer to this question matters enormously. If assisted living is defined as housing *with* services, the implication is that housing is a distinct component, the cost of which should be calculated separately. If it is defined as housing *and* services, the implication is that like services, housing is integral to assisted living and that both housing and services should factor jointly into the calculation of cost.

Senior housing, as opposed to health care, has traditionally been funded through federal government housing programs or by individuals themselves with whatever income or assets they possess, whereas community-based services have been funded though Medicare, Medicaid, or state and local funds using provider service contracts. Assisted living advocates have been hesitant to demand consolidation of these costs under Medicaid, as there is a concern that, if assisted living is funded like nursing homes, it will be regulated in the same way (see chapter 11).

When long-term care—primarily nursing homes—was conceived and implemented on a disease-based or illness model no one was thinking much about the cost of the shelter component for those who had extended stays. Payment covered bed, board, and whatever care was required, regardless of amount or type. With the advent of Medicaid, the funding structure changed. Although bed and board are covered at fixed rates, Medicaid's reimbursement structure permits variable payments for the care component depending on case mix and diagnostic related groups (DRGs), and offers reimbursements keyed to the required level of skilled nursing or rehabilitative services. This strategy worked relatively well as long as choices were limited and access was tightly controlled, as was the case before the explosion of interest in community-based care during the past 20 years.

As early as 1975, however, states began to be alarmed about rising costs of long-term care and their impact on state budgets (Kane & Ladd, 1997). In 1981 this led to a series of initiatives to provide home-and community-based care funded by Medicaid (under sections 2176 and 1915[c] of Public Law 97-35). Because some early arguments for public funding of community-based care rested on cost savings, many of these initiatives pegged reimbursements for programs such as assisted living to a percentage, typically 50–80 percent, of reimbursement rates for nursing home care.

Meanwhile, policy for shelter has been tied to supplement security income (SSI) benefits, which are used to pay for bed and board. While the care needs of residents have been changing, the range of boarding services has remained constant, including food, laundry, and housekeeping. Linking payment for shelter to SSI benefits made it easier to administer Medicaid as a joint program for subsidizing health-related services in which states must match federal dollars, but rental fees have risen well above what current SSI benefits can cover. As a result, many states opt to provide a state supplement to SSI, but this amount is still generally insufficient to pay for needed basic bed and board services. Thus, the stage has been set for those who cannot afford to pay out of pocket for their care to experience a significant financial disconnect when they seek both shelter and care.

Setting Criteria for Environment and Services

The task of defining assisted living does not end with answering the question of whether shelter and care components should or should not be costed out separately for policy purposes. The second definitional aspect has to do with which services and environmental features are necessary to make assisted living a reimbursable service. Unlike nursing home care, which is defined by the federal government, what is considered assisted living is usually defined by states, and it is clear from examining state statutes and regulations that there is no single, shared definition (Hyde & Mollica, 2002; Mollica, 2005a). In some states—Oregon, for example—regulations restrict the label "assisted living" to those facilities that meet specific criteria for the design of the physical environment and the range of offered services, and mandate choice, dignity, and privacy as principles to which assisted living must adhere. Other states, such as Maryland, lump together all settings providing any personal care that are not nursing homes under the heading of assisted living. Many states fall somewhere between these two approaches.

Although some progress has been made in addressing this problem, two major efforts to establish workable, universal criteria have failed in the past decade. The Assisted Living Quality Coalition (ALQC), a group of leading private organizations involved with services for the aging, attempted to achieve consensus in 1998 (ALQC, 1998). More recently the Assisted Living Work Group (ALWG, 2003), convened in 2001 by the U.S. Senate Special Committee on Aging, struggled to craft a common definition. The fissures fell along predictable lines. Some viewed attempts to include "philosophical" statements—such as promoting residents' independence, autonomy, and dignity (ALQC, 1998)—as unnecessary and impossible to regulate. Others argued that prescribing a range of available services or defining service capacity inhibited innovation. Most involved in these attempts agreed that the type of prescriptive regulations used to define nursing homes had not worked very well but recognized that the lack of a common definition posed problems for consumers, providers, and regulators. A viable solution remains a distant prospect for multiple reasons.

First, the cost of oversight is a significant challenge to establishing a universal definition of what service and housing combination(s) should count as assisted living. If there are rules, there must be a system of oversight. Effective oversight is a cost few states have been willing to fund adequately in past years to monitor other combinations of housing and services.

Second, the fear is real among providers that such oversight will be subsidized by private pay residents and result in operating restrictions of the same type that drove private pay clients to assisted living in the first place. For providers, the prospect of being more heavily regulated without a guaranteed source of reimbursement for residents who cannot pay at market rates themselves is not particularly appealing.

The perspective of providers is that the documentation burden, potential restrictions on the freedom to respond to market demands, the possibility of increasing liability, and the cost of regulatory mandates are too high a price to pay given the proposed benefits to them. Thus, it is likely only significant sustained public outrage or sufficient dollars to which strings can be attached would result in additional movement to define assisted living more explicitly unless there are also fundamental changes in how we think about how we provide long-term care.

Private Space as an Index Feature

Much of the debate around setting specific criteria for assisted living has coalesced around the need to insure private living arrangements—that is, bedrooms and bathrooms that are not shared. The perceived importance of privacy when creating a homelike residential setting is reflected, in part, by new construction codes and market conditions that mandate private space. Arguments once advanced that shared space offers a psychological benefit and is attractive to consumers are now often challenged; at the same time, efforts to achieve consensus about the defining features of assisted living have foundered on the question of privacy.

From a policy perspective, one can argue that, although privacy might be highly prized, it is not essential for adequate and safe shelter. Furthermore, its critics are not convinced that the added value it generates relative to its increased provision cost is either an individual—or more important in view of competing demands for government dollars—a public benefit, even though studies of consumers regularly highlight its importance. For their part, providers argue that the amount of reimbursement for shelter available through SSI is far from adequate, so it is possible to provide private space only in settings that are debt free, have additional sources of support, or where inventive definitions of care translate into higher reimbursement rates.

Of course, such arguments do not take account the hidden costs of *not* providing private space. Much anecdotal evidence abounds regarding the management challenges and lost income faced by providers when they cannot match the gender or personalities of shared occupants; to the additional expenses they incur when dealing with the housekeeping costs generated by roommates with different lifestyles; to pay for more staff interventions to address the unfavorable behavioral consequences of two strangers forced to live intimately with one another; and the increased risk that shared accommodations help spread infectious diseases.

Nonetheless, without a universal definition, at the end of the day what assisted living means depends on where you live and on who pays the bill. Defining assisted living as broadly as we do creates a big box—but because assisted living mostly accommodates private pay residents, those who can pay out of pocket arguably have more choices for places that provide both housing and services.

Public Policy: A Subsidy for Assisted Living

For individuals who cannot afford to pay privately—and this will characterize a sizable share of tomorrow's seniors given the shrinking private retirement resources described above—the picture is different. The more broadly assisted living is defined, the more hard fought will be the assisted living funding policy battles on the ground as states face budget shortfalls for essential services like schools, infrastructure repair, and other public needs.

Recent experience in Oregon is illustrative. Known since the early 1980s as a hotbed of innovation in the area of services for older and disabled adults, Oregon's much-vaunted integrated approach to service delivery is at serious risk. For years, Oregon has been recognized for its statewide case management system that uses a single assessment to determine and establish priority for services. Elders, including Medicaid clients, were able to select from a wide array of service options in a variety of settings with multiple price points even when their service needs were similar. Now suffering from leadership exhaustion, a series of "little cuts" threaten the state's ability to maintain seamless access to a wide variety of long-term care services. Oregon has addressed budget woes in the past; indeed a serious financial depression in the late 1970s actually provided impetus for the development of the current community-based system of care. The last several budget cycles, however, have been particularly fraught with angst as the state struggled to determine how to cut more in order to balance the budget.

As a result, reimbursement rates did not keep pace with the inflated costs of providing services. In response, some providers reduced their

Medicaid participation. This limited client choices and increased the use of lower cost residential care alternatives. When this cost savings mechanism proved inadequate, the state government developed various scenarios to reduce caseload by tightening eligibility criteria. Existing clients received letters warning of potential loss of benefits, which generated a massive increase in workload for state case managers assigned to reevaluate eligibility on the new, more stringent criteria. In the end, few clients were declared ineligible for services, and, despite the drama, few elderly were actually cut from service. The level of reimbursement, however, was cut for individual Medicaid clients residing in assisted living and providers had to cushion the consequences. (A much more serious impact was seen in other services, particularly to an already weakened Oregon Health Plan.) When the reclassification of elderly clients to lower levels of service and frozen payment rates failed to contain costs sufficiently, other measures were hotly debated. A number of rather Byzantine strategies were floated, including one that taxed nursing home providers in an effort to stave off deeper cuts in community-based care programs such as assisted living.

Most other states are feeling the financial pinch as well. Growing numbers of seniors are in need of shelter, require assistance to perform their instrumental activities of daily living (IADLs), and manage their chronic health problems. Some in particular have more complicated health issues, which provokes uncertainty, and sometimes fierce battles, about who should be financially responsible. Is the older adult who has bipolar disorder and diabetes unable to live independently because of the mental illness or because of the diabetes? The answer matters enormously to those responsible for allocating budgets, but the answer varies widely from state to state. Similarly, who is eligible for nursing home care and Medicaid services in any given residential or group setting is largely a function of each state's willingness and ability to match federal Medicaid dollars. Assisted living policy becomes easily entangled in these questions.

Fixing the System: Four Scenarios for Public Policy

The looming financial crisis in long-term care may be bringing the United States closer than many can imagine possible to radical change. If this is indeed the case, current circumstances suggest four possible scenarios for configuring how we provide the services needed by older adults.

Scenario 1: And the Band Played On

In the first scenario, the United States would continue to use the current fee-for-service system with the government setting reimbursement rates for the care that providers offer. Individuals would continue to enroll in various programs according to established eligibility criteria. The current mix of funding mechanisms would continue, with some programs under federal and some under state jurisdiction, and some, like Medicaid, jointly administered. Eligibility, benefits, and co-pay amounts would continue to vary, with some means tested, some not. Individuals who did not meet eligibility criteria for publicly subsidized services would continue to purchase care privately. Those with the resources to do so would continue to be urged to purchase supplemental or gap insurance as a way to avoid impoverishment in the face of catastrophic and long-term care costs.

Those who could not afford to purchase supplemental insurance or pay market rate for services would continue to receive charity care (public or private). Or their care would be "invisibly" subsidized through cost-shifting (to private payers), despite the fact that the subsidies built into the rates paid by others is likely to increase the cost of urgent care or lead to greater subsequent costs when individuals delay or forgo needed treatment they cannot pay for. Perversely, the net effect would still be lower aggregate costs, since providing no care at all costs less than any other intervention. (Some have argued that this is effectively the current modus operandi of the Medicaid long-term care system: make it hard to apply, make it undesirable to receive care this way, and only those who are very poor and most desperate will use the system.) The major difference going forward would be widespread public acceptance and support of an overt multitiered system of health-related services—dependent on who can pay out of pocket or who has private insurance coverage—as the status quo.

Scenario 2: Patch the Gap

A different response to the growing concerns about the number of people who do not have access to either private or public services could parallel the approach of the age-entitled Medicare Part D program, which requires seniors to select and enroll in a plan to receive prescription drug benefits. Although the program has received mixed reviews regarding its operation and benefits, something similar might be developed to bridge the gap—better, chasm—between the financial eligibility criteria and market rates for long-term care. In this scenario, carefully defined, less stringent eligibility criteria would create a new category of public beneficiary, although the program would continue to be a fee-for-service arrangement for individual enrollees.

The cost of a given service (minus a co-pay) would be covered as long as it was used and individuals maintained their qualifying status. Alternatively, the eligibility requirements could remain income and asset based, as Medicaid now is, but allow limits to be adjusted by means of a formula that allowed greater variation based on some form of means testing. Receipt of the benefit would be predicated on submission of pre-authorized expenses or services, much like the current practice of some insurance plans or utilization management so common in "managed care" programs. Once the deductible, based on documented income and expenses, had been met, individuals would receive the covered service. Florida, in some respects, is currently pursuing a course not unlike this.

This plan would require more integration among all potential funding sources, and significantly more centralized assessment and record keeping than currently exists. Although this would potentially enable the growing numbers of lower income seniors to access assisted living, it might bring with it a level of government oversight that would fundamentally change the relationship between resident and provider, and dampen efforts to expand consumer satisfaction demands for quality. Further, it might result in few direct care dollars with higher administrative costs per client that could be particularly hurtful in balanced budget environments.

Scenario 3: Defined Lifetime Benefit for Adults

Under this scenario, once individuals reached a particular age, they would have access to a personal health account established over their lifetime. Such accounts would be established to receive regular, restricted "cash" deposits or credits to be used as vouchers for individual-designated health-related services. Allowable amounts would be calculated based on annualized projections of care costs, adjusted for location, health conditions, and risk factors, with a lifetime cap. Some portion of the contribution might be mandatory, like current Medicare contributions. Individuals could supplement their personal health account with tax-free personal contributions in the form of payroll deductions, insurance supplements, or cash donations from third parties. Cap adjustments would be permitted for certain events, such as permanent disability or catastrophic illness. While coverage would be universal, individual beneficiaries would determine how to use the benefit. This plan is similar in many ways to the "Cash and Counseling" experiment (Doty, 2004), touted as a great success, except it would be expanded to include a lifetime cap.

Although beneficiaries would be permitted to determine how to spend the benefit, certain choices would result in the reduction or elimination of other benefits, much the way Medicare's hospice benefit currently works. Fees would largely be driven by the market, with no constraint on supply. Incentives to reduce use of health services could be built in—for example, cash rebates for "healthy" lifestyle choices, such as participation in exercise or weight-control programs. Older adults might be permitted to include unused personal contributions in their estates. A healthy spouse might be permitted to "lend" excess credits to a sick partner. For each use, a statement would be generated indicating the amount of remaining benefits, helping to increase individual awareness of the cumulative cost of health services. This scenario could support the assisted living philosophy by giving seniors choices about the extent to which they access needed services.

Scenario 4: A Socially Defined Minimum Benefits Package

This final scenario envisions a form of universal health care. From birth, every individual would have coverage for all services in a socially defined minimum benefit package. Anything outside of this plan would be the financial responsibility of the individual. The benefits included in the package would be defined through a process of collective prioritization like that employed by the acclaimed, but ill fated, Oregon Health Plan. Initially hailed as a great success not only in health planning but in participatory democracy and fair resource allocation as well, the Oregon plan solicited public input to prioritize treatment-condition pairs for the purposes of defining the state's Medicaid benefits package for those not covered by existing programs, particularly "poor working adults." It should be noted that this was for acute care benefits and so would require considerable thought if it were to include long-term care benefits. Each year, the cut-off point for services is adjusted based on negotiated vendor rates for a defined benefit and the dollars allocated by the legislature.

The plan has fallen on hard times as prolonged budget woes beginning in 2000 have reduced the scope of covered services and led to more restrictive eligibility criteria. With reimbursement caps set at rates that discourage provider participation, the program is but a shell of what it once was. The obvious lesson is that however great the collective buy-in, nothing can work without the money to pay for it.

A plan that permitted individuals to buy additional health services out of pocket would not provoke the same negative response as a single payer system or the same visions of bureaucratic foul-ups, but it would put limitations on both clients and providers of care insofar as available services would be adjusted based on the ability or willingness of the public to pay for them. The lower on the list a requested service, the longer the wait for assistance, and in lean times assistance may never come. Thus, seniors with need for IADL support may not be eligible for the supports, such as healthy meals and socialization, that are available in assisted living and that can prevent further decline.

Alas, this outcome feels uncomfortably close to the dreaded "socialized medicine." It is also a reminder that authorizing something and actually getting it are not even close to the same thing. Looming crisis aside, Americans are reluctant to endorse any plan that does not enhance their individual access and personal benefits, much less an approach that might reduce them for selected individuals for the benefit of all. Without careful thought, assisted living might suffer under this option unless it was treated in policy much like nursing homes are today. The investment required for purpose built shelter with limited conversion capacity requires significant thought about how to adequately motivate providers and investors to respond to a demand where adequate return on investment carries a higher than ordinary risk.

Conclusions and Implications for the Future

It is difficult to know whether any of these approaches would meet the demands of the diverse constituencies who have a stake in whatever health services are made available or what mechanism is used to pay for them. Sad as it may be, it is not the individual's best interest that matters most in solutions at the policy level. This is true, of course, whenever the needs of one are weighed against the needs of many, but it is particularly the case in representative democracies in which decisions are not made by consensus but by majority rule involving a certain amount of "horse-trading" for votes or agreement.

The inability to respond effectively to concerns about the health care system is reflected in the continuing increase in the numbers of Americans who do not believe the system is working. In fact, it could be argued the increasingly fevered discussion about health care signals an impending collision of sizable force. This collision is made more likely by increasingly polarized views of government, particularly about its rightful role and its responsibility to those who live under it. This crisis has been brought on, in part, by an unwillingness to confront reality and manage expectations in light of those realities.

As gerontologist Robert Applebaum once noted in another context, Americans "want autonomy for themselves and safety for those they love," and they tend to want both without regard for cost. Reluctance to accept limits—such as means testing, managed care, co-pays, preauthorization, capped benefits, and noncovered services—suggests that it will not be easy to cut the pie into smaller slices so that all might have a piece. The road ahead promises to be bumpy for those who seek "a little help."

REFERENCES

Assisted Living Quality Coalition. 1998. *Assisted living quality initiative: Building a structure that promotes quality.* Washington, DC: Public Policy Institute, American Association of Retired Persons.

Assisted Living Quality Coalition. No date. Report from the outcome measurement summit, July 1999. Unpublished manuscript.

Assisted Living Workgroup. 2003. *Assuring quality in assisted living: Guidelines for federal and state policy, state regulation, and operations.* Washington, DC: American Association of Homes and Services for the Aging.

Ball, M. M., Whittington, F. J., Perkins, M. M., Patterson, V. L., King, S. V., Combs, B. L. 2000. Quality of life in assisted living facilities: Viewpoints of residents. *Journal of Applied Gerontology 19* (3), 304–325.

Branigin, W. 2000. Va. nursing home dispute highlights industry issues. *Washington Post,* April 10, B2.

Chisholm, J. F. 1999. The sandwich generation. *Journal of Social Distress and the Homeless 8* (3), 177–191

Commission on Health Care Facilities in the Twenty-first Century. 2006. *Report of the Commission on Health Care Facilities in the Twenty-first Century.* http://www.nyhealthcarecommission.org/index.htm

Consumer Reports. 2004. Many of the nation's nursing homes continue to have problems and offer questionable care. *Consumer Reports,* September 21.

Decker, F. 2006. Nursing staffs and the outcomes of nursing home stays. *Medical Care 44* (9), 812.

Diamond, P., & Orszag, D. 2005. Saving Social Security. *Journal of Economic Perspectives 19* (2), 11–32.

Doty, P. 2004. *Consumer-directed home care: Effects on family caregivers: Policy brief.* San Francisco: Family Caregiver Alliance.

Finkelstein, K. 2001. Man to pay $48 million in Medicaid fraud scheme. *New York Times,* April 7.

Hanoch, Y., & Rice, T. 2006. Can limiting choice increase social welfare? The elderly and health insurance. *Milbank Quarterly 84* (1), 37–73.

Harris Interactive. 2002. *Harris Interactive health care news 2* (17). www.harris interactive.com/news/newsletters/healthnews/HI_HealthCareNews2002Vol2_Iss17.pdf.

Harris Interactive. 2004. Americans rate Canadian health care system better than U.S. system, according to Harris interactive survey. Harris Poll Online. www.harrisinteractive.com/news/allnewsbydate.asp?NewsID=837.

Hyde, J., & Mollica, R. 2002. The Medicaid program and assisted living properties: How the rules stymie government and industry needs. *Seniors Housing and Care Journal 10* (1) 45–54.

Institute of Medicine. 2000. *America's health care safety net: Intact but endangered.* Washington, DC: Institute of Medicine.

Kane, R., & Wilson, K. B. 2001. *Assisted living at the crossroads: Principles for its future.* Portland, OR: Jessie F. Richardson Foundation.

Kane, R. L., & Kane, R. A. 2001. What older people want from long-term care, and how they can get it. *Health Affairs 20* (6), 114–127.

Kane, R. L., Kane, R. A., & Ladd, R. L. 1998. *The heart of long-term care.* New York: Oxford University Press.

Kemper, D. W., Lorig, K., & Mettler, M. 1993. The effectiveness of medical self-care interventions: A focus on self-initiated responses to symptoms. *Patient Education Counseling 21,* 29–39.

Mahoney, K. J., Simon-Rusinowitz, L., Loughlin, D. M., Desmond, S. M., & Squillace, M. R. 2004. Determining personal care consumers' preferences for a consumer-directed cash and counseling option: survey results from Arkansas, Florida, New Jersey, and New York elders and adults with physical disabilities. *Health Services Research 39,* 643–664.

Mollica, R. 2005a. *Aging in place in assisted living: State regulations and practice.* Prepared for American Senior Housing Association. Portland, ME: National Academy for State Health Policy.

Mollica, R. 2005b. *Informing Consumers about Assisted Living: State Practices.*

Prepared for American Senior Housing Association. Portland, ME: National Academy for State Health Policy.

Mollica, R. L. 2002. *State assisted living policy, 2002.* Portland, ME: National Academy for State Health Policy.

Mollica, R. L., & Johnson-Lamarche, H. 2005. *State residential care and assisted living policy, 2004.* Portland, ME: National Academy for State Health Policy.

Norton, S., & Lipson, D. 1998. *Public policy, market forces, and the viability of safety net providers.* Washington, DC: Urban Institute.

Nursing home abuse seldom reported: Study also finds that safeguards are insufficient. 2002. *USA Today,* March 4.

Pension Benefit Guaranty Corporation. 2005. *Companies report a record $353.7 billion pension shortfall in latest filings with PBGC.* Washington, DC: Department of Public Affairs, Pension Benefit Guaranty Corporation. www.pbgc.gov/media/news-archive/2005/pr05-48.html.

Pew Research Center. 2005. *Baby boomers approach 60: From the age of Aquarius to the age of responsibility.* Washington, DC: Pew Research Center.

Pro Matura. 1998. *National survey of adults 60+.* Annapolis, MD: National Investment Center.

Seidman BDO, LLP. 2005. *A report on shortfalls in Medicaid funding for nursing home care.* Washington, DC: American Health Care Association. www.ahca.org/brief/bdo_seidman_study.pdf.

Smith, D. B. 2001. *Long-term care in transition: The regulation of nursing homes.* Frederick, MD: Beard Books.

Spector, W. D., Fleishman, J. A., Pezzin, L. E., & Spillman, B. C. 1998. The characteristics of long-term care users. Paper prepared for the Institute of Medicine Committee on Improving the Quality of Long-Term Care, Washington DC.

Trapps, T. E. 2001. Nursing home abuse rising across nation. *Wall Street Journal,* July 31, A8.

Weiner, J., Sullivan, C., & Skaggs, J. 1996. *Spending down to Medicaid: New data on the role of Medicaid in paying for nursing home care.* Washington, DC: American Association of Retired Persons.

Wilson, K. B. 2003. *Assisted living: Evolving model for a new generation of elderly. Testimony given June 11, 2003, before the Federal Trade Commission.* Washington, DC: Government Printing Office.

Ziemba, S. 2004. Nursing home fined $10,000: Security is cited after man wanders off, dies of cold. *Chicago Tribune,* June 3, 4.

CHAPTER 15

Assisted Living

What It Should Be and Why

LARRY POLIVKA, PH.D.
JENNIFER R. SALMON, PH.D.

Before 1990, one of the biggest gaps in our long-term care system across the country was the absence of a congregate care program that would allow frail elderly people to "age in place" and offer them the same freedom (personal control, privacy) and level of service that many had been able to receive in their own homes since the 1970s. As counterintuitive as it may seem today, the publicly supported in-home long-term care program initiated in the 1970s and 1980s served persons with more functional impairment and greater care needs than were permitted to be admitted to or remain in congregate settings. Today this kind of community residential care has been substantially achieved through the growth of the assisted living industry for private-pay residents and is arguably the most positive development in long-term care in recent decades.

Although what constitutes an assisted living residence cannot always be stated simply and concisely, this option for long-term care has been associated with a set of core values and goals focused on residents' quality of life that have guided its development over the past 20 years. These include the philosophical values of respect for resident autonomy and choice, privacy and dignity, and the goal of enabling residents to age in place in the most homelike and least-restrictive environment possible.

A focus on the philosophy of care that informs practice in assisted living residences is now especially important because of its role in distinguishing the appeal of assisted living to older residents and their family members—why they choose assisted living and why they leave.

Although overall, residents in assisted living residences and nursing homes have quite different impairment profiles and health care needs, for many residents assisted living is a substitute for nursing home care. As is discussed in chapter 2, assisted living residents increasingly have serious cognitive and physical impairments. A recent analysis of nationwide Medicare data from 1992 to 1998 for beneficiaries older than 65 found that assisted living may be an alternative to nursing home care for many of those with serious long-term care needs (U.S. Department of Health and Human Services, 2003). The principle difference between the two populations was that assisted living residents have significantly higher incomes than nursing home residents. More recent data from Florida show that among demographically similar individuals with comparable levels of impairment and health status, those entering assisted living residences were 47 percent less likely ultimately to end up in a nursing home (Andel, Hyer, & Slack, 2005).

As a substantial portion of the assisted living population is beginning to resemble the nursing home population, some nursing homes have adopted the core values of assisted living. Examples include the Eden Alternative, with its emphasis on residents' quality of life and mutually supportive relationships (Thomas, 2003), and the Nursing Home Pioneers' model of care, which promotes change in the institutional culture and physical environment of nursing homes (Fagan, 2003).

The fact that assisted living residences can now provide much of the care once available only in nursing homes, however, does not mean that assisted living should be seen as a comprehensive alternative for those who are now admitted to nursing homes—at least, not if the goal is to ensure that assisted living remains true to its core values. Nor do we mean to suggest that nursing homes should not focus on quality of life as well as specialized care—there is no reason that nursing homes cannot become "cozier," less institutionalized, more resident-centered, assisted-living-like places while serving a qualitatively more impaired, higher-need population. Although the number of more seriously impaired residents in assisted living will continue to increase for the foreseeable future, we expect that nursing homes will continue to play a unique role in our system of long-term care by serving a greater number of seriously impaired residents (those who need assistance with four or more activities of daily living [ADLs]). Assisted living has its own role to play in complementing, not in fully substituting for nursing home care.

The fundamental message of this chapter is quite different. Our argument is that the gap between the original vision for assisted living and the extent to which that vision is actually realized is not as wide as skeptics thought it would become, nor as narrow as many consumers and their advocates would like. Many challenges lie ahead that threaten to widen rather than close the gap, evidenced in part in the growing convergence between populations and levels of care across nursing homes and assisted living. Policy makers, providers, and advocates will be especially pressed to ensure that the needs of larger populations of residents with serious chronic conditions and impairments are met, while adhering to the core values of assisted living. We examine these core values, assess the extent to which they now guide the care practices of assisted living residences, and identify the major features needed in a regulatory framework that would support putting the ideals of assisted living into practice.

Core Values

The original vision for assisted living was largely a product of a philosophical commitment to the widely recognized values of respect for autonomy, choice, privacy, and dignity, and to the deep preference of most impaired persons to "age in place" in the least-restrictive environment possible. These core values emerged as guiding policy principles in the independent living movement in the 1970s (Scala & Nerney, 2000), which primarily affected younger adults living with disabilities in their own dwellings. They were later adopted for older adults with disabilities in assisted living residences or through consumer-directed in-home programs of long-term care (Polivka & Salmon, 2003). Underlying these values was the distinction between the "medical model" of care that is typical of nursing home care and a new, more "social model" of care that can be provided in settings that are more homelike and less closely regulated than nursing homes. The medical model focuses on the delivery of appropriate health care services; the social model places at least equal emphasis on such quality-of-life criteria as autonomy and privacy.

Autonomy and Choice

Autonomy, or self-rule, is based on the societal values of freedom and choice and is the cornerstone of democratic institutions (Kapp, 2000). Autonomy encompasses both negative and positive rights. What has been called "negative autonomy" (Collopy, 1998) is the power to keep others from intervening in one's life without one's fully informed, voluntary (non-coerced) consent. Positive autonomy is the power of an individual, however dependent, to communicate freely with others, to give and to receive affection, and to initiate actions that are consistent with the person's sense of self. This positive autonomy is closely related to choice, privacy, and dignity, and is especially important in the development of an ethic for long-term care (Collopy, 1988). Positive autonomy preserves a person's sense of self and extends the boundaries of her own volitional capacities by providing the assistance she needs to live as she chooses to, or to approximate her choices as closely as possible (Polivka & Salmon, 2003).

Historically, however, policy makers have not prioritized autonomy as an achievable goal for frail older adults in long-term care (Polivka & Salmon, 2003). To formulate an ethical standard for the care of people who are dependent, policy makers and caregivers must marry the concept of positive autonomy to the realities of day-to-day life for recipients of long-term care. They must view the world of long-term care from the perspective of frail elders and support the individual's need to define and make a world that is consistent with her own preferences and identity, developed over her lifetime as a unique individual.

Assisted living residences can offer frail elders greater opportunity to exercise meaningful personal control than many would otherwise have. By providing the kinds of resources, especially staff services, transportation, and social activities, that are too great a burden on informal caregivers and beyond the means of many individuals and the public sector to provide as home care, assisted living can make achieving autonomy more feasible.

Given its role in shaping the philosophy of assisted living, the significance of autonomy in determining quality of life in long-term care is just beginning to receive the attention it merits in long-term care research and policy development. Much of the current research is designed to provide insight into of the meaning of autonomy from the perspectives of both residents and staff (Ball et al., 2000; Carder & Hernandez, 2004; Utz, 2003), as well as the role of autonomy in supporting choice and control over one's social and physical environments (Parker et al., 2004; Yee et al., 1999). For example, a study of quality of life in nursing homes, assisted living residences, and long-term home care programs in Florida found that elders who were in assisted living and who had high levels of personal control experienced the highest levels of life satisfaction (Salmon, 2001).

The importance of autonomy and personal control is not limited to those who are cognitively intact. In a study of 427 residents in 15 Alzheimer's special care units, Zeisel and colleagues found that control over their environment reduced residents' aggressive and agitated behavior and psychological problems (Zeisel et al., 2003). Privacy, a homelike atmosphere, varied ambience in common areas, and camouflaged exit doors also contributed to lower incidence of depression, social withdrawal, and hallucinations. The authors conclude that "the design features [of the assisted living residences studied], by providing residents with greater control over their own lives, empower them, and thus reduce their tendency to withdraw and even to be situationally depressed" (p. 709).

Respecting and supporting resident autonomy also entails allowing a resident to take risks in order to maintain acceptable quality of life. For example, a resident with diabetes may choose a less-restrictive diet than has been prescribed for her to increase her dining pleasure and improve her quality of life, even though she risks shortening her life, or a physically impaired resident may choose to preserve her privacy and dignity by showering alone despite her risk of falling. At the same time, however, assisted living providers have a responsibility to safeguard residents' well-being. One method of balancing the competing goals of promoting autonomy and protecting from harm is to negotiate with the resident what risks the residence will permit the individual to take in the interest of quality of life. Such negotiated risk agreements articulate the nature of the risk(s) residents may choose to take, the resident's rationale for running those risks, and the actions both parties will take to reduce the potential for harm. By entering into a risk agreement, the resident accepts responsibility for potential consequences of taking risks and the assisted living provider agrees to abide by the resident's expressed choices. Negotiated risk is likely to become increasingly salient as the number of more seriously impaired residents who want to age in place with as much autonomy as possible grows. As the concept of negotiated risk evolves in assisted living, we can anticipate the emergence of legislation and case law that will help clarify the appropriate boundaries and procedures for negotiated risk agreements.

Privacy and Dignity

Privacy is a necessary but not always sufficient condition for the effective exercise of autonomy, for maintaining interpersonal relationships, and for achieving a sense of self-efficacy and dignity (Polivka & Salmon, 2003). For many people this means maintaining a modicum of control over one's personal space and how one spends one's time. So too is bodily privacy—that is, maintaining modesty and controlling access to one's body to the extent compatible with one's needs for assistance.

Assisted living residents and potential residents place a high priority on privacy as a quality-of-life value (Kane et al., 1998). As a practical matter, this translates into a strong preference for private rooms and bathrooms and, to a lesser extent, private kitchenettes. The significance of privacy and dignity in the context of assisted living is evident from a national survey of residents in the 41 percent of U.S. assisted living buildings that provide high levels of service, private rooms, or both. The vast majority (85 percent) of respondents reported that their top two priorities on entering the assisted living residence were the availability of a private bathroom and of a private bedroom (Hawes & Phillips, 2000a).

Many providers and policy makers believe this level of privacy is not affordable for many assisted living residents, especially those who are publicly supported. Others argue that private rooms are not necessarily more costly than shared space. According to Kane and colleagues, the difference in construction costs between 39 private units versus 39 shared units ranges from $3.20 to $6.30 a day per tenant (Kane, Kane, & Ladd, 1998). But these higher construction costs for private units are offset by their lower operational costs, and shared space is vulnerable to higher operational costs generated by vacancies and roommate matching. The authors state, "If a unit is vacant for a week more because of the difficulty in finding a new occupant, a whole year's savings on the development and construction costs are more than wiped out" (p. 182).

The debate between these two perspectives is illustrated in the struggle over the role of private rooms in defining assisted living (Assisted Living Workgroup, 2003). Those who supported defining assisted living units as private occupancy argued that the requirement is "critical to realizing the goals of assisted living—resident control, autonomy, and dignity" (p. 16). Those who questioned privacy as a standard for assisted living argued that requiring private rooms would preclude allowing residents to choose whether they wished to share a room and would deny providers the flexibility of offering consumers more, rather than fewer options.

Aging in Place in the Least-Restrictive Environment

One of the principal reasons for the creation of home-based programs for seniors in the late 1970s was that older people wanted to have their long-term care needs met in their own homes for as long as possible to preserve their quality of life. Before the development of assisted living, that option was not available to residents of congregate housing. Residents who required a substantial level of assistance with a number of ADLs could not be admitted to or remain in congregate housing. This meant that moderately impaired residents were not allowed to age in place—they had to enter a nursing home or find an unlicensed residence that would accept them (Golant, 1999).

Policy analysts and advocates concluded that the community-residential part of the long-term care system was seriously handicapped by the absence of a program for those who could not remain in their own home and who needed substantial levels of personal or home health care, but did not need the level of 24-hour skilled nursing care provided in nursing homes (Polivka, Sims & Salmon, 1996). Assisted living bridges that gap between home and nursing home, assuring that older persons who need care can receive it in the least-restrictive environment possible.

For any individual, the "least-restrictive environment" is the one that supports autonomy, privacy, and dignity to the greatest extent possible. The rapid growth of assisted living as a long-term care option reflects the fact that many older persons with higher incomes are willing to pay substantial fees ($2,500 to $5,000 monthly) to receive the services they need in such an environment (most private-pay residents in assisted living choose private apartments).

How well does assisted living support the goal of aging in place? A variety of factors can affect whether residents in assisted living can successfully age in place, especially the level of services assisted living is able to provide, which varies geographically. In a relatively mature market, such as Oregon (where regulation and public funding strategies governing long-term care are designed to minimize nursing home admissions in favor of assisted living), assisted living does well in enabling residents to age in place. For example, Frytak and colleagues found that assisted living residences and nursing homes achieved comparable outcomes in terms of trajectories of activities of daily living (ADL), levels of pain and discomfort, and psychological well-being (Frytak et al., 2001), after controlling for the fact that nursing home residents were, on average, substantially more impaired than residents in assisted living. These findings are encouraging in terms of the capacity of assisted living residences to accommodate aging in place by providing necessary health care services.

In a study comparing assisted living and adult foster care (small providers with five or fewer residents, usually operated by individual providers in their own homes) in Washington state, Hedrick and colleagues found that persons at every level of impairment reside in assisted living (Hedrick et al., 2003). Assisted living residences were able to provide the services needed even by individuals who required assistance with all six activities of daily living (ADLs). The study also found very high levels of satisfaction among residents in assisted living, with 92 percent reporting that moving to the setting was a good decision, and that they were very satisfied with every aspect of their care.

Data from Florida indicate that in 1995 about 25 percent of all residents in assisted living required assistance with three or more ADLs or had serious cognitive impairments (Polivka, Dunlop & Brooks, 1997). By 2003, impairment levels were even higher among residents in Florida's Medicaid waiver-funded assisted living program. A higher percentage of these residents had a dementia diagnosis than residents in nursing homes (Mitchell, Salmon, Chen & Hinton, 2003).

When they compared assisted living and nursing homes in New Jersey, North Carolina, Florida, and Maryland, Zimmerman and colleagues found that location (state), type of ownership (for-profit versus not-for-profit) and age of building were significant factors in accounting for whether residents could age in place. They stratified their assisted living sample into small, traditional, and "new model" properties—purpose-built buildings that generally offer more services, amenities, and private apartments than other small or traditional properties and tend to be part of multiple-site corporations. Residents were more likely to be discharged to a higher level of care in Florida, as were residents of for-profit and older residences in all four states.

In a second study, Zimmerman also found that assisted living residences that have more restrictive admission policies, are affiliated with another higher level of care program, or have registered or licensed practical nurses (RNs or LPNs) on staff are more likely to transfer residents to nursing homes. They also found, however, that residents were less often hospitalized when the provider offers more RN care.

In a national survey of high-end assisted living, Hawes and colleagues found that during a 12-month period, of the residents who were discharged (19 percent of the total sample population), 60 percent moved to receive a higher level of care, usually a nursing home. The most common reason for entering a nursing home was a decline in cognitive status or need for the services of a full-time registered nurse that could not be met at the original assisted living residence. When the assisted living building had a registered nurse on staff, residents were not only less likely to be discharged to a nursing home but also less likely to be hospitalized.

Although these data indicate that, overall, assisted living is effectively supporting residents as they age in place, some residents do pose special challenges. Assisted living has great potential to serve residents with dementia or other cognitive impairments and indeed is already serving many people with moderate to serious dementia. There is a danger, however, that as a consequence of serving this cognitively impaired population, states will impose restrictive regulations that will unnecessarily limit the capacity of assisted living to serve this population (Chapin & Dobbs-Kepper, 2001).

Regulating Assisted Living to Support Its Core Values: Excerpts from the ALW Report to the U.S. Senate

Our notion of the "ideal" assisted living model is based on a continuing commitment to a set of core values which we think the available research literature shows is achievable and should be embedded in the regulatory framework for assisted living. The ideal model can be applied across many types of congregate housing with services and supported by regulations explicitly designed to express the values of autonomy, privacy, and the capacity of assisted living to allow residents to age in place in an affordable setting. In thinking about how the regulatory framework can advance the ideal model of assisted living, we draw on some of the recommendations and reflections of the Assisted Living Workgroup (2003).

The workgroup, made up of some 48 organizations involved with aging services, was formed in 2001 in response to congressional concerns about the regulation of assisted living. The perspectives of the participating organizations constitute an informed commentary on current stakeholder views of assisted living policy. The workgroup's recommendations and members' responses to them reflect philosophical differences among trade and professional associations and advocacy organizations about how best to regulate assisted living. Although the workgroup was not of one mind in formulating regulatory guidelines, its work played an important role in framing the debate about how assisted living should be regulated.

Many of the workgroup's recommendations for oversight of assisted living strongly support resident autonomy and choice (Assisted Living Workgroup, 2003). They were framed with the goal of designing a regulatory system for assisted living that would abate harm while supporting the resident's decision-making control and ensuring meaningful resident and family participation. Like the workgroup, we maintain that regulations should specify the practices, protocols, and methods by which services that are provided are respectful of, and responsive to, individual residents' preferences, needs, and values. We also agree with the workgroup's view that assisted living regulation should remain with state regulatory agencies. We need to learn a lot more about the relative efficacy of different regulatory policies and practices before imposing a national scheme that would prematurely end the opportunities to learn more about the costs and outcomes of different policies for different groups of residents. We draw on the insights of the workgroup in suggesting the following guidelines for a regulatory framework that is most consistent with the ideal model of assisted living.

Disclosure

Residents and their families should not be surprised by provider decisions. Every prospective resident and her family should be fully informed about the services the facility offers, how much they cost and how costs change in response to changes in resident need, institutional policies regarding aging in place, physical environments, and other issues identified by the General Accounting Office (1999) as full disclosure problems in assisted living. Adequate disclosure of services available for dementia patients is particularly important and should be addressed explicitly in regulation.

The Assisted Living Workgroup's (2003) recommendations regarding disclosure for specialized programs, such as dementia care, provide an effective framework for developing regulations in this area. The workgroup recommended that assisted living providers disclose the philosophy guiding their dementia care program and describe their placement process, individualized service plans and costs, staff training, and environmental support. This is especially important, given the growing number and proportion of assisted living residents who have cognitive impairments and the fact that program and environmental features can have positive outcomes for these residents (Zeisel et al., 2003).

Regulatory attention should focus on disclosure by requiring that residences clearly indicate what consumers can expect in terms of services and the provider's capacity to meet the needs of seriously impaired or sick residents. Policy makers, however, must be careful to avoid heavy-handed regulatory intrusion into the provider-resident relationship. Providers should be granted the flexibility to address individual resident's changing needs and personal preferences as he or she ages in place.

Admission and Retention Criteria and Staffing Levels

To maximize consumer choice and fulfill the preference of many residents to age in place as long as possible, admission and retention criteria should be inclusive and flexible.

Regulation that imposed highly specific, restrictive criteria for admission and retention would keep many frail elders out of assisted living, forcing them into nursing homes, and diminish the quality of life for those who no longer would be allowed to remain in assisted living. Ball and colleagues note that aging in place is a complex phenomenon and suggest that there may be as many ways of aging in place as there are assisted living residents (Ball et al., 2004). They conclude that resident pathways to aging in place are influenced by a wide range of dynamic and interacting factors that determine "the 'fit' between the capacity of both the facility and the resident to manage resident decline" (p. 205). Mandating uniform admission and retention criteria could also have the unintended consequence of increasing cost, adversely affecting the ability of seniors with lower incomes to afford assisted living.

Negotiated Risk

If clear, noncoercive conditions are met, negotiated risk agreements should be widely permitted in assisted living. These agreements have the potential to become an important vehicle for consumer choice, giving residents greater opportunity to define for themselves the conditions for their aging in place. Special provisions must be made for those who are cognitively impaired.

The Assisted Living Workgroup argued that "shared responsibility agreements" offer a tool for communicating a resident's preferences and a "systematized method of accommodating individual resident choices, or finding acceptable alternatives to those choices" (p. 153). Although it was not unanimously endorsed, the recommendation provides a workable framework for developing equitable agreements between residents and providers that support resident choice without relieving residences of responsibility to safeguard resident safety. The workgroup outlined a detailed process of negotiation to guide state regulation. It recommended that shared responsibility agreements: clearly describe what the resident wants and the cause for concern; identify probable consequences of the resident's choice(s) and possible alternatives; and document the process of negotiation and the final agreement between resident and assisted living provider. Added commentary noted that the process is designed to recognize that some courses of action may not be feasible, but that the resident's choices should be honored, even when the provider thinks they are not in the resident's best interests.

Dementia Care

The assisted living industry, the Alzheimer's Association, and other advocates should collaborate in the development of model guidelines for dementia care for states to use in developing regulatory standards for ensuring an acceptable level of care for residents with dementia.

Together, the Assisted Living Workgroup's recommendations regarding care for residents with cognitive impairment and recent guidelines by the Alzheimer's Association provide an effective framework for serving this population. Good care for persons with dementia or other cognitive impairment builds on the strengths, values, and choices of these individuals. Dementia care programs must be prepared to address the resident's evolving needs as her cognitive condition changes and deteriorates. These preparations should include: staff training about cognitive impairment and procedures for assessing and reassessing the resident's cognitive status, abilities, and needs; direct care staff who are able to understand and respond effectively to residents' behavioral symptoms; specialized activities that are appropriate for residents with cognitive impairment or dementia; procedures for designating and working with a surrogate decision maker if residents are not capable of making decisions for themselves; policies and procedures to protect residents who wander or are at risk of physical harm; regular monitoring to assure resident safety and health care status, consistent with impairment; and policies and procedures for involving and supporting family members.

Physical Plan/Environmental Design

Regulations governing physical plant and environmental design should focus on creating as homelike a living environment as possible, assuring privacy, and enhancing autonomy.

Many current and prospective residents of assisted place a high priority on privacy as a quality-of-life value (Hawes, 2000; Kane, 1998). To the extent that privacy is important for exercising one's autonomy, maintaining dignity, and achieving an acceptable quality of life, whatever the level or type of one's impairment, regulations governing the physical plant and environment of assisted living buildings should support the provision of private space as a value. Oregon and Washington have demonstrated that such regulation is not prohibitively costly—in both states, costs are within industry norms despite requirements for resident privacy. And although privacy provisions were hotly debated, a majority of participant organizations in the Assisted Living Workgroup supported a recommendation that single occupancy rooms be included as a defining criterion of assisted living.

Staffing Levels and Training

Staffing should be sufficient to meet the needs of each resident. Staffing levels should be based on assessed resident needs and regulated accordingly. Training provisions should support cross training to enable staff to perform as "generalists."

To support providers in realizing the core values of assisted living, regulation should grant reasonable discretion with respect to staffing. Regulations that mandated uniform staffing levels would adversely affect cost, making assisted living less affordable. As the Assisted Living Workgroup noted, there is no compelling evidence that permitting assisted living residences to staff at levels commensurate with the needs of their resident populations (as many states, in fact, do) jeopardizes resident safety or systematically threatens quality of care. Staffing at assessed need levels is a more challenging regulatory approach than relying on simple, uniform staffing standards; however, the affordability benefits of this approach outweigh downside risks at this point.

The industry tendency to have employees play multiple roles is generally positive in that it can help dilute the stifling effects of hierarchy and avoid the alienation and detachment of command and control structures and so help to maintain staff morale, creativity, and commitment. The tendency toward "generalist worker" roles can also contribute to a more integrated, familial, homelike environment and help contain staff costs. It does, however, create a greater need for cross training, both pre- and in-service, especially for workers in residences serving more physically and cognitively impaired residents. Staff training should be designed to focus on the values of assisted living in all phases of caregiving and interaction with residents. The industry can expect more regulatory activity in this area and should create guidelines in anticipation of state initiatives.

Quality-of-Life Outcome Measures

Priority should be given to the development and use of resident-oriented outcomes measures based on quality-of-life considerations.

Outcome measures for assisted living should reflect its fundamental values: autonomy, privacy, dignity, and the experience of as full a life as possible, however impaired one may be. This approach to performance accountability would emphasize systematic consumer feedback on indicators such as enjoyment, opportunity for meaningful activity, quality of relationships, spiritual well-being, autonomy, privacy, dignity, security, and physical comfort (Kane et al., 2004). Quality-of-life standards related to enjoyment should also include measures designed to increase the availability of good-tasting food (just as important as nutrition), especially for residents with dementia. Even in the absence of regulatory requirements, assisted living providers should use these measures (as some already are) as essential components of an internal quality-monitoring program.

Nurse Delegation and Medication Management

Allow non-nursing staff, when supervised by nurses, to assist in administering medications.

Nurse delegation refers to training and permitting unlicensed personnel to administer medications with ongoing RN oversight and supervision (Reinhard et al., 2003). One of the principal purposes of nurse delegation in assisted living is to create an effective balance between cost and risk in medication management. Three-fifths of states provide for some form of delegated nurse supervision of unlicensed staff or the use of trained aides to administer oral medications in assisted living, and some also allow these staff to administer injections. Most informants from state boards of nursing report few consumer complaints concerning nurse delegation, although there are no formal mechanisms for reporting errors (Reinhard et al., 2003).

Sikma and Young found great enthusiasm among registered nurses for supervised delegation (Sikma & Young, 2001; as cited in Munroe, 2003). In addition, the fact that many assisted living residents who have serious chronic conditions have been found to be undermedicated or not to be receiving appropriate medications (Sloane et al., 2004) indicates a need for better medical assessments and medication management protocols. Regulation should address such concerns, which also arise in nursing home and home care settings (Munroe, 2003), including mandating periodic (e.g., quarterly) evaluations by pharmacists or physicians for certain residents. The Assisted Living Workgroup (2003) developed several medication management recommendations, most of which focus on the roles, training, and monitoring of medication management assistants working under the supervision of a nurse according to the provisions of nurse delegation acts.

Accommodating Small Facilities

Policies, financing, and regulatory strategies should reflect our awareness of and support for the different forms of assisted living and the need to provide the consumers with as many options as possible to choose from, consistent with the values of the assisted living philosophy and basic safety requirements. Small residences should not be held to precisely the same standards, which they are not as likely to meet as the larger, purpose-built, "new model" properties.

The value of small residences is evident in the findings of two recently reported studies, which found that larger and newer properties are better able to provide services and meet the privacy and autonomy desires of residents, but small residences may provide more familial, homelike settings, which many impaired elderly seem to prefer and for which they are willing to give up some privacy, autonomy, and level of services (Morgan, Eckert, Gruber-Baldini, & Zimmerman, 2004; chapter 5).

In a follow-up study, Zimmerman and colleagues found that small properties (average 8.9 beds) fared as well as "new model" properties in terms of medical outcomes and nursing home transfers, and better in terms of reducing or maintaining functional and social decline and social withdrawal (Zimmerman et al., 2005). Other studies have found that small or mid-size properties are often more willing to accept Medicaid and SSI-supported residents than are larger properties (Salmon, 2003; Stearns, 2001), a finding that has major implications for state long-term care policy and the use of Medicaid-waiver funds to expand community-based alternatives to nursing homes.

Staffing issues generally, and nurse delegation in particular, are critical to the expansion and possibly even the survival of small assisted living residences. Staffing is a major cost factor for all assisted living providers and plays an important role in determining affordability. In the absence of the economies of scale that benefit larger buildings, however, small providers are especially vulnerable to the costs of regulations that prescribe staffing levels and preclude or greatly limit the delegation of certain nurse practices, including medication management.

Zimmerman and colleagues (2002) note that, if regulation and funding turn on adherence to the parameters of "new model" residences, it may mean the demise of smaller properties. Eschewing uniform standards for assisted living regardless of size will undoubtedly complicate the way assisted living is regulated, but if it results in supporting the expansion of the range of community-based options available to consumers of housing with services, it should be considered worth the additional complexity. An appropriate regulatory framework would recognize the unique value of small residences through supportive initiatives designed to prevent abuse or neglect without imposing standards that would force the closing of residences favored by many consumers for their affordability and home-like features. The affordability issue is also important from the perspective of policy makers and advocates interested in expanding the availability of publicly supported assisted living for lower-income residents and maximizing the potential of assisted living to help contain the use of nursing homes. In short, small residences are too important to let them become extinct without a comprehensive and committed effort to save them.

Conclusions and Implications for the Future

The best available information indicates that with the support of policy makers and the regulatory community, the assisted living industry has built a sound foundation for serving residents who have a wide range of long-term care needs, in a manner largely consistent with the values of the original vision for assisted living. Continuing skepticism about the capacity of assisted living to achieve these values will help policy makers, providers, advocates, and residents keep their eyes on the prize. A sense of fatalism about the practical ability of assisted living to achieve the original vision on a continuing basis, however, is simply *not* justified. The record shows that the growth of assisted living has helped to promote the preferences and interests of consumers to prominence across the entire spectrum of long-term care.

The biggest problem for the future of assisted living is not insufficient regulation, but rather the lack of access for less affluent seniors who require public support, have limited access to community resources, and want to avoid the constraints on personal freedoms common in nursing homes. For many of these individuals, assisted living offers the optimal long-term care setting, not only for receiving the physical care they need, but also for achieving a quality of life that may not be available to them in their own homes. Our primary goals for assisted living should be to expand access for publicly supported residents and avoid regulatory schemes that would undermine the quality of life features that constitute the fundamental appeal of assisted living as a long-term care program.

The Assisted Living Workgroup recognized the critical challenge that access poses for assisted living and developed several recommendations designed to increase the affordability of assisted living for low-income persons, including expansion of the assisted living Medicaid waiver and HUD-funded programs related to assisted living. The workgroup also recommended increasing SSI spending to cover the room and board costs of assisted living and allowing family members to provide supplemental support for assisting living residents.

Research on assisted living has grown along with the industry. Although there are still major gaps in our knowledge, we now have a good deal of information that provides an informed perspective on the extent to which the values of assisted living have been achieved and the service needs of residents met. More broadly, this information can help us to understand what we can realistically expect from assisted living in the future in regard to such issues as quality of life and appropriate regulation.

Research findings demonstrate the importance of assisted living goals and values (privacy, autonomy, dignity, homelike ambiance) to residents and the capacity of assisted living to achieve outcomes that reflect these values more often than not. Consumer advocates and policymakers have a responsibility to recognize and respect resident-oriented outcomes, and to resist regulatory interventions that would make assisted living significantly less affordable and less livable in terms of quality of life.

Assisted living is sustained largely by the fact that many older people very much prefer it to nursing home care and may, in many cases, find it preferable to home care. It would not take the application of very many nursing home style regulations, however, to make assisted living substantially less affordable *and* far less attractive than it has proven to be during the past ten years. Every effort should be made to contain these risks by putting the perspective of the consumer foremost in developing regulation and by supporting rigorous research to support the development of sound, rational policy.

REFERENCES

ADVANCE and Case Management Society of America. 2005. *2005 case management salary survey results.* King of Prussia, PA: Advance for Providers of Post-Acute Care. http://post-acute-care.advanceweb.com/resources/pp050105_p53 salsurvey.pdf.

Andel, R., Hyer, K., & Slack, A. 2005. The effect of health and functional factors on the risk of nursing home placement in frail older adults. Unpublished paper, School of Aging Studies, University of South Florida, Tampa.

Assisted Living Workgroup. 2003, April. *Assuring quality in assisted living: Guidelines for federal and state policy, state regulation, and operations. A report to the U.S. Senate Special Committee on Aging.* Washington, DC: Government Printing Office.

Ball, M., Whittington, F., Perkins, M., Patterson, V., Hollingsworth, C., King, S., et al. 2000. Quality of life in assisted living facilities: Viewpoints of residents. *Journal of Applied Gerontology 19* (3), 304–325.

Ball, M., Perkins, M., Whittington, F., Connell, B., Hollingsworth, C., & King, S. 2004. Managing decline in assisted living: The key to aging in place. *Journal of Gerontology: Social Sciences 59B* (4), S202–212.

Carder, P., & Hernandez, M. 2004. Consumer discourse in assisted living. *Journals of Gerontology: Series B: Psychological Sciences and Social Sciences 59B* (2), S58–67.

Callopy, B. 1998. Autonomy in long term care: Some crucial distinctions. *Gerontologist 28* (supplement), 10–17.

Chapin, R., & Dobbs-Kepper, D. 2001. Aging in place in assisted living: Philosophy versus policy. *Gerontologist 41* (1), 43–50.

Fagan, R. 2003. Pioneer network: Changing the culture of aging in America. *Journal of Social Work in Long-Term Care 2* (1/2), 125–140.

Frytak, J., Kane, R., Finch, M., Kane, R., & Maude-Griffin, R. 2001. Outcome trajectories for assisted living and nursing facility residents in Oregon. *Health Services Research 36* (1, part 1), 91–111.

Golant, S. 2004. Do impaired older persons with health care needs occupy U.S. assisted living facilities? An analysis of six national studies. *Journals of Gerontology: Social Sciences 59B,* S68–79.

Golant, S. 2003. *The ability of U.S. assisted living facilities to accommodate impaired older persons with health care needs: A meta-analysis.* University of Florida, Department of Geography and Institute on Aging, Gainesville.

Hawes, C., Rose, M., & Phillips, C. 1999. *A national study of assisted living for the frail elderly: Results of a national survey of facilities.* Prepared by the U.S. Department of Health and Human Services. Washington, DC: U.S. Department of Health and Human Services.

Hawes, C., & Phillips, C. 2000a. *A national study of assisted living for the frail elderly: Final summary report.* Prepared by the U.S. Department of Health and Human Services. Washington, DC: U.S. Department of Health and Human Services.

Hawes, C., & Phillips, C. 2000b. *High service or high privacy assisted living facilities, their residents and staff: Results from a national survey.* Prepared by the U.S. Department of Health and Human Services. Washington, DC: U.S. Department of Health and Human Services.

Hedrick, S., Sales, A., Sullivan, J., Gray, S., Tornatore, J., Curtiz, M., et al. 2003. Resident outcomes of Medicaid-funded community residential care. *Gerontologist 43* (4), 473–482.

Kane. R. A., Kane., R. L., & Ladd, R. C. 1998. *The heart of long-term care.* New York: Oxford University Press.

Kane, R. A. Olsen Baker, M., Salmon, J., & Veazie, W. 1998. *Consumer perspectives on private versus shared accommodations in assisted living settings.* Washington, DC: American Association of Retired Persons.

Kane, R. L., Bershadsky, B., Kane, R. A., Degenholtz, H., et al. 2004. Using resident reports of quality of life to distinguish among nursing homes. *Gerontologist 44* (5), 624–632.

Kane, R. L., Bershadsky, B., Kane, R. A., Degenholtz, H. Liu, J. Giles, K., & Kling, K. 2004. Using resident reports of quality of life to distinguish among nursing homes. *Gerontologist 44* (5), 624–632.

Kapp, M. 2000. Health care in the marketplace: Implications for decisionally impaired consumers and their surrogates and advocates. In M. Kapp (Ed.), *Ethics, law and aging review: Consumer-directed care and the older person* (vol. 6, pp. 3–52). New York: Springer.

MetLife Mature Market Institute. 2004. *The mature market survey of assisted living costs.* Westport, CT: The Institute.

Mitchell, G., Salmon, J., Chen, H., & Hinton, S. 2003. *Florida's Medicaid waiver programs and demonstration projects serving the older long-term care population: A preliminary look at five outcomes.* Prepared by the Florida Policy Exchange Center on Aging at the University of South Florida for the Florida Department of Elder Affairs (#S-6500-050392), Tallahassee.

Morgan, L., Eckert, K., Gruber-Baldini, A., & Zimmerman, S. 2004. The methodologic imperative for small assisted living facilities. Paper presented at the 55th meeting of the Gerontological Society of America, Boston.

Munroe, D. 2003. Assisted living issues for nursing practice. *Geriatric Nursing 24* (2), 99–105.

Parker, C., Barnes, S., McKee, K., Morgan, K., et al. 2004. Quality of life and building design in residential and nursing homes for older people. *Ageing and Society 24* (6), 941–962.

Polivka, L., Sims, V. M., & Salmon, J. R. 1966. *Assisted living and extended congregate care: The Florida experience.* Tampa: Florida Policy Exchange Center on Aging.

Polivka, L, Dunlop, B., & Brooks, M. 1997. *Project two: The Florida long-term care elder population profiles survey.* Tampa: Florida Policy Exchange Center on Aging.

Polivka, L., & Salmon, J. R. 2003. Autonomy and personal empowerment: Making quality-of-life the organizing principle for long-term care policy. In J. L. Ronch & J. A. Goldfield (Eds.), *Mental wellness in aging: Strengths-based approaches* (pp. 27–52). Baltimore: Health Professions Press.

Reinhard, S., Young, H., Kane, R. A., & Quinn, W. 2003. *Nurse delegation of medication administration for elders in assisted living.* New Brunswick, NJ: Rutgers Center for State Health Policy.

Salmon, J. R. 2001. The contribution of personal control and personal meaning to quality of life in home care, assisted living facility, and nursing home settings. Doctoral dissertation, University of South Florida.

Salmon, J.R. 2003. The diversity of assisted living: One size does not fit all. Paper presented at the 56th annual meeting of the Gerontological Society of America, San Diego, CA.

Scala, M., & Nerney, T. 2000. People first: The consumers in consumer direction. *Generations 24* (N3), 55–59.

Sikma, S., & Young, H. 2001. Balancing freedom with risks: The experience of nursing task delegation in community-based residential care settings. *Nursing Outlook 49,* 193–201.

Sloane, P., Gruber-Baldini, A., Zimmerman, S., Roth, M., Watson, L., Boustani, M., et al. 2004. Medication undertreatment in assisted living settings. *Archives of Internal Medicine 168* (18), 2031–2037.

Stearns, S., & Morgan, L. A. 2001. Economics and financing. In Zimmerman, S., Sloane, P. D. & Eckert, J. K. (Eds.), *Assisted living: Needs, practices and policies in residential care for the elderly* (pp. 271–291). Baltimore: Johns Hopkins University Press.

Thomas, W. H. 2003. Evolution of Eden. In A. S. Weiner & J. L. Ronch (Eds.), *Culture change in long-term care* (pp. 146–157). New York: Haworth Press.

U.S. Department of Health and Human Services. 2003. *Estimates of the risk of long-term care: Assisted living and nursing home facilities.* Prepared by the Assistant Secretary for Planning and Evaluation Office of Disability, Aging and Long-Term Care Policy, Washington, DC.

Utz, R. 2003. Assisted living: The philosophical challenges of everyday practice. *Journal of Applied Gerontology 22* (3), 379–404.

Yee, D., Capitman, J., Leutz, W., & Sceigaj, M. 1999. Resident-centered care in assisted living. *Journal of Aging and Social Policy 10* (3), 7–26.

Zeisel, J., Silverstein, N., Hyde, J., Levkoff, S., & Lawton, M. 2003. Environmental correlates to behavioral health outcomes in Alzheimer's special care units. *Gerontologist 43* (5), 697–711.

Zimmerman, S., Sloane, P. D., & Eckert, J. K. 2001. Emerging issues in residential care/assisted living. In S. Zimmerman, P. D. Sloane & J. K. Eckert (Eds.), *Assisted living: Needs, practices, and policies in residential care for the elderly* (pp. 317–331). Baltimore: Johns Hopkins University Press.

Zimmerman, S., Eckert, J., Morgan, L. Gruber-Baldini, A., Mitchell, C., & Reed, P. 2002. Promising directions in assisted living research. Paper presented at the 55th annual meeting of the Gerontological Society of America, Boston.

Zimmerman, S., Sloane, P., Eckert, J., Gruber-Baldini, A., Morgan, L., Hebel, J., et al. 2005. How good is assisted living? Findings and implications from an outcomes study. *Journal of Gerontology: Social Sciences 60B* (4), S195–204.

INDEX

Page numbers in *italics* refer to illustrations and tables.